Radiographic Interpretation for the Dentist

Editor

MEL MUPPARAPU

DENTAL CLINICS OF NORTH AMERICA

www.dental.theclinics.com

July 2021 • Volume 65 • Number 3

ELSEVIER

1600 John F. Kennedy Boulevard • Suite 1800 • Philadelphia, Pennsylvania, 19103-2899

http://www.dental.theclinics.com

DENTAL CLINICS OF NORTH AMERICA Volume 65, Number 3
July 2021 ISSN 0011-8532, ISBN: 978-0-323-81303-7

Editor: John Vassallo; j.vassallo@elsevier.com
Developmental Editor: Ann Gielou M. Posedio

Dental Clinics of North America (ISSN 0011-8532) is published quarterly by Elsevier Inc., 360 Park Avenue South, New York, NY 10010-1710. Months of issue are January, April, July, and October. Business and Editorial Offices: 1600 John F. Kennedy Boulevard, Suite 1800, Philadelphia, PA 19103-2899. Periodicals postage paid at New York, NY and additional mailing offices. Subscription prices are $313.00 per year (domestic individuals), $846.00 per year (domestic institutions), $100.00 per year (domestic students/residents), $366.00 per year (Canadian individuals), $888.00 per year (Canadian institutions), $100.00 per year (Canadian students/residents) $428.00 per year (international individuals), $888.00 per year (international institutions), and $200.00 per year (international students/residents). International air speed delivery is included in all *Clinics* subscription prices. All prices are subject to change without notice. **POSTMASTER:** Send address changes to *Dental Clinics of North America*, Elsevier Health Sciences Division, Subscription Customer Service, 3251 Riverport Lane, Maryland Heights, MO 63043. **Customer Service (orders, claims, online, change of address): Elsevier Health Sciences Division, Subscription Customer Service, 3251 Riverport Lane, Maryland Heights, MO 63043. Tel: 1-800-654-2452 (U.S. and Canada). Fax: 314-447-8029. E-mail: journalscustomerservice-usa@elsevier.com (for print support); journalsonlinesupport-usa@elsevier. com (for online support).**

Reprints. For copies of 100 or more, of articles in this publication, please contact the Commercial Reprints Department, Elsevier Inc., 360 Park Avenue South, New York, NY 10010-1710. Tel.: 212-633-3874; Fax: 212-633-3820; E-mail: reprints@elsevier.com.

The Dental Clinics of North America is covered in *MEDLINE/PubMed (Index Medicus), Current Contents/Clinical Medicine, ISI/BIOMED* and *Clinahl*.

Contributors

EDITOR

MEL MUPPARAPU, DMD, MDS
Diplomate, American Board of Oral and Maxillofacial Radiology; Professor and Director of Radiology, Department of Oral Medicine, Director of Oral and Maxillofacial Radiology Fellowship, University of Pennsylvania School of Dental Medicine, Philadelphia, Pennsylvania, USA

AUTHORS

SUNDAY O. AKINTOYE, BDS, DDS, MS
Associate Professor, Department of Oral Medicine, University of Pennsylvania School of Dental Medicine, Philadelphia, Pennsylvania, USA

ANWAR A.A.Y. ALMUZAINI, DDS, MS, BDM, MSOB
Dental Specialist, Ministry of Health, Kuwait City, Kuwait

EVA ANADIOTI, DDS, MS, FACP
Assistant Professor of Clinical Restorative Dentistry, Department of Preventive and Restorative Sciences, University of Pennsylvania School of Dental Medicine, Philadelphia, Pennsylvania, USA

MARIA JOSE CERVANTES MENDEZ, DDS, MS, FAAPD
Department of Developmental Dentistry, University of Texas Health San Antonio School of Dentistry, San Antonio, Texas, USA

JULIAN CONEJO, DDS, MSc
Clinical CAD/CAM Director, Department of Preventive and Restorative Sciences, University of Pennsylvania School of Dental Medicine, Robert Schattner Center, Philadelphia, Pennsylvania, USA

ADRIANA G. CREANGA, BDS, MS
Diplomate, American Board of Oral and Maxillofacial Radiology; Assistant Professor, Department of Diagnostic Sciences, Rutgers School of Dental Medicine, Newark, New Jersey, USA

ADEYINKA F. DAYO, BDS, MS
Assistant Professor of Radiology, Department of Oral Medicine, University of Pennsylvania School of Dental Medicine, Robert Schattner Center, Philadelphia, Pennsylvania, USA

JOSEPH P. FIORELLINI, DMD, DMSc
Professor, Department of Periodontics, University of Pennsylvania School of Dental Medicine, Philadelphia, Pennsylvania, USA

BRIAN FORD, DMD, MD
Assistant Professor, Department of Oral and Maxillofacial Surgery and Pharmacology, University of Pennsylvania School of Dental Medicine, Philadelphia, Pennsylvania, USA

KATHERINE FRANCE, DMD, MBE
Assistant Professor of Oral Medicine, University of Pennsylvania School of Dental Medicine, Philadelphia, Pennsylvania, USA

EVLAMBIA HAJISHENGALLIS, DDS, DMD, MSc, PhD
Division of Pediatric Dentistry, University of Pennsylvania School of Dental Medicine, Philadelphia, Pennsylvania, USA

ANGELA HOIKKA, DDS
Department of Comprehensive Dentistry, The University of Texas Health San Antonio School of Dentistry, San Antonio, Texas, USA

DEREK J. HONG, BA
Research Associate, Division of Oral and Maxillofacial Radiology, University of Pennsylvania School of Dental Medicine, Philadelphia, Pennsylvania, USA

JAYAKUMAR JAYARAMAN, BDS, MDS, MPed Dent RCS, FDSRCS, PhD
Department of Developmental Dentistry, The University of Texas Health San Antonio School of Dentistry, San Antonio, Texas, USA

NADEEM KARIMBUX, DMD, MMSc
Dean and Professor, Department of Periodontics, Tufts University School of Dental Medicine, Boston, Massachusetts, USA

IRENE H. KIM, DMD, MPH
Clinical Professor of Oral Medicine, University of Pennsylvania School of Dental Medicine, Philadelphia, Pennsylvania, USA

EUGENE KO, DDS
Assistant Professor of Oral Medicine, Department of Oral Medicine, University of Pennsylvania School of Dental Medicine, Philadelphia, Pennsylvania, USA

HEIDI KOHLTFARBER, DDS, MS, PhD, FADI, FICD
Adjunct Assistant Professor, Division of Diagnostic Sciences, University of North Carolina School of Dentistry, Chapel Hill, North Carolina, USA

SU-MIN LEE, DDS, MSD, DScD
Assistant Professor, Department of Endodontics, School of Dental Medicine, University of Pennsylvania, Philadelphia, Pennsylvania, USA

KEVIN W. LUAN, BDS, MSOB, MEd
Clinical Assistant Professor, Department of Periodontics, University of Illinois at Chicago College of Dentistry, Chicago, Illinois, USA

MEL MUPPARAPU, DMD, MDS
Diplomate, American Board of Oral and Maxillofacial Radiology; Professor and Director of Radiology, Department of Oral Medicine, Director of Oral and Maxillofacial Radiology Fellowship, University of Pennsylvania School of Dental Medicine, Philadelphia, Pennsylvania, USA

TEMITOPE OMOLEHINWA, BDS, DScD
Assistant Professor, Department of Oral Medicine, University of Pennsylvania School of Dental Medicine, Philadelphia, Pennsylvania, USA

HECTOR SARIMENTO, DMD, MSOB
Clinical Assistant Professor, Department of Periodontics, University of Pennsylvania
School of Dental Medicine, Philadelphia, Pennsylvania, USA

FRANK C. SETZER, DMD, PhD, MS
Assistant Professor, Department of Endodontics, School of Dental Medicine, University of
Pennsylvania, Philadelphia, Pennsylvania, USA

STEVEN R. SINGER, DDS
Professor and Chair, Department of Diagnostic Sciences, Rutgers School of Dental
Medicine, Newark, New Jersey, USA

DENNIS SOURVANOS, BsDH, DDS
Periodontics Resident, Department of Periodontics, University of Pennsylvania School of
Dental Medicine, Philadelphia, Pennsylvania, USA

ALI Z. SYED, BDS, MHA, MS
Diplomate, American Board of Oral and Maxillofacial Radiology; Oral and Maxillofacial
Radiologist, Assistant Professor and Director, Admitting and Oral and Maxillofacial
Radiology Clinics, Internship Program Director, Oral and Maxillofacial Radiology,
Department of Oral and Maxillofacial Medicine and Diagnostic Sciences, CWRU School
of Dental Medicine, Cleveland, Ohio, USA

NIPUL K. TANNA, DMD, MS
Clinical Associate Professor of Orthodontics, Director, Postdoctoral Periodontics/
Orthodontics Program, University of Pennsylvania School of Dental Medicine,
Philadelphia, Pennsylvania, USA

STEVEN WANG, DMD, MD, MPH
Assistant Professor, Department of Oral and Maxillofacial Surgery and Pharmacology,
University of Pennsylvania School of Dental Medicine, Philadelphia, Pennsylvania, USA

MARK S. WOLFF, DDS, PhD
Morton Amsterdam Dean, University of Pennsylvania School of Dental Medicine,
Philadelphia, Pennsylvania, USA

Contents

Radiographic imaging is an integral part of the diagnostic process in clinical dentistry. This article provides the fundamentals of radiographic interpretation beginning with evidence-based guidelines on dental radiographic selection criteria and cone beam computed tomography use. The goal is to present to the reader with a systematic approach to radiographic interpretation such that no significant features are overlooked and an optimal differential diagnosis can be achieved. In addition, medicolegal considerations of radiographic acquisition, interpretation, and storage are discussed.

Dental caries is a dynamic, preventable, reversible, complex biofilm–mediated, multifactorial disease that involves a series of demineralization/neutrality/remineralization of dental hard tissue in primary and permanent dentition. An imbalance in the continuum with a net demineralization over time results in the initiation of caries lesions. Visual inspection and intraoral radiographs are vital in caries detection, although they are of suboptimal sensitivity for early caries lesions. Shifting toward a conservative, noninvasive approach to caries management has resulted in the development of innovative-sensitive technologies. These newer techniques may serve as adjunct for the dental practitioner in detecting earliest changes in tooth structure.

Dental radiography can be used to detect alveolar bone levels around periodontal and peri-implant structures. Periodontal radiographic images can assess alveolar bone height, periodontal ligament, furcation involvement, and evidence of bone destruction. Peri-implant radiographic images can assess the alveolar bone height in relation to the implant structure. As an adjunct to patient care, radiography can aid in the diagnosis of non-health.

Endodontics requires radiographic imaging for diagnosis, treatment planning, therapy, and follow-up. Dental radiography allows for the identification of pathologic changes in the periradicular tissues that cannot be visualized by clinical inspection. For the precise execution of endodontic therapy, regular radiographic verification of individual treatment steps is necessary. As a review for clinicians, normal and pathologic findings relevant to Endodontics are presented. Key radiographic imaging techniques, such as the paralleling and bisecting techniques, as well as horizontal and vertical eccentric radiographs, are discussed. The increasing utilization and impact of cone-beam computed tomography providing 3-dimensional volume imaging are reviewed.

The scope of oral and maxillofacial surgery treatment and care is very broad, from dentoalveolar surgery, to pathology and reconstruction, to treatment of craniofacial deformities. The effective surgical treatment of patients requires appropriate and accurate diagnostic imaging. The various imaging modalities used in oral and maxillofacial surgery are typically for diagnostic and treatment planning purposes. With the improvements of three-dimensional imaging and software programs, surgical treatment and care have been enhanced with patient-specific guides, hardware, and implants. This article discusses the various imaging modalities used for a variety of typical oral and maxillofacial surgery procedures.

Oral medicine practice includes the diagnosis and nonsurgical treatment of oral and orofacial diseases and oral manifestations of systemic conditions. Oral medicine specialists in medical and dental settings often require imaging in assessment and treatment of these conditions. This article reviews imaging that may be used in practice, particularly as relevant for facial pain, bone conditions, and salivary gland disease. It reviews imaging that may be considered in a hospital setting for assessment of admitted patients, patient evaluation before surgical procedures, and provision of dentistry in a hospital setting for patients who cannot submit to treatment in an outpatient setting.

The purpose of this article is to synthesize different technologies that are available for the creation of a virtual patient, "the digital clone" because the data can be used for diagnosis as well as treatment planning. The role of facial scans, 3-dimensional intraoral scans as well as the cone beam computed tomography in the creation of a digital clone is discussed in detail. A step-by-step guide is created for the reader for integration of the intraoral scan data with the cone beam computed tomography Dicom data to create a digital clone.

This article aims to help the practitioner identify structures found in routine three-dimensional imaging studies of the head and neck region and understand their significance and possible need for intervention. The prevalence of advanced imaging in dental practice, especially cone beam computed tomography, highlights the need to recognize and identify various high-density structures that are, in fact, soft tissue calcifications or alterations of normal bony anatomy. The wide range of these findings includes both benign and malignant pathologic entities as well as age-related calcifications and remodeling of normal anatomic structures and dystrophic calcifications.

Radiographic changes of the oral and maxillofacial hard tissues can be an indication of an underlying systemic disease. In this article, the range of individual disease entities that have both systemic and dental manifestations are reviewed. Images for many conditions are provided to illustrate the radiographic changes. A summary of the most common jaw affected, radiographic and pathognomonic findings, and management aspects is listed in a table format within this article for quick reference.

This article focuses on radiographic imaging with regard to planning, treating, and maintaining partially and completely edentulous prosthodontic patients with dental implants. Cone-beam computed tomography (CBCT) is the preferred imaging method for pretreatment dental implant treatment planning. Radiographic guides containing radiopaque materials and/or fiducial markers transfer both the proposed prosthesis design and desired implant location for appropriate radiographic evaluation. The three-dimensional CBCT analysis provides information on the adjacent relevant anatomy, bone volume of the edentulous sites, and restorative space assessment.

Imaging in orthodontics has evolved from cephalometric and extraoral films, manual cephalometric tracings, to digital imaging and intraoral scanners. Software-assisted cephalometric tracings and three-dimensional image analysis have become routine in orthodontic diagnosis and treatment planning. Determination of biologic boundaries of orthodontic treatment and evaluation of temporomandibular joints and airway became part of orthodontic assessment. Use of advanced imaging and software to digitally plan the orthognathic surgery and accurately predict a successful outcome are now integral to orthodontic practice. This article discusses radiographic methods used in cephalometric analysis and craniofacial growth and development for a predictable orthodontic assessment and treatment planning.

Jayakumar Jayaraman, Angela Hoikka, Maria Jose Cervantes Mendez, and Evlambia Hajishengallis

This article emphasizes the selection criteria for radiographic acquisition in children due to the greater sensitivity of children for radiation compared with adults. Diagnosis of common pediatric dental conditions, including dental caries, periodontitis, dental anomalies, cysts, tumors, and traumatic dental conditions, are discussed with relevant clinical scenarios.

DENTAL CLINICS OF NORTH AMERICA

SERIES OF RELATED INTEREST

Atlas of the Oral and Maxillofacial Surgery Clinics
http://www.oralmaxsurgeryatlas.theclinics.com

Oral and Maxillofacial Surgery Clinics
http://www.oralmaxsurgery.theclinics.com

THE CLINICS ARE AVAILABLE ONLINE!
Access your subscription at:
www.theclinics.com

Preface

Oral and Maxillofacial Radiographic Data: A Multidisciplinary Diagnostic, Presurgical, and Virtual Tool for the Twenty-First Century

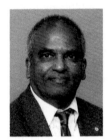

Mel Mupparapu, DMD, MDS, DABOMR
Editor

Until recently, radiographic data have primarily been used as a diagnostic tool, but such use only skims the surface of the data's full potential. While imaging still has its diagnostic value, clinical applications of radiographic data have evolved, especially since the advent of cone-beam computed tomography (CBCT). Combined with other forms of imaging, like intraoral scanners and Three-dimensional (3D) facial photographs, CBCT data have become a formidable driver in the creation of surgical guides, presurgical templates, tools for mock surgeries, and creation of the "virtual patient."

This issue of *Dental Clinics of North America* presents to the readers the value of diagnostic imaging and attempts to familiarize them with the aforementioned uses. Radiographic data, especially from a 3D perspective, have taken on a far greater role in the integration of clinical concepts and delivery of dental care. Individual articles in this issue deal with diagnostic tasks in various specialties apart from general dentistry (oral medicine, oral and maxillofacial radiology, endodontics, periodontics, prosthodontics, oral and maxillofacial surgery, pediatric dentistry) in terms of the utilization of radiographic data. The articles detail the use of radiographic data in understanding the pulp morphology in endodontics, in the creation of implant-supported crowns and bridges as well as their use as a reliable presurgical tool for advanced orthognathic and maxillofacial surgery. 3D data of the patient have never been more anatomically accurate, functional, and visually reliable.

Dent Clin N Am 65 (2021) xiii–xiv
https://doi.org/10.1016/j.cden.2021.03.001
0011-8532/21/© 2021 Published by Elsevier Inc.

The next revolution of imaging data might investigate concepts such as ironing out the differences in pixel resolution, seamless data acquisition, and integration of photographic, radiographic, and scanning data within the dental practice. For some of these, the tools may already be available, but wide applications of these concepts are still emerging.

The radiographic data, of course, have been a key factor in many medicolegal issues. As we continue to utilize these data, we must remain cognizant of having adequate checks and balances for technology transfer, radiation dose reduction, and affordable and patient-friendly dentistry. This will ensure a win-win for both providers and patients.

This issue wouldn't have been possible without the consistent and crucial help of many people. John Vassallo, the associate publisher of *Dental Clinics of North America*, who advances global education, reference, and continuity, was instrumental in driving the idea behind this issue. I appreciate the developmental editors, Laura Fisher and Anngie Posedio, for their immense help in getting this issue published on time. All of my authors and coauthors worked tirelessly to gather the most current and reliable information and present the material in a concise way, and I sincerely thank them for their help. My children, Vamsee and Archana, helped me in many ways by encouraging me to become a better writer and editor, helping me channel my thoughts, and being there for me all the time. I also want to thank Dr Kalpana Vaidya and Arun Vaidya for their constant guidance, mentorship, and inspiration. Finally, I would not be who I am today without the influence of my late beloved wife, Anitha Vuppalapati, MD, a great physician and a loving and caring mom, who constantly encouraged and supported me in all my endeavors. I would like to dedicate this issue to her memory!

Mel Mupparapu, DMD, MDS, DABOMR
Department of Oral Medicine
University of Pennsylvania
School of Dental Medicine
240 South 40th Street, Suite 240
Philadelphia, PA 19104, USA

E-mail address:
mmd@upenn.edu

Fundamentals of Radiographic Interpretation for the Dentist

Irene H. Kim, DMD, MPH[a], Steven R. Singer, DDS[b],
Derek J. Hong, BA[c], Mel Mupparapu, DMD, MDS, DABOMR[a],*

KEYWORDS

- Radiology • Digital radiography • Cone beam computed tomography
- Selection criteria • Diagnosis • Medicolegal

KEY POINTS

- Dental radiographs are an integral part of the diagnostic process in clinical dentistry.
- Radiographs aid in the diagnosis and characterization of the type and extent of disease, but care must be taken to minimize the radiation exposure to the patient.
- Selection guidelines help the practitioner choose the appropriate radiographs as an adjunct to their professional judgment.
- Two-dimensional or plain radiography is the first choice of imaging in many clinical scenarios; cone beam computed tomography should be used when 2-dimensional imaging cannot answer the clinical question.
- It is best to use a systematic method of reading and interpreting radiographs each time so that no significant features are overlooked. Knowledge of normal radiographic anatomy is paramount.

INTRODUCTION

The diagnostic process consists of a patient interview, clinical examination, and the ordering of tests to help the practitioner make a sound diagnosis. In dentistry, the most common test ordered in a preliminary examination is radiographic imaging (Fig. 1). The patient is interviewed to determine the patient's chief complaint, the history of the present illness, and the patient's medical history. A systematic clinical examination of the patient is then performed and, based on the information collected, the practitioner will order diagnostic imaging. After reviewing the images, the dentist may

[a] University of Pennsylvania School of Dental Medicine, 240 South 40th Street, Suite 214, Philadelphia, PA 19104, USA; [b] Department of Diagnostic Sciences, Rutgers School of Dental Medicine, 110 Bergen Street, Room D-885A, Newark, NJ 07103, USA; [c] Division of Oral and Maxillofacial Radiology, University of Pennsylvania School of Dental Medicine, 240 South 40th Street, Suite 214, Philadelphia, PA 19104, USA
* Corresponding author.
E-mail address: mmd@upenn.edu

Dent Clin N Am 65 (2021) 409–425
https://doi.org/10.1016/j.cden.2021.02.001

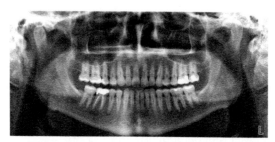

Fig. 1. Panoramic radiograph showing dentition along with maxillofacial structures. Although this radiograph is acquired using rotation tomography, it is still a 2D image, hence the third dimension is not noted in the radiograph.

perform further clinical examinations and order further testing to assist in formulating a differential diagnosis. Dental radiographs are an integral part of the diagnostic process in clinical dentistry. Appropriate radiographic selection and interpretation along with clinical information and other tests are essential for the formulation of a strong differential diagnosis.

EVIDENCE-BASED SELECTION CRITERIA

After a history and clinical examination are performed, a decision must be made about whether or not to order radiographs to aid in the diagnosis. Radiographs aid in the diagnosis and characterization of the type and extent of disease, but care must be taken to minimize the radiation exposure to the patient using the as low as diagnostically acceptable principle.[1] The Canadian Dental Association's position paper concluded that the frequency of radiographic examinations is a matter of clinical judgment.[2] The Food and Drug Administration and the American Dental Association as well as the US Department of Health and Human Services have issued guidelines to help the practitioner choose the appropriate radiographs as an adjunct to their professional judgment.[3–8] The efficacy of these guidelines has been demonstrated by White and colleagues.[9] Among 500 new adult patients, the guidelines resulted in a 43% decrease in the number of radiographs ordered and only 3.3% of carious lesions were missed. The guidelines have also been shown to be effective in the diagnosis of periodontal disease[10] and defective restorations.[11]

Recommended Radiographic Selection Criteria

New patient
Primary dentition. If the proximal surfaces cannot be probed, then select periapicals, occlusal, and/or bitewing radiographs should be taken. If there is no evidence of disease, no radiographs are recommended.[12]

Transitional dentition. Either bitewing radiographs and a panoramic radiograph or bitewing and select periapical radiographs should be taken.

Permanent dentition. If there is no clinical evidence of disease or extensive dental treatment, individual radiographic examinations are recommended. Such examinations would include either bitewing and panoramic radiographs or bitewings and select periapical radiographs. If there is evidence of dental disease or extensive dental treatment, a full mouth series of radiographs should be taken.

Edentulous. In an edentulous patient, an individual radiographic examination based on clinical signs and symptoms is recommended.

Recall patient
Clinical caries or increased risk for caries. In a patient with clinical caries or an increased risk for caries, who has primary, transitional, or permanent dentition (before the eruption of third molars), and whose proximal surfaces cannot be probed, bitewing radiographs at 6- to 12-month intervals should be taken. In a patient with clinical caries or an increased risk for caries who has adult dentate or partially edentulous dentition, bitewing radiographs at 6- to 12-month intervals are recommended.

No clinical caries, not at increased risk for caries. In a patient with no clinical caries and who is not at increased risk for caries, and has primary, transitional, or permanent dentition (before the eruption of third molars), and the proximal surfaces cannot be probed, bitewing radiographs at 12- to 24-month intervals should be taken. For patients with no clinical caries and no increased risk for caries, with permanent dentition before the eruption of third molars, bitewing radiographs at 18- to 36-month intervals are recommended. Patients with no clinical caries and no increased risk for caries with adult dentate or partially edentulous dentition, should have bitewing radiographs exposed at 24 to 36-month intervals.

Periodontal disease. In a recall patient with clinical signs and symptoms of periodontal disease, the radiographic examination is based on clinical judgment to select the radiographs necessary to evaluate the presence and extent of periodontal disease. The recommendation is to take select vertical bitewing and periapical radiographs of the areas with periodontal disease.

Monitoring growth and development
To monitor growth and development in the primary dentition, choosing radiographs based on the practitioners' clinical judgment of prior caries experience, oral hygiene, orthodontic treatment, and impending eruption of third molars should dictate the need for bitewing, periapical, and panoramic examinations. When evaluating implants, pathology, restorative/endodontic needs, periodontitis, and caries remineralization, clinical judgment of the need for radiographs needed is recommended. Practitioners should be mindful of the increased risks of radiation for growing children.

EVIDENCE BASED CONE BEAM COMPUTED TOMOGRAPHY GUIDELINES

Although two-dimensional (2D) or plain radiography is the first choice of imaging in many clinical cases, cone beam computed tomography (CBCT) can be used when 2D imaging alone cannot answer the clinical question. As with plain radiography, guidelines have been established to aid the dental practitioner using their best clinical judgment.[13] In all cases, the smallest possible field of view, the smallest voxel size, the lowest mA setting, and the shortest exposure time in conjunction with the pulsed exposure mode should be used.[14] In addition, the use of CBCT should be implemented only after the patient's health history and imaging history have been carefully reviewed, a thorough clinical examination has been performed, and the diagnostic yield has been determined to improve the patient care, enhance patient safety, and significantly improve clinical outcomes.[15]

Endodontics

In endodontic cases, the use of CBCT should be limited to the assessment and treatment of complex conditions.[14]

- To identify potential accessory canals in teeth with suspected complex morphology as shown on plain radiography

- To identify root canal system anomalies and determine root curvatures
- To diagnose periapical pathoses:
  - With contradictory or nonspecific clinical signs and symptoms
  - With poorly localized symptoms associated with no evidence of pathosis by conventional imaging
  - Where anatomic superimposition of roots or areas of the maxillofacial skeleton may interfere with adequate visualization of areas in question
- To diagnose periapical pathosis of a nonendodontic origin to determine the extent of a lesion and its effect on surrounding structures
- To assess intraoperative or postoperative endodontic treatment complications
  - Overextended root canal obturation material
  - Separated endodontic instruments
  - Calcified canals
  - Perforations
- To diagnose and manage dentoalveolar trauma
  - Root fractures
  - Luxation and/or displacement of teeth
  - Alveolar fractures
- To localize and differentiate
  - External from internal root resorption
  - Invasive cervical resorption from other conditions
- For presurgical case planning
  - To determine the exact location of root apex/apices
  - To evaluate proximity to anatomic structures

Implantology

In dental implant cases, panoramic radiography is the imaging modality of choice for the initial evaluation, and intraoral periapical radiography should supplement panoramic radiography.[16] It is not recommended to use CBCT as the initial diagnostic examination. However, owing to inaccurate distance measurements and the lack of three-dimensional visualization, panoramic radiographs are extremely limited in usefulness in final implant planning.

- Preoperative site-specific imaging
  - CBCT should be considered as the imaging modality of choice for preoperative cross-sectional imaging of potential implant sites
  - CBCT should be considered if there is a clinical need for augmentation procedures or site development before implant placement
    - Sinus augmentation
    - Block of particulate bone grafting
    - Ramus or symphysis grafting
    - Assessment of impacted teeth in the field of interest
    - Evaluation of previous traumatic injury
  - CBCT should be considered if bone reconstruction and augmentation procedures have been performed to treat bone volume deficiencies before implant placement
- Postoperative imaging
  - CBCT is recommended immediately postoperatively only if the patient presents with implant mobility or altered sensation, especially if in the posterior mandible

- o Intraoral periapical and panoramic radiographs are recommended in the absence of signs or symptoms
- o CBCT may be considered if implant retrieval is anticipated

Periodontics

In periodontology, experts have addressed the use of CBCT in three specific areas: placement of implants, interdisciplinary dentofacial therapy involving orthodontic tooth movement in the management of malocclusion associated with risk to the supporting periodontal tissues, and the management of marginal periodontitis.[17]

Placement of implants

- o To evaluate root morphology and associated pathology for extractions and reconstruction
- o To locate relevant anatomic structures and their relation to the planned implant
- o For the preimplant evaluation of sinus grafting
- o To evaluate the autogenous bone donor site
- o To fabricate static surgical guides and dynamic navigation of implant placement
- o For postbone augmentation implant planning
- o To evaluate complications from previous implants
    - ■ Risk to supporting periodontal structures in tooth movement
- o In a skeletally mature patient with malocclusion in need of fixed orthodontic appliance for decompensation
- o When thin dentoalveolar phenotype and dentoalveolar bone deficiencies are suspected
- o In patients with malocclusion requiring advanced tooth movement and there is an increased risk for positioning the roots outside the orthodontic boundary
- o In a skeletally immature orthodontic patient requiring an interdisciplinary approach to treatment
- o In an orthodontic patient with concomitant mucogingival deformities
- o Other treatment considerations requiring global analysis, such as
    - ■ Temporomandibular disorders
    - ■ Dentofacial disharmonies requiring orthodontic-periodontal-orthognathic management
    - ■ Congenitally missing teeth
    - ■ Skeletal anchorage requirements
    - ■ Management of periodontitis
- o Advanced furcation lesions with dental implants being considered as an alternative treatment option
- o Advanced bone loss encroaching on anatomic structures such as sinus cavities or the inferior alveolar nerve
- o Questionable root fracture, root resorption, or periodontal lesions confluent with apical inflammatory lesions that cannot be identified by 2D imaging and/or clinical evaluation
- o Management and diagnosis of peri-implantitis when necessary

Cone Beam Computed Tomography Summary

- • A 2D or plain radiograph is the first choice of imaging in many clinical scenarios, and CBCT should be used when 2D imaging alone cannot answer the clinical question.[13]
    - o A comprehensive clinical examination must precede use of CBCT, and caution must be exercised to use dose-sparing techniques.
    - o Preimplant imaging using CBCT is more useful than postimplant imaging.

- ○ The effective doses for dentoalveolar CBCT range from 11 to 674 μSv. The effective doses for craniofacial CBCT range from 30 to 1073 μSv.
- ○ CBCT is indicated in situations where a tooth is impacted, infected, or missing, and 2D radiography did not reveal pathosis. Preimplant planning, preoperative evaluation, postsurgical evaluation in a variety of oral surgical, periodontal, endodontic, restorative, and prosthodontic conditions can be performed using CBCT.

INTERPRETATION
Quality of the Image

Initially, the radiograph must be of diagnostic quality. It should have the correct contrast and density where the region of interest or lesion is clearly visible. The surrounding normal tissue should be approximately 2 to 3 mm, and there should be no geometric distortion. Based on the initial radiographs, a clinical determination is made as to the necessity of additional radiographs or different projections, such as periapical, bitewing, occlusal, and panoramic radiographs. The clinician may also try to obtain prior radiographs for comparison even if they are not of highest quality (**Fig. 2**). When deciding to expose the patient to additional radiation, the expected diagnostic yield from the radiographs should be taken into consideration.

Systematic Reading of Radiographs

It is best to use a systematic method of reading radiographs each time so that nothing is overlooked. A knowledge of normal radiographic anatomy for each projection is paramount. Anatomic landmarks such as canals, foramina, and cortices should be identified first by viewing the radiographs quadrant by quadrant while also checking for symmetry. The clinician then should review again by quadrant the trabecular

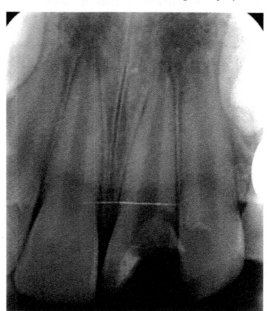

Fig. 2. Intraoral maxillary central incisor periapical radiograph. Although the radiograph shows artifacts from the scratched phosphor plate, it is clinically useful and hence need not be repeated unless a third dimension is required for diagnosis.

pattern of the bone noting whether it is spare or dense, symmetric to the contralateral side, aligned with the direction of anatomic stress, or any other altered patterns. The interdental bone is studied next, again quadrant by quadrant in the same systematic pattern. Additionally, the heights, cortication, and shape of the bony crest of the interdental bone should be noted. Bitewing radiographs are the optimal projection of proximal bone heights (**Fig. 3**). Finally, the clinician should return to the systematic quadrant review and examine the teeth, checking the enamel, dentin, pulp, and anatomy for any changes as well as checking the number of teeth and restorations using the best projections for each evaluation.

Appropriate Use of Terminology

Why describe the lesion?
A thorough and accurate description of a lesion on a radiograph can give indications of the tissue of origin, biological behavior, and prognosis of the pathology. For example, if the epicenter of the lesion is above the mandibular canal or below the maxillary sinus, the lesion is likely to be odontogenic in origin, whereas if the epicenter is in the sinus it is likely not to be odontogenic in origin. Cartilaginous lesions are found nearer the condyles and, sometimes, the mandibular symphysis. The location of the lesion can also give insight into any treatment concerns and aid with formulation of the differential diagnosis.

Describing the lesion
Similar to reading radiographs in a systematic manner, it is best to consistently and systematically describe each lesion such that no significant features are overlooked. Every description should always include the following:

- Size
  - Measure in two dimensions, width and height in millimeters or centimeters as appropriate.
  - Three-dimensional measurements should be obtained where advanced imaging is available.
- Shape
  - Regular
    - Round, triangular, ovoid, etc
  - Irregular
- Location

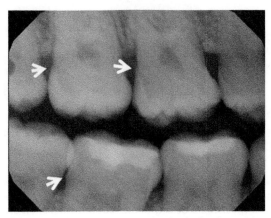

Fig. 3. Right molar bite wing showing interproximal calculus (*arrows*).

- o Localized or generalized
- o Unilateral or bilateral
- o Relation to other structures and anatomic landmarks
- o Use terms such as mesial/distal, anterior/posterior, inferior/superior
- Density
  - o Radiopaque, radiolucent, or mixed density. The terms "high-density" and "low-density" are preferred when describing CBCT images. "Homogenous" or "heterogenous" are again CBCT terms used to represent uniform or mixed density appearance based on the attenuation properties of a structure. The term lytic is often used as a CT or CBCT terminology to represent significant loss of osseous component within bone.
  - o Peel
- Effect on adjacent structures
  - o Is the lesion causing
    - ▪ Resorption (see **Fig. 5**)
    - ▪ Displacement
    - ▪ Scalloping
    - ▪ Effacement or destruction
    - ▪ Destruction (see **Fig. 5**)
    - ▪ Space occupation
      - • Displacement of other structures
      - • Creates its own space by displacing teeth, maxillary sinus, inferior alveolar nerve, etc
    - ▪ Remodeling (see **Fig. 5**)
  - o Expansion
  - o Opacity, if relative to adjacent structures (**Fig. 4**)

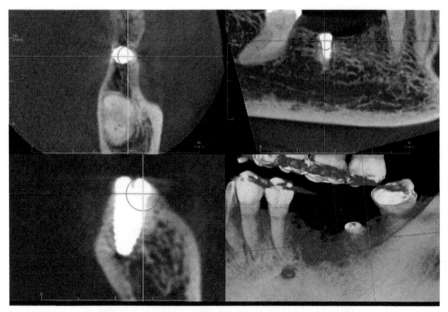

Fig. 4. CBCT axial, sagittal, coronal, and three-dimensional renderings of a patient's mandibular left molar region. The metallic density of the root form implant is distinct from the rest of the anatomy.

- o If mixed density, describe appearance
- o Well or poorly demarcated (**Fig. 5**)
- o Punched out (no bony reaction)
- o Corticated (thin opaque border) (see **Fig. 5**)
- o Sclerotic (wide, uneven, opaque border)
- o Hyperostotic (increased density or trabeculation)
- Internal architecture
  - o Uniformity of lesion (see **Fig. 5**)
  - o Internal structures such as septae (bony walls) or loculations (individual compartment)
  - o Tooth-like elements
    - Use terms such as cotton wool, ground glass, wispy, orange
    - Thinning or thickening

Radiographic Interpretation

Once the radiographic image is described systematically, all the radiographic findings will have been collected in an organized manner. With this information, along with the clinical data, the clinician can often arrive at a reasonable diagnosis or differential diagnosis of the abnormality (**Fig. 6**).[18,19]

Normal versus abnormal

In some cases, what may appear as an abnormality could be merely be a normal anatomic variation that was not seen before. The knowledge of regional anatomy as

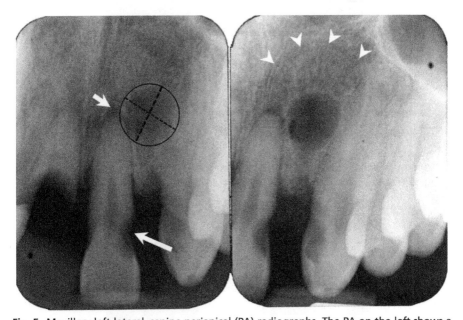

Fig. 5. Maxillary left lateral–canine periapical (PA) radiographs. The PA on the left shows a deep carious lesion (*long arrow*) and an apical rarefying osteitis on the left central incisor (*short arrow*), along with a residual cyst in the region of left lateral incisor. The trabecular bone is either resorbed or lost. The PA on the right demonstrates that the lesion is well-defined, somewhat round in nature, well corticated, with significant amount of bone re-modeling superiorly where the rest of the cystic lesion and surgical defect is now scarring. This is considered a bone scar (*arrowheads*).

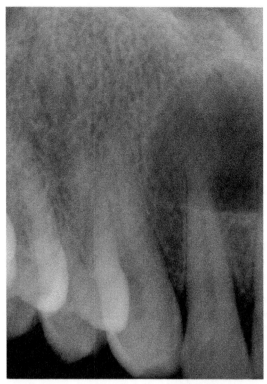

Fig. 6. Maxillary right lateral–canine periapical radiograph showing a well-defined, enlarged and corticated radiolucent area consistent with an incisive canal cyst. All anterior teeth are vital.

well as the myriads of variations that the region could present to the clinician is important.

Developmental or acquired

An abnormality could be developmental or acquired, and that assessment can often be made based on its presentation. Further, if the abnormality is acquired, placing the entity in a category is the most important task the clinician must do before coming a diagnosis (**Fig. 7**).

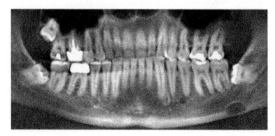

Fig. 7. A CBCT image cropped panoramic reconstruction showing Stafne's developmental salivary gland defect in the left body of the mandible at the angle inferior to the mandibular canal. This is radiographically consistent with Stafne's bone defect.

Categorization

Identifying the suspected lesions as belonging in one category leads to a good differential diagnosis. A series of similar appearing lesions, perhaps belonging to one or more categories, would comprise the differential diagnosis. By the process of elimination, the more improbable lesions are eliminated first, followed by lesions that are rarer, the lesions that are not likely to be in that location, and so on. Eventually, the patient's age and sex must be considered before coming to a tentative radiographic diagnosis. For instance, the lesion apical to maxillary left central incisor (**Fig. 8**) seems to be inflammatory based on the clinical and radiographic features of an endodontic lesion.

MEDICOLEGAL CONSIDERATIONS
Acquisition

The proper acquisition of radiographs can be informed by its legal implications. For example, it is known that any ionizing radiation has potential carcinogenic effect,[20] and therefore the radiation protection principle of as low as diagnostically acceptable should be considered for all radiation are exposed. Consequently, the dentist should ensure that only the necessary number of radiographs, and not more, are taken to minimize radiation exposure. Excessive radiograph taking may be an unexpected issue in digital radiography, but the ease of generating an immediate image with the technology means that retakes are more common thus increasing radiation exposure.[21] Furthermore, one should ensure that assistants, technologists, and the

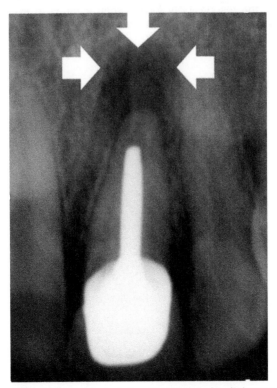

Fig. 8. Maxillary central incisor periapical showing an apical radiolucency (*arrows*) in relation to the left maxillary central incisor radiographically consistent with an apical rarefying osteitis (inflammatory).

dentists themselves are competently trained and, in the case of auxiliaries, supervised to avoid technical errors (**Fig. 9**) that can result in radiograph retakes or missed pertinent information.

In addition to adhering to the as low as diagnostically acceptable principle, the dentist should be careful to ensure that the patient is able to make an informed choice. In the case that there are multiple diagnostic procedure options, the dentist must describe the ideal diagnostic procedure as well as alternate and less-than-ideal options, regardless of financial cost.[22] Informing the patient of all treatment options ensures that the dentist meets a standard of care. Failure to meet or exceed a standard of care is considered professional negligence. In malpractice lawsuits, the patient is required to provide evidence of negligence,[22] which could be thusly argued from the standpoint of excessive radiograph retakes, inadequate training, or being incompletely informed about the best treatment option.

Interpretation

Another important facet of radiographic practice is the degree to which a dentist or radiologist is responsible for the interpretation of a scan.[23] Fundamentally, the dentist who orders the imaging study is responsible for making sure that the entire study is interpreted. This does not mean that the dentist themselves needs to personally read the scan, only that the dentist who orders the scan is responsible for having it read completely by a competent individual.[23] The onus of responsibility on the dentist is the same whether the dentist takes the scan or has their scans taken somewhere else. Furthermore, the responsibility for the scan extends to everything within the scan, not just the anatomic region for which the scan was taken.[23] Therefore, if the

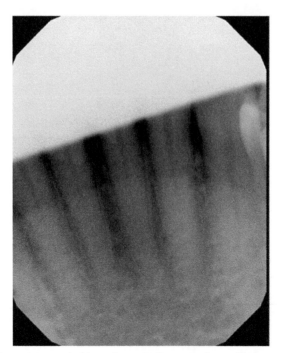

Fig. 9. A collimator cut was noted in an improperly exposed mandibular central incisor periapical radiograph. Significant collimator cuts render the radiographs useless and many times would require a re-exposure adding to the patient radiation dose.

dentist is not able to interpret the whole scan, they must refer to a radiologist who can do so. Needless to state, there should be a complete written record of the findings and other data related to the study.

If a dentist takes a scan for a patient other than their own, that dentist should make clear to the referring dentist and to the patient that only the technical service of taking the scan is being offered and that no diagnostic service was done. Many facilities that offer scanning services have such a disclaimer and furthermore require the ordering dentist to obtain a reading from the scans to limit liability.[23] It should be noted that in some states, California for example, there exist "scan reading" services by imaging centers. These imaging centers may employ lay people who, although being well trained in the technical aspects of taking radiographs, are otherwise untrained to interpret them. Although the radiographs taken at such centers should be of diagnostic quality, a dentist who also relies on such scan reading services may be vulnerable to liability issues based on the legal concept of negligent referral[23] because the dentist may not know the reader's qualifications. Although such situations are rare and considered a gray area,[23] the dentist should be aware of their existence and vet their referred radiologists to avoid liability.

In the United States, state-by-state licensing laws complicate the issue of out-of-state referrals for reading radiographs. Fundamentally, licensing laws exist to protect the citizens of a state, so a radiologist who provides services for patients in a state must be licensed to practice in that state and only in that state.[23] Therefore, a radiologist who reads the radiograph of an out-of-state patient must be licensed in the state of that patient.[23] However, this is not to say that the radiologist who reads from out-of-state is necessarily exempt from also having a license in their own state. The constitutional standard that a state needs to meet to justify requiring licensure is extremely low,[23] and it is possible that the radiologist could be required to carry a license for state in which they reside even if the radiologist reads no scans for patients within their own state. This licensing pitfall affects both the radiologist who reads the scan and the dentist who refers to the radiologist. If the radiologist fails to obtain the necessary licenses, they could be charged with practicing without a license. Consequently, the referring dentist may be guilty of aiding and abetting the practice of unlicensed dentistry.[23] Because licensing laws vary state by state, the dentist who refers to an out-of-state radiologist should consult both the board of their own state as well as the board where the radiologist is located. These licensing pitfalls increase potential liability for a suit based on negligent referral which, although rare, should be kept in mind.

Storage

Most directives that dictate the handling of digital radiographs stem from the idea that the standard for radiographic image quality is film when viewed on a standard illumination viewer under reduced ambient lighting.[21] Thus, digital technology has a few caveats of which the dentist must be aware to ensure that the digital image quality does not fall below that of film.

With respect to storage, the electronic record should be complete and accurate to the original content.[21] The electronic files generated by a CBCT scan are quite large and so it may be tempting to compress the file to save storage space. There are two ways to compress data; by lossless or by lossy algorithms. Lossless compression does not involve any data loss, but lossy compression involves irrevocable loss of data.[21] To ensure that the electronic record is in fact complete and accurate, lossy compression should be avoided at all costs. Furthermore, the computer program chosen to view digital radiographs should prevent the erasure or alteration of images that, on principle, serves as a software fail safe to help prevent the dentist from accidently losing or inappropriately modifying scans.

The digital display should have a resolution high enough to display digital radiographs of diagnostic quality, to prevent misdiagnosis.[21] Similarly, hard copies of digital radiographs must be of diagnostic quality; to this end, appropriate software and printers must be used. If scans of film are created, the original films must be kept for legal purposes because scanned copies do not produce images of diagnostic quality.[21] The laws that dictate the length of time that film must be stored vary from state to state.

Medicolegal Considerations that Are Considered Fraudulent

The following dental practice or service-related acts could result in criminal charges if discovered. Lewis and Farragher[24] wrote about the most common situations that are considered fraudulent related to dental practice billing.

Misrepresenting dates of service

Lewis and Farragher articulated that, "Misrepresenting the date of service in a dental practice is fraudulent. This makes a difference to insurance companies as there may be a waiting period before benefits being available or benefits may have ended before the day of service. Sometimes the date of service is changed to take advantage of any early deductible requirement"[24] (**Fig. 10**).

Performing unnecessary procedures

Lewis and Farragher[24] defined these procedures as the "performance and billing for treatments not needed or providing additional services or procedures beyond what was required, to increase billings and claims amounts."

Billing for services not rendered

Similar to issues seen in many professions, billing for services not provided happens in dentistry as well. For instance, when a dentist examines a patient and then bills for other preventive procedures such as sealants or fluorides without actually performing them, it is defined as fraudulent billing.[24]

Waiving of copayments

If dentists inflate their charges for procedures and do not collect any necessary copayments, it is considered a billing fraud.

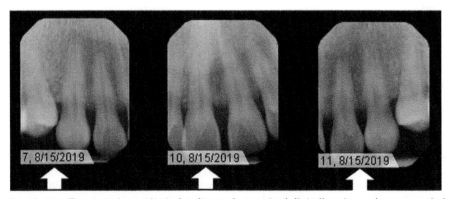

Fig. 10. Maxillary anterior periapical radiographs acquired digitally using a charge-coupled device sensor. Note the acquisition dates (*white arrows*) automatically populated on the images.

Misrepresentation of services

Diagnosing or coding procedures incorrectly is fraudulent and can cause liability. In 1 case as per Lewis and Farragher,[24] "a provider was performing routine dental extractions and using the procedure code for impacted teeth. The insurance company noticed that the same radiograph was being provided for each patient with the name being changed." In some instances, dentists who are not oral and maxillofacial radiologists may bill for acquisition and reading of CBCT volumes as two 2D images instead of one 3D volume because the patient's insurance may not have covered the 3D volume for either acquisition or interpretation or both. This is a classic example of misrepresentation of services. The oral and maxillofacial radiologists could have billed for services if he or she had hospital privileges and the service would have been covered completely. Although these situations are rare, they happen sporadically.

Unbundling of procedures

The American Dental Association defines unbundling of procedures as "the separating of a dental procedure into component parts with each part having a charge, so that the cumulative charge of the components is greater than the total charge to patients who are not beneficiaries of a dental benefit plan for the same procedure."[24]

Upcoding

Defined by the American Dental Association as "reporting a more complex and/or higher cost procedure than was actually performed,"[24] upcoding increases the limits set by insurance companies, and hence dental offices collect more money from the patient that is not covered by the insurance. This is considered a fraudulent behavior.

Although most dentists are honest, sincere, and law abiding, there might be a small percentage of them or their office staff who may resort to some unethical behavior discussed here but, thankfully, it is rare. Dental practitioners always try to uphold the values of the profession and live up to the expectations of the people who trust them for their health care needs.

CLINICS CARE POINTS

- Care should be taken to minimize radiation exposure to the patient using the as low as diagnostically acceptable principle.
- As an adjunct to professional judgment, evidence based guidelines help the practitioner choose the appropriate radiographs.
- Plain radiography is the first choice in most scenarios.
- CBCT should be used when 2D imaging alone cannot answer the clinical question
- Knowledge of normal radiographic anatomy is paramount.
- Radiographs serve as evidence in investigations of suspected medical or dental malpractice.

DISCLOSURES

The authors have nothing to disclose.

REFERENCES

1. Bushberg JT. Eleventh annual Warren K. Sinclair keynote address-science, radiation protection and NCRP: building on the past, looking to the future. Health Phys 2015;108(2):115–23.

2. Canadian Dental Association. Position paper on "Control of X-Radiation in Dentistry.". Available at: http://www.cda.adc.ca/files/position_statements/xradiation.pdf. Accessed August 12, 2020.

3. Brooks SL, Joseph LP. Basic concepts in the selection of patients for dental x-ray examinations. Rockville (MD): U.S. Department of Health and Human Services; FDA. HHS Publication 85-8249; 1985.

4. US Department of Health and Human Services. The selection of patients for x-ray examinations: dental radiographic examinations. Washington, DC: HHS Publ (FDA); 1987. p. 88–8273.

5. American Dental Association Council on Dental materials instruments and equipment. Recommendations in radiographic practices: an update, 1988. J Am Dent Assoc 1989;118:115–7.

6. American Dental Association Council on Scientific Affairs. An update on radiographic practice: information and recommendations. J Am Dent Assoc 2001; 132:234–8.

7. American Dental Association council on scientific affairs and the U.S. Department of Health and Human Services. The selection of patients for dental radiographic examinations. Available at: http://www.ada.org/prof/resources/topics/topics_radiography_examinations.pdf. Accessed August 12, 2020.

8. American Dental Association Council on Scientific Affairs. The use of dental radiographs: update and recommendations. J Am Dent Assoc 2006;137:1304–12.

9. White SC, Atchison KA, Hewlett ER, et al. Efficacy of FDA guidelines for ordering radiographs for caries detection. Oral Surg Oral Med Oral Pathol 1994;77: 531–40.

10. Atchison KA, White SC, Flack VF, et al. The efficacy of FDA guidelines for ordering radiographs to diagnose periodontal disease. J Dent Res 1994;73:2413.

11. Hewlett ER, Atchison KA, White SC, et al. Efficacy of FDA guidelines for detecting restoration defects. J Dent Res 1994;73:2412.

12. Kim IH, Mupparapu M. Dental radiographic guidelines: a review. Quintessence Int 2009;40:389–98.

13. Kim IH, Singer SR, Mupparapu M. Review of cone beam computed tomography guidelines in North America. Quintessence Int 2019;50:136–45.

14. American Association of Endodontists; American Academy of Oral and Maxillofacial Radiology. Use of cone beam computed tomography in endodontics Joint Position Statement of the American Association of Endodontics and the American Academy of Oral and Maxillofacial Radiology. Oral Surg Oral Med Oral Pathol Oral Radiol Endod 2011;111:234–7.

15. The American Dental Association Council on Scientific Affairs. The use of conebeam computed tomography in dentistry, an advisory statement from the American Dental Association Council on Scientific Affairs. J Am Dent Assoc 2012;143: 899–902.

16. Tyndall D, Price J, Tetradis S, et al. Position statement of the American academy of oral and maxillofacial radiology on the selection criteria for the use of radiology in dental implantology with emphasis on cone beam computed tomography. Oral Surg Oral Med Oral Pathol Oral Radiol Endod 2012;113:817–26.

17. Mandelaris GA, Scheyer ET, Evans M, et al. American academy of periodontology best evidence consensus statement on selected oral applications for conebeam computed tomography. J Periodontol 2017;88:939–45.

18. Mupparapu M, Nadeau C. Oral and maxillofacial imaging. Dent Clin North Am 2016;60(1):1–37.

19. Mupparapu M, Creanga AG, Singer SR. Interpretation of cone beam computed tomography volumetric data. How to report findings? Quintessence Int 2017; 48:733–41.
20. Zinman E, White SC, Tetradis S. Legal considerations in the use of cone beam computer tomography imaging. CDA J 2010;38(1):49–56.
21. MacDonald-Jankowski DS, Orpe EC. Some current legal issues that may affect oral and maxillofacial radiology: part 1. Basic principles in digital dental radiology. J Can Dent Assoc 2007;73(5):409–14.
22. Curley A, Hatcher DC. Cone beam CT – anatomic assessment and legal issues: the new standards of care. CDA J 2009;37(9):653–62.
23. Friedland B, Miles DA. Liabilities and risks of using cone beam computed tomography. Dent Clin North Am 2014;58:671–85.
24. Dental health-care fraud and abuse. Available at: https://www.dentaleconomics.com/practice/article/16393378/dental-healthcare-fraud-and-abuse.   Accessed August 30, 2020.

Radiology of Dental Caries

Adeyinka F. Dayo, BDS, MS[a],*, Mark S. Wolff, DDS, PhD[b],
Ali Z. Syed, BDS, MHA, MS, DABOMR[c], Mel Mupparapu, DMD, MDS, DABOMR[b]

KEYWORDS

- Dental caries • Biofilm • Ecosystem • Caries detection • Sensitivity • Radiography
- Reflectance • Fluorescence

KEY POINTS

- Dental caries is a preventable, reversible, multifactorial, complex biofilm disease that progresses with time.
- Dental caries is a dynamic continuum of tooth demineralization/neutrality/remineralization with a net demineralization initiating caries lesion.
- Visual examination and intraoral radiographs are still vital in diagnosis of dental caries.
- Early caries detection is paramount to effective chemotherapeutic, noninvasive management.
- Sensitive caries detectors serve as adjuncts for early caries detection that help to shift the dental practitioner toward minimal intervention dentistry.

DENTAL CARIES

Dental caries is a complex biofilm disease that creates prolonged periods of low pH in the mouth, resulting in a net mineral loss from the teeth.[1] Dental caries forms through a complex interaction over time between acid-producing bacteria and fermentable carbohydrate, and many host factors, including teeth and saliva. The disease develops in the crowns and roots of teeth, and it can arise in early childhood as an aggressive tooth decay that affects the primary teeth of infants and toddlers.

CARIES PROCESS AND CURRENT CONCEPTS

Cariogenic bacteria are essential to the disease process. At least 2 major groups of bacteria, namely, the *streptococci* species (chiefly *Streptococcus mutans*) and the *lactobacilli* species (chiefly *Lactobacillus fermentum*, *Lactobacillus casei/paracasei*,

[a] Department of Oral Medicine, University of Pennsylvania School of Dental Medicine, 240 South 40th Street, Philadelphia, PA 19104, USA; [b] University of Pennsylvania School of Dental Medicine, 240 South 40th Street, Philadelphia, PA 19104, USA; [c] Department of Oral and Maxillofacial Medicine and Diagnostic Sciences, CWRU School of Dental Medicine, Office # 245 C, 9601 Chester Avenue, Cleveland, OH 44106, USA
* Corresponding author.
E-mail address: dayoad@upenn.edu

Dent Clin N Am 65 (2021) 427–445
https://doi.org/10.1016/j.cden.2021.02.002
0011-8532/21/© 2021 Elsevier Inc. All rights reserved.

and *Lactobacillus salivarius*),[2] can produce organic acids during metabolism of fermentable carbohydrates and are known as acidogenic. Acids produced by these bacteria include lactic, acetic, formic, and propionic acid, all of which readily dissolve the mineral content of enamel and dentin.

FROM HISTORICAL DEFINITION TO CURRENT EVIDENCE

The definition of dental caries has expanded to a more complex discussion of the caries process that represents a continuum of tooth demineralization/remineralization. This "modern" view started with the definition by Miller[3] 1890 of a 2-step process whereby bacteria on the tooth, exposed to fermentable carbohydrates, produce acid, and in a second step, dissolve the surface of the tooth. Stephan[4] demonstrated that this production of acid after exposure to fermentable carbohydrate resulted in a localized drop in pH within the plaque followed by a subsequent return to the baseline pH over time hence establishing the concept of caries being a cyclic event of demineralization/neutrality/remineralization. Englander and colleagues[5] demonstrated the role of saliva in neutralizing the decrease in plaque pH after exposure to fermentable carbohydrate. Although considerable attention has been placed on a few bacterial species as the cause of dental caries (eg, *S mutans*, *Lactobacillus*), there is general agreement today that the dental biofilm exists as a complex ecosystem that can shift from a neutral pH to a more acidic ecosystem.[6] Today, dental caries is accepted as an imbalance in the biofilm-induced cyclic process of demineralization and remineralization of tooth structure, by the acidic by-products resulting in a pH maximal drop followed by the return of the pH to initial pH modulated by saliva. The mixed ecology of the biofilm may be naturally shifted in composition to a more acidic ecology by repeated exposure to fermentable carbohydrate.[3,5,7] Saliva helps modulate both the composition of the biofilm and the recovery of the biofilm pH after sugar challenge.[5] The susceptibility of tooth to demineralization may be modulated by the incorporation of fluoride in the tooth structure.[7] Dental caries is a continuum of demineralization and remineralization with a net demineralization resulting in tooth surface alterations that eventually result in cavitation. The caries process is influenced by several factors, such as increase in frequency of sugar consumption and increase in sugar retention time, which directly relates to an increase in demineralization of teeth resulting in cavitation, measured clinically as decay/missing/filled/teeth.[8] However, it must be remembered that in this balance, frequent/longer acid cycles result in a shift in the biofilm flora in favor of acidogenic bacteria.[6] Importantly, an increase in the quantity of sugar consumed alone is not a predictor of increased caries, as many communities around the world have increased caries preventive strategies over the same time period as sugar consumption has increased.[9] Decreases in saliva flow can also favor a shift in the caries balance toward demineralization, resulting in an increase in caries progression. The caries balance is affected by multiple social determinants favoring demineralization. Research has demonstrated that acid is not the only product of the mixed ecology. Alkali production has potential in changing the pH of the oral biofilm, which impacts demineralization.[10]

INTRAORAL RADIOGRAPHY

Intraoral radiography has been an integral part of the diagnostic arsenal for more than 100 years. Intraoral radiographs typically consist of periapical and bitewing radiographs, and both have excellent spatial resolution. Periapical means surrounding the apex of the root of a tooth (**Fig.1**); hence it captures the complete crown and root of a tooth with about 2mm beyond the root apex. On the other hand, bitewing

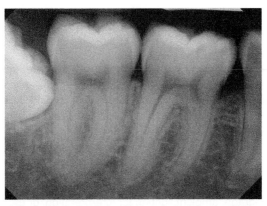

Fig. 1. Mandibular right molar periapical radiograph showing both the erupted molars and the partially visible impacted third molar.

radiographs capture the crown and a third of the root of the maxillary and mandibular teeth with its accompanying interalveolar bone (**Fig. 2**) and are used in clinical practice to evaluate interproximal caries; crestal bone height in the interproximal region; calculus; and periodontal disease.

Bitewing radiographs are obtained for examination of interproximal surfaces as well as crestal bone levels. Based on the orientation of the detector in the mouth, they can be either vertical (see **Fig. 2**) or horizontal. Technological innovations and advancement in radiography with a focus on minimizing the amount of radiation to the patient when acquiring radiographs led to a shift of radiographic image receptors from analog films to direct digital sensors. Analog films are still being used in clinical practice; however, it is recommended that no dental radiographic film with speeds lower than E- or F-speed shall be used for intraoral radiography, as the dose is essentially halved from

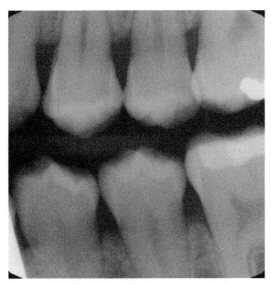

Fig. 2. A vertical left premolar bitewing showing interproximal contacts and crestal bone levels.

the older D-speed to E-plus or F-speeds.[11] Phosphor plates may be compared with analog films in terms of flexibility and is suitable for pediatric and special needs patients. One major disadvantage of the phosphor plates is that after extensive usage, they sustain irreversible damage because of their susceptibility to scratches, bite marks, and creasing. Solid-state sensors, also known as direct digital sensors, are of 2 types depending on how the image is captured: charge coupled device (CCD) and complementary metal oxide semiconductors. Alcaraz and colleagues[12] showed dose reduction using direct digital sensors in comparison with the analog films. Digital radiographic sensors are an objective and reproducible technique; however, its sensitivity for detection of early and recurrent caries is suboptimal,[13,14] with reported sensitivity being as low as 0.30.[13,15] Caries detection can be affected by a variety of factors during acquisition or interpretation, such as variation in image capture, detector placement, status of the detector, focus to object distance, kilovolt or milliampere used for capture of the radiograph, ambient lighting for interpretation, or the experience of the clinician.

EXTRAORAL BITEWING RADIOGRAPHY (USING PANORAMIC RADIOGRAPHS)

Initial ex vivo studies have shown that intraoral bitewing radiography (IOBWR) is superior to extraoral bitewing radiography (EOBWR).[16] Another study compared the detection accuracy of proximal caries and crestal bone loss using EOBWR or IOBWR and concluded that although EOBWR has promise, clinicians should be aware of the false positive diagnoses of proximal caries and crestal bone loss when using EOBWR.[17] Despite these diagnostic issues, during the COVID-19 pandemic, the use of EOBWR (**Fig. 3**) was recommended as a guideline, because of the possibility of creation of aerosols during intraoral procedures, more so in exaggerated gag and cough reflex cases (Personal communication from Dr. David MacDonald, University of British Columbia (UBC), Vancouver, Canada - Oral and Maxillofacial Imaging guidelines during COVID-19 pandemic. Submitted to Oral Surg Oral Med Oral Pathol oral Radiol, 2020).

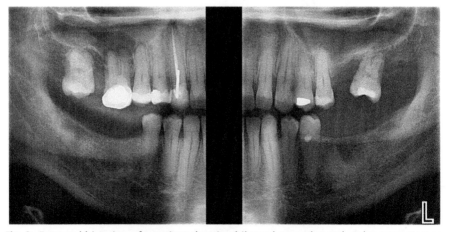

Fig. 3. Extraoral bitewing of a patient showing bilateral premolar and molar contact areas. There are other significant periapical findings in this radiograph, especially apical regions of maxillary right canine, premolars, and molars.

CARIES DETECTION: DIGITAL VERSUS CONVENTIONAL RADIOGRAPHY

Sensitivity and specificity values for direct digital radiography were 73% and 95% at the buccal and lingual line angles, and 29% and 90% at the midgingival floor, respectively.[18] Corresponding values for conventional radiography were 63% and 93% at the buccal line angle, 61% and 93% at the lingual line angle, and 44% and 95% at the mid-gingival floor, respectively.[18] The total sensitivity and specificity values were 58% and 93% for digital radiography and 56% and 93% for conventional radiography with no significant difference ($P = .104$). The sensitivity and specificity of film, CCD, and photostimulable phosphors (PSP) for the detection of enamel caries were 38% and 98%; 15% and 96%; and 23% and 98%, respectively. The sensitivity and specificity of film, CCD and PSP for the detection of both dentin and enamel caries, were 55% and 100%; 45% and 100%; and 55% and 100%, respectively.[19] Sensitivity of all 3 receptors (CCD, PSP, film) for detection of enamel lesions was low (5.5%–44.4%), but it was higher for dentin lesions (42.8%–62.8%); PSP with 70 kVp and 0.03-second exposure time had the highest sensitivity for enamel lesions, but the difference among receptors was not statistically significant ($P>.05$). PSP with 60 kVp and 0.07-second exposure time had higher sensitivity and lower patient radiation dose for detection of cavitated and noncavitated lesions, but the difference was not significant ($P>.05$).[20]

RADIOGRAPHIC INTERPRETATION OF CARIES

Imaging is an integral component of caries detection. Radiographically, dental caries is essentially a process of demineralization leading to density changes within the enamel or dentine and hence detectable using radiographic imaging. Radiographic detection of dental caries and the methods used for detection have changed over the years. In the early days, the focus of radiographic imaging was on the periapical areas of teeth, as the investigation was based on pain or infection, which was the late stage of dental caries that had led to cavitation and pulp exposure with tracking of bacteria through pulpal blood vessels to the periapical region causing an inflammatory process. Currently, there is a shift toward early detection and minimal intervention dentistry (MID).

INTERPRETATION OF CARIES

Accurate interpretation of carious lesions starts with accurate radiographic depiction of adjacent contact points of teeth using bitewing radiography. To obtain bitewing radiographs that are of optimum diagnostic values, contacts should be opened using appropriate horizontal angulation and XCP positioning device. Appropriate kilovolt and milliampere as well as standardized exposure time are essential for optimally exposed radiographs. A good contrast is essential for the diagnosis of dental caries, as both underexposures and overexposures will lead to erroneous interpretation of dental caries, as demonstrated in **Fig. 4**.

Radiographically, dental caries appears as radiolucency leading to loss of normal homogeneity of the enamel, as the lesion extends further toward the dentino-enamel junction (DEJ), the DEJ line loses its continuity in the region. The inherent low-contrast resolution of plain radiographs makes it impossible to determine the full extent of dentin involvement. The line pair resolution of digital dental radiographs is about 20 line pairs per millimeter.[21] Small occlusal lesions, buccal and lingual pit cavities, are better studied clinically, as radiography plays a small role in the detection of these lesions.[22] Dental caries recurs if not completely excavated before restoration, and lesions appear as radiolucency adjacent to or beneath the restoration. Because

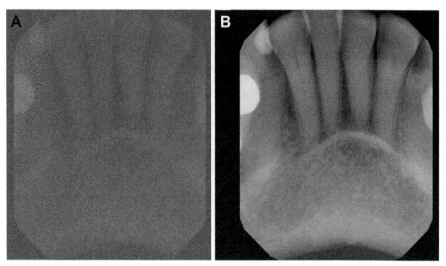

Fig. 4. Mandibular central incisor periapical radiograph. Poor contrast (A); appropriate contrast (B).

radiographs are a 2-dimensional representation of a 3-dimensional tooth structure, it is not always possible to determine caries extension to the pulp chamber or pulp horn because of anatomic variations and presence of radiopaque restorations in the crowns. In the presence of caries, pulp is generally reactive and lays down new dentin called, "secondary dentin," which functions to wall off the receding pulp from the carious attack. The only radiographically certain way of determining pulp exposure is the visualization of secondary caries and periapical changes in the alveolar process, such as widened periodontal ligament space or lack of continuity of lamina dura. Rarely, cavitated dental caries undergoes spontaneous arrest.[22]

RADIATION CARIES

Radiotherapy for head and neck cancers lead to decreased salivation especially if the salivary glands are in the "direct path of radiation." It is known that the short-term loss of function in the salivary glands leads to clinical xerostomia, which further accentuates clinical caries, especially rapidly advancing root caries. The lack of lubrication and buffering action from saliva, increased salivary pH (acidic), and increased colonization of acidogenic bacteria (especially S mutans) all lead to caries of smooth surfaces, and this is termed "radiation caries," although it not directly caused by radiation. Advanced radiation-induced hyposalivation may lead to tooth fracture, dental abscess, tooth loss, or osteoradionecrosis. Direct-acting cholinergic parasympathomimetic agents, such as Pilocarpine hydrochloride, or muscarinic agonist, like Cevimeline, are used for treatment of xerostomia. A thiol-containing agent, like Amifostine, has been used for its radioprotective properties in the prevention of radiation-induced changes by scavenging free radicals.

CLASSIFICATION OF CARIES ACTIVITY AND RADIOGRAPHIC DETECTION

Caries is a dynamic disease that requires a classification system that is sensitive enough to monitor the disease activity, the surface of involved teeth, and the depth of caries penetration. There are several caries classification systems, and the American Dental Association Caries Classification System[23] is as follows:

- Sound surface: Healthy sound enamel with no detectable lesion with normal glossy surface.
- Initial caries lesion: Early lesions that demonstrate net mineral loss in enamel or exposed dentin that may only be visible when the tooth is dried by air or color change toward white.
- Moderate caries lesion: Moderate mineral loss with loss of tooth surface integrity/anatomy with deeper demineralization. There may be shallow or microcavitation. There may be color changes in enamel with brown or gray shadows and/or translucency.
- Advanced caries lesion: Advanced mineral loss with cavitation through enamel. Dentin is exposed.

Caries activity is defined as active or inactive/arrested. Active lesions are shiny/glossy and smooth to touch; inactive/arrested lesions are frosty/matte in luster with a roughened surface. Caries can also be detected radiographically by looking at the approximal surface of teeth. Lesions are classified based on the depth of demineralization detected on the approximal surface. The stage of the lesion is based on depth of penetration from the outer tooth surface, as follows:

- E0: Intact tooth surface (see **Fig. 2**)
- E1: Radiographic penetration less than halfway into enamel, initial lesion (**Fig. 5**)

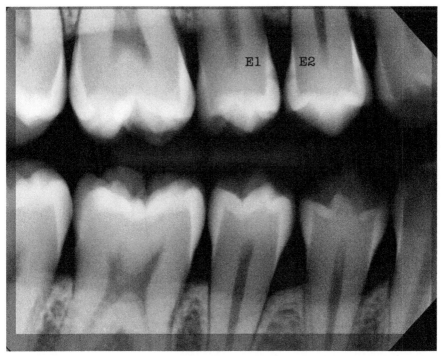

Fig. 5. Right premolar bitewing showing carious lesions (E1, E2) in the maxillary right premolars.

- E2: Radiographic penetration more than halfway into enamel but not penetrating the dentin, initial lesion (see **Fig. 5**)
- D1: Radiographic penetration to the outer one-third of the dentin, initial lesion **(Fig. 6)**
- D2: Radiographic penetration to the middle one-third of the dentin, moderate lesion **(Fig. 7)**
- D3: Radiographic penetration to the inner one-third of the dentin, advanced lesion (see **Fig. 7**)

Teeth with E1 lesions do not have cavitation; E2 lesions demonstrate surface cavitation less than 11% of the time, and D1 lesions demonstrate surface cavitation 41% of the time.[24]

Appropriate classification of the caries lesion is needed for adequate treatment planning and restoration of the affected tooth. In addition, what was previously termed "preeruptive caries" is now thought to be either progressive or nonprogressive. "Preeruptive intracoronal radiolucency (PEIR)" **(Fig. 8)** has been studied extensively, and in 1 study, for 9 years clinically and radiographically. They are generally noted just below the DEJ within dentin with no direct communication to either enamel or pulp. All nonprogressive lesions are managed nonoperatively by sealants.[25] There is evidence to support use of silver diamine fluoride to treat dentine caries in primary teeth and in also preventing recurrence.[26]

EVOLUTION OF CARIES DETECTION TECHNIQUES (OVERVIEW)

Current understanding of the dynamic caries process has led to a paradigm shift in dentistry from Black's model of "extension for prevention" to the concept of MID.

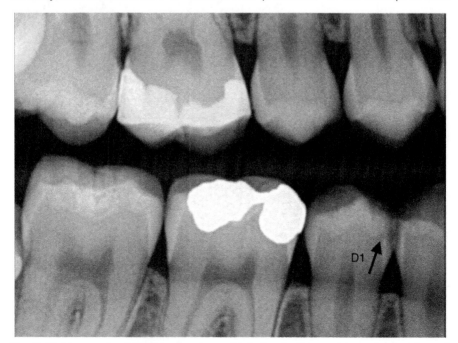

Fig. 6. Right premolar bitewing showing a D1 lesion in the mesial proximal surface of mandibular right second premolar.

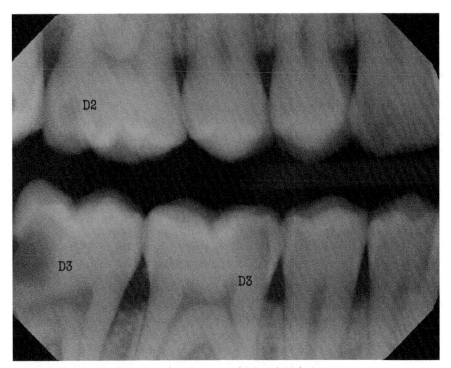

Fig. 7. Right premolar bitewing showing several D2 and D3 lesions.

Caries detection is a process of recognizing and recording in a standardized format, changes in dental hard tissues that are caused by the caries process. Sensitive caries-detecting techniques allow monitoring of dental caries, which involves the assessment of the severity, extent, or activity of caries over time. Clinical visual inspection and intraoral radiographs are vital for caries diagnosis and management,

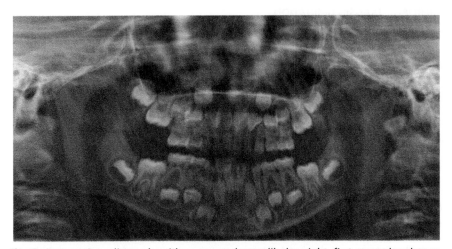

Fig. 8. Panoramic radiograph with unerupted mandibular right first premolar demonstrating the pre-eruptive intracoronal radiolucency.

although not a sensitive modality for early caries detection.[13–15,27] Approximately 30% to 40% of mineral loss is necessary before an early enamel caries lesion is visible radiographically,[28] and bitewing radiographs are associated with a relatively high proportion of false positive and negative scores.[29] Meja're and colleagues[29] reported 203 white spot lesions out of 305 being incorrectly scored as sound on radiographs. At the stage of cavitation, dental caries cannot be controlled by chemotherapeutic treatments or noninvasive procedures. Visual inspection is based on changes in color, transparency, and hardness of the dental tissue; however, it is a subjective method with low reproducibility in detecting occlusal caries, because it is influenced by the knowledge and clinical experience of the examiner.[23,24] Adjunctive modalities are needed for early caries detection, especially in an "at-risk" population.[27,30,31]

CURRENT TRENDS OF CARIES DETECTION

Globally, it is recognized that the development of new technologies that are sensitive for early caries detection is essential to quantitatively and qualitatively monitor dental decay.[30–32] Gomez and colleagues[33] in a systematic review on the performance of caries detection methods reported a sensitivity ranging from 0.12 to 0.84 and 0.20 to 0.96 for radiographic and visual diagnosis of caries, respectively; this lower limit is suboptimal. Early detection of dental caries will ultimately provide health and socioeconomic benefits through timely preventive interventions, reduced treatment cost, and facilitation of clinical dental research on potential anticaries agents. Here, the authors describe some of the advanced, sensitive, nonionizing radiation technologies available to the dental practitioner as an adjunct to clinical visual examination and radiographic evaluation for early detection of dental caries and possible monitoring of interventional treatment over time. Dental caries is a dynamic process, and at any point in time, it may be in the active, inactive (arrested), or reversed phase of development. Subclinical and early clinical stages can be reversed by nonsurgical modalities, such as fluoride application, diet modification, antimicrobials, sealants, and no treatment.[30,32] Hence, the evolution of new sensitive technologies can qualitatively detect and monitor the activity of caries lesion by quantification of changes in mineral content of the lesion over time. Some of these technologies are as follows (**Table 1**).

FIBEROPTIC TRANSILLUMINATION

Fiberoptic transillumination uses the principle of light transmission using a narrow beam of intense white light to illuminate the tooth. Carious enamel has a lower index of light transmission than sound enamel, so more light is absorbed because of changes in the light scattering and absorption properties. Demineralized areas in dentin or enamel appear as darkened areas. DiagnoCam is a digitalized and computed version of fiberoptic transillumination (FOTI), replacing white light with near infrared (NIR; 780 nm) and adding a digital CCD camera. It images the light emerging from the surface closest to the CCD camera.

MIDWEST CARIES I.D.

The Midwest caries ID is a small, battery-operated piece of equipment that emits a soft light-emitting diode (LED) light between 635 nm and 880 nm to measure the reflectance and refraction of light from the tooth surface for detecting and quantifying caries. Demineralized or carious areas turn the LED from green to red, which is converted by fiberoptics into an audible signal. A buzzer beeps with different frequencies to indicate the intensity of demineralization detected. Sensitivity and specificity are reported to be

Table 1
The salient features of various caries detection systems

Type of System	FOTI	DIAGNOCam	Diagnodent	ECM	QLF	OCT	PTR-LUM
Technique	High-intensity white light via fiberoptic illuminator	High-intensity white light via fiberoptic illuminator and CCD camera	Laser diode (generates a pulsed 655-nm laser beam)	Weak alternating current	Optical imaging system (488 nm)	Low coherence interferometry Uses infrared and red LED	Combination of laser light-induced LUM and heat (659 and 830 nm)
Mechanism	Carious enamel has a lower index of light transmission than sound enamel (scattering from the porous enamel and absorption in demineralized dentin)	Carious enamel has a lower index of light transmission than sound enamel (scattering from the porous enamel and absorption in demineralized dentin)	Stimulated fluorescence due to demineralization and presence of bacteria and their metabolites	• Measures the electrical resistance or impedance • Decrease in electrical resistance seen as lesions increase in porosity and become water filled	• Assessment of the lesion based on loss of a fluorescence signal • Decrease in fluorescence is related to the scattering properties of carious enamel	• Illuminates tissue with low-power NIR light, collects the backscattered light, and analyzes the intensity • The interference signal is acquired by a photodiode or CCD	Measures the modulated thermal infrared radiation (PTR) and modulated LUM of tooth surface
Usage	Proximal and occlusal caries	Caries on all tooth surfaces	Smooth and occlusal surface caries	Incipient and occlusal caries	Incipient and smooth surface caries	Incipient enamel and root caries	Quality, depth characterization, monitoring caries progression

(continued on next page)

Table 1
(continued)

Type of System	FOTI	DIAGNOCam	Diagnodent	ECM	QLF	OCT	PTR-LUM
Best application	Assessment of the depth of occlusal lesions	Incipient caries, depth of occlusal caries, fractures, cracks, secondary caries	DIAGNOdent pen for proximal caries	Can monitor lesion progression, arrest, or remineralization	Assessment of smooth surface lesions, enamel fluorosis	Interproximal and margins of restorations	Depth profilometric technique Permit detection up to 5 mm from tooth surface
Other uses	N/A	• Quantitative method • Patient education and motivation	• Quantitative method • Convenient and fast	• Quantitative method • Objective reading	• Quantitative method • Monitor tooth whitening	• Quantitative method • Assess periodontal tissues, implants, versatile • Not affected by staining or calculi	• Quantitative method • Can assess caries under restorations, sealants • Not affected by staining or calculi
Appearance	Enamel and dentine caries appear as shadows	• Enamel and dentine caries appear as shadows • Create high-resolution digital images	• Infrared fluorescence of caries • Score of 0–99.9	Score of 0–9: directly proportional to the degree of demineralization	Caries lesions appear dark surrounded by highly luminescent sound enamel	Cross-sectional images	Canary numbers from 1 to 100: 1–20 (healthy), 21–70 (early caries lesion), 71–100 (decay)

Disadvantage	• Nonquan-titative method • Cannot assess all surfaces or early caries • False negative	• Limited depth of detection • Stains or calculi can give false positives	Organic and nonorganic materials (stains, plaque, calculus, amalgam overhang, and hypoplasia) fluoresce giving false positives	• It is time consuming • Limited scan area • Sensitive to saliva or temperature changes	Stains on tooth surface and fluorosis give false positives	Penetration depth and scanning range are limited	Sensitive to angulation
Cost	Low cost	Low cost	Low cost	—	—	High cost	High cost

higher than that of DIAGNOdent.[32] It has good reproducibility but false positive signals from malformed teeth, dark stains, dental fluorosis, hypoplasia, plaque, and calculus, because of alteration in the translucency of enamel caused by these conditions.

ELECTRICAL CARIES MONITOR

The technology of the electrical caries monitor (ECM) is based on the electrical conductivity differences between sound and carious dental tissues. Caries causes demineralization of enamel and results in increased porosity of the enamel with the influx of saliva into its pores forming conductive pathways for electrical transmission. There is increased conductivity with increased demineralization. ECM measures the electrical resistance or impedance of an area on the tooth; high measurements indicate well-mineralized tissue, whereas low values indicate demineralization. The tooth is dried to avoid electrical conductance via saliva.

ALTERNATING CURRENT IMPEDANCE SPECTROSCOPY, CarieScan PRO

This technology, alternating current impedance spectroscopy, CarieScan pro, uses alternating current impedance spectroscopy involving the passing of an insensitive level of electrical current through the tooth to identify and localize decay. Healthy or sound enamel exhibits high electrical resistance (impedance), and demineralized areas have lower resistance. CarieScan is not affected by optical factors, such as staining or discoloration of the tooth. A green color display indicates sound tooth tissue; a red color indicates deep caries requiring invasive treatment, and a yellow color is associated with a range of numerical figures from 1 to 99, depicting varying severity of caries that can be treated via noninvasive techniques. The device is indicated for the detection, diagnosis, and monitoring of occlusal and accessible smooth surface dental caries. It cannot be used to assess secondary caries or the integrity of a restoration.

QUANTITATIVE LIGHT-INDUCED FLUORESCENCE, QUANTITATIVE

This technology of quantitative light-induced fluorescence (QLF), quantitative was introduced in 1995.[34] QLF uses the natural fluorescence of teeth (light absorption and scattering properties) and its ability to differentiate between caries and sound enamel. A broad beam of blue-green light from argon laser of 488-nm wavelength is used to induce fluorescence. The QLF system is made up of an intraoral camera device connected to a computer fitted with a frame grabber with the QLF software. Any area with a drop in fluorescence radiance of more than 5% is a lesion.[35] It can detect and monitor caries in real time, both in children and in adults with high sensitivity.[35]

DIAGNOdent LASER SYSTEM

The DIAGNOdent laser system technique is based on the resultant increase in the fluorescence of demineralized tooth at specific excitation wavelengths. DIAGNOdent has a laser diode that generates a pulsed 655-nm red laser beam via a central fiber, which is transported to the tip of the device and into the tooth. The intensity of fluorescence is directly proportional to the degree of demineralization or bacterial concentration in the area scanned. This infrared fluorescence corresponds to a numerical value between zero and 99 that represents lesion severity. A laser fluorescence pen, DIAGNOdent Pen, is also available.

POLARIZATION-SENSITIVE OPTICAL COHERENCE TOMOGRAPHY

The polarization-sensitive optical coherence tomography (OCT) was first demonstrated in 1991.[36] OCT creates a cross-sectional, 2-dimensional map of tissue microstructure by illuminating the tissue with low-power NIR light, collecting the backscattered light, and analyzing the intensity. It provides high spatial resolution (10–20 μm) and real-time, 2-dimensional depth visualization.[32] It has been used to image tooth structure.[37] Factors, such as lesion staining, ambient lighting, and the presence of saliva or bacterial plaque, which have been identified to adversely affect other technologies, do not influence OCT imaging and measurements.

FREQUENCY-DOMAIN INFRARED PHOTOTHERMAL RADIOMETRY AND MODULATED LUMINESCENCE

Frequency-domain infrared photothermal radiometry (PTR) and modulated luminescence (LUM) is a noninvasive energy conversion technology that measures 2 different signals: modulated thermal infrared radiation (PTR) and modulated LUM; thus, it measures the heat and light responses[38] (**Figs. 9** and **10**). The first response signifies the conversion of absorbed optical energy into thermal energy that results in a modulation in the temperature of tooth structure (PTR). The second response signifies the conversion of absorbed optical energy to radiative energy (LUM). It enables the clinician to examine lesions up to 5 mm below the surface.[39] Dayo and colleagues,[13] in their study comparing intraoral radiograph (IR), cone-beam computed tomography (CBCT), and PTR/LUM for detection of recurring caries lesion, reported sensitivity for PTR/LUM as 0.89 (0.78–0.99), whereas the average sensitivity among 6 observers was 0.38 (0.31–0.44) for IR. Training and calibration are required because it is sensitive to angulation.

Other techniques using fluorescence and inherent properties of the teeth include the Spectra Caries Detection System, endoscopically viewed filtered fluorescence, videoscope, and intraoral television camera among others.

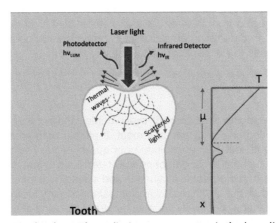

Fig. 9. The PTR/LUM technology. The radiative orange arrow is the laser light. Radiated energy in the PTR/LUM technology can be related by Planck constant "h" and emitted photon frequency "v" (hv). The plot is illustrating the progress of temperature (T) as a function of depth (X) from the tooth surface.

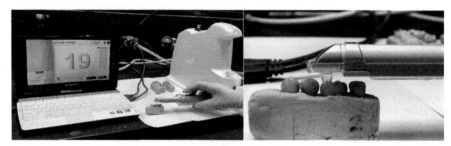

Fig. 10. Canary system (Quantum Dental Technologies, Toronto, Ontario, Canada) with the probe positioned perpendicular to the tooth surface to be scanned. (*From* Dayo, A., Amaechi, B., Noujeim, M., Deahl, T., Gakunga, P. And Katkar, R., 2019. Comparison Of Photothermal Radiometry And Modulated Luminescence, Intraoral Radiography, And Cone Beam Computed Tomography For Detection Of Natural Caries Under Restorations. *Oral Surgery, Oral Medicine, Oral Pathology and Oral Radiology*, 128(4), p.e153; with permission)

SPECIES SPECIFIC MONOCLONAL ANTIBODIES

Shi and colleagues[40] in 1998 identified specific monoclonal antibodies that recognize the surface of cariogenic bacteria. Three highly species-specific monoclonal immunoglobulin G antibodies targeted against *S mutans* were used, and the probes are tagged with fluorescent molecules that measure quantitatively with a spectrometer. It can be used chairside by the dentist, giving quick results, and an overall risk assessment can be made. It also provides useful information for analyzing the role of *S mutans* in dental caries.

ARTIFICIAL INTELLIGENCE

Advances in digital radiography with computer-assisted diagnostic systems that can read and interpret radiographs have been explored. In radiology, a rapidly evolving new area of medical research is deep convolutional neural networks (CNNs) used in diagnosis and prediction.[41–44] Deep CNN algorithm has been documented to be an effective, efficient, and accurate modality for detection and diagnosis after image processing and pattern recognition training. Lee and colleagues[45] have reported a diagnostic accuracy ranging from 82% to 89% and stated that it provided considerably good performance in detecting dental caries in periapical radiographs. This field is exciting and promises to yield adaptable techniques that can be helpful to the dental practitioner.

SUMMARY

Dental caries is a globally widespread, preventable, and reversible condition with detrimental socioeconomic and mental impact. It affects both young and adult and can lead to early tooth loss with a resultant poor quality of life. The dental practitioner can use adjunctive techniques to detect noncavitated lesions that are hidden from visual inspection and/or radiographic evaluation and a candidate for chemotherapeutic/noninvasive procedures of MID, thereby avoiding unnecessary tooth tissue loss. Early caries detection ultimately positively impacts general well-being of an individual. However, care should be taken in the use of these sensitive systems as adjuncts to visual inspection and IR because false positives may result in overtreatment. CBCT demonstrated a significantly lower specificity for detection of recurrent caries compared with intraoral radiography and PTR and modulated LUM in 1 ex vivo study.[13]

CLINICS CARE POINTS

- Caries is a dynamic pathologic process that can be prevented, arrested, or treated.
- Proper staging of dental caries is needed for appropriate management of the disease.
- Sensitive caries diagnostic tools can serve as adjuncts to radiographs for early detection and the opportunity for minimally invasive treatment.

REFERENCES

1. Kutsch VK. Dental caries: an updated medical model of risk assessment. J Prosthet Dent 2014;111:280–5.
2. Caufield PW, Schön CN, Saraithong P, et al. Oral lactobacilli and dental caries: a model for niche adaptation in humans. J Dent Res 2015;94:110S–8S.
3. Miller WD. The microorganisms of the human mouth. Philadelphia (PA): SS White and Co Reprinted; 1973. Basel:Karger; 1890.
4. Stephan RM. Intra oral hydrogen ion concentrations associated with dental caries activity. J Dent Res 1944;23:257–66.
5. Englander HR, Shklair IL, Fosdick LS. The effects of saliva on the pH and lactate concentration in dental plaques. I. Caries-rampant individuals. J Dent Res 1959; 38:848–53.
6. Marsh PD. Dental plaque as a biofilm: the significance of pH in health and caries. Compend Contin Educ Dent 2009;30:76–8, 80,83-7.
7. Pitts NB, Zero DT, Marsh PD, et al. Dental caries. Nat Rev Dis Primers 2017; 3(17030):1–17.
8. Bernabe E, Vehkalahti MM, Sheiham A, et al. Sugar-sweetened beverages and dental caries in adults: a 4-year prospective study. J Dent 2014;42:952–8.
9. Konig KG. Diet and oral health. Int Dent J 2000;50:162–74.
10. Bowen WH, Burne RA, Wu H, et al. Oral biofilms: pathogens, matrix, and polymicrobial interactions in microenvironments. Trends Microbiol 2018;26:229–42.
11. NCRP Report No. 177 – radiation protection in dentistry and oral & maxillofacial imaging. Bethesda (MD): National Council on Radiation Protection and Measurements; 2019.
12. Alcaraz M, Parra C, Martínez Beneyto Y, et al. Is it true that the radiation dose to which patients are exposed has decreased with modern radiographic films? Dentomaxillofac Radiol 2009;38:92–7.
13. Dayo AF, Amaechi BT, Noujeim M, et al. Comparison of photothermal radiometry and modulated luminescence, intraoral radiography, and cone beam computed tomography for detection of natural caries under restorations. Oral Surg Oral Med Oral Pathol Oral Radiol 2020;129:539–48.
14. Schwendicke F, Tzschoppe M, Paris S. Radiographic caries detection: a systematic review and meta-analysis. J Dent 2015;43:924–33.
15. Jeon RJ, Sivagurunathan K, Garcia J, et al. Dental diagnostic clinical instrument. J Phys Conf Ser 2010;214:012–23.
16. Kamburoglu K, Kolsuz E, Murat S, et al. Proximal caries detection accuracy using intraoral bitewing radiography, extraoral bitewing radiography and panoramic radiography. Dentomaxillofac Radiol 2012;41:450–9.
17. Chan M, Dadul T, Langlais R, et al. Accuracy of extraoral bite-wing radiography in detecting proximal caries and crestal bone loss. J Am Dent Assoc 2018; 149:51–8.

18. Anbiaee N, Mohassel AR, Imanimoghaddam M, et al. A comparison of the accuracy of digital and conventional radiography in the diagnosis of recurrent caries. J Contemp Dent Pract 2010;11:E025–32.

19. Abesi F, Mirshekar A, Moudi E, et al. Diagnostic accuracy of digital and conventional radiography in the detection of non-cavitated approximal dental caries. Iran J Radiol 2012;9:17–21.

20. Dehghani M, Barzegari R, Tabatabai H, et al. Diagnostic value of conventional and digital radiography for detection of cavitated and non-cavitated proximal caries. J Dent (Tehran) 2017;14:21–30.

21. Mupparapu M, Nadeau C. Oral and maxillofacial imaging. Dent Clin North Am 2016;60:1–37.

22. Worth HM. Principles and practice of oral radiographic interpretation. Chicago (IL): Year Book Medical Publishers; 1963. p. 150–63.

23. Young DA, Nový BB, Zeller GG, et al. The American Dental Association caries classification system for clinical practice. J Am Dent Assoc 2015;146:79–86.

24. Pitts NB, Rimmer PA. An in vivo comparison of radiographic and directly assessed clinical caries status of posterior approximal surfaces in primary and permanent teeth. Caries Res 1992;26:146–52.

25. Manmontri C, Mahasantipiya PM, Chompu-Inwai P. Preeruptive intracoronal radiolucencies: detection and nine years monitoring with a series of dental radiographs. Case Rep Dent 2017;2017:6261407.

26. Crystal YO, Niederman R. Evidence-based dentistry update on silver diamine fluoride. Dent Clin North Am 2019;63:45–68.

27. Bader JD, Shugars DA, Bonito AJ. Systematic reviews of selected dental caries diagnostic and management methods. J Dent Educ 2001;65:960–8.

28. Wenzel A. Radiographic display of carious lesions and cavitation in approximal surfaces: advantages and drawbacks of conventional and advanced modalities. Acta Odontol Scand 2014;72:251–64.

29. Meja're I, Gröndahl HG, Carlstedt K, et al. Accuracy at radiography and probing for diagnosis of proximal caries. Scand J Dent Res 1985;93:178–84.

30. Pretty A, Ekstrand KR. Detection and monitoring of early caries lesions: a review. Eur Arch Paediatr Dent 2016;17:13–25.

31. Srilatha A, Doshi D, Kulkarni S, et al. Advanced diagnostic aids in dental caries – a review. J Glob Oral Health 2019;2(2):118–27.

32. Amaechi BT. Emerging technologies for diagnosis of dental caries: the road so far. J Appl Phys 2009;105:102047–9.

33. Gomez J, Tellez M, Pretty IA, et al. Non-cavitated carious lesions detection methods: a systematic review. Community Dent Oral Epidemiol 2013;41:54–66.

34. de Jong J, Sundström F, Westerling H, et al. A new method for in vivo quantification of changes in initial enamel caries with laser fluorescence. Caries Res 1995;29:2–7.

35. Amaechi BT, Higham SM. Quantitative light-induced fluorescence: a potential tool for general dental assessment. J Biomed Opt 2002;7:7–13.

36. Huang D, Swanson EA, Lin CP. Optical coherence tomography. Science 1991;254:1178–81.

37. Feldchtein FI, Gelikonov GV, Gelikonov VM, et al. In vivo OCT imaging of hard and soft tissue of the oral cavity. Opt Express 1998;3:239–50.

38. Kim J, Mandelis A, Matvienko A, et al. Detection of dental secondary caries using frequency-domain infrared photothermal radiometry (PTR) and modulated luminescence (LUM). Int J Thermophys 2012;33:1778–86.

39. Silvertown JD, Wong BP, Sivagurunathan KS, et al. Remineralization of natural early caries lesions in vitro by P11 -4 monitored with photothermal radiometry and luminescence. J Investig Clin Dent 2017;8(4). https://doi.org/10.1111/jicd. 12257.
40. Shi W, Jewett A, Hume WR. Rapid and quantitative detection of Streptococcus mutans with species-specific monoclonal antibodies. Hybridoma 1998;17: 365–71.
41. Hosny A, Parmar C, Quackenbush J, et al. Artificial intelligence in radiology. Nat Rev Cancer 2018;18:500–10.
42. Li S, Fevens T, Krzyzak A, et al. Toward automatic computer aided dental X-ray analysis using level set method. Med Image Comput Comput Assist Interv 2005;8:670–8.
43. Ekert T, Krois J, Meinhold L, et al. Deep learning for the radiographic detection of apical lesions. J Endod 2019;45:917–22.
44. Setzer FC, Shi KJ, Zhang Z, et al. Artificial intelligence for the computer-aided detection of periapical lesions in cone-beam computed tomographic images. J Endodontics 2020;46(7):987–93.
45. Lee JH, Kima DH, Jeonga SN, et al. Detection and diagnosis of dental caries using a deep learning-based convolutional neural network algorithm. J Dent 2018; 77:106–11.

Periodontal and Implant Radiology

Joseph P. Fiorellini, DMD, DMSc[a],*, Dennis Sourvanos, BsDH, DDS[a],
Hector Sarimento, DMD, MSOB[a], Nadeem Karimbux, DMD, MMSc[b],
Kevin W. Luan, BDS, MSOB, MEd[c]

KEYWORDS

- Alveolar bone loss/classification • Periodontal diseases • Periodontitis
- Peri-implantitis/ classification • Peri-implant mucositis

KEY POINTS

- Radiographs can be use to aid with identifying sites of periodontal and peri-implant health, nonhealth, and progression of disease.
- Radiographs can monitor evidence of changes in the underlying alveolar structures, because this indication can aid in the diagnosis of a site of nonhealth.
- Accepted forms of radiographic assessment of periodontal and peri-implant hard and soft tissues include periapical and bitewing radiographs and cone beam computed tomography.
- The progression from a state of health to periodontitis and peri-implantitis can present as radiographic bone loss, which may be site specific and pattern specific, depending on the etiology.

INTRODUCTION

In the field of periodontics, radiography can be used to detect alveolar bone levels with respect to the pattern and extent. Crestal bone levels and osseous defects can be measured from the cementoenamel junction (CEJ) to the crest of the alveolar bone and from the CEJ to the osseous defect base, respectively. Through radiographs, the periodontal ligament (PDL) space, periapical region, and lamina dura can be viewed and are adjunctively useful to help identify risk factors, such as defective restorations and calculus. The value of radiographs for periodontal disease diagnosis lies in the ability to estimate severity and degree of progression, determine prognosis, and evaluate treatment outcomes. Radiographs, however, cannot replace the need for

a Department of Periodontics, University of Pennsylvania, School of Dental Medicine, 240 South 40th Street, Philadelphia, PA 19104, USA; b Department of Periodontics, Tufts University School of Dental Medicine, 1 Kneeland Street, Boston, MA 02111, USA; c Department of Periodontics, University of Illinois at Chicago College of Dentistry, 801 South Paulina, Chicago, IL 60612, USA
* Corresponding author.
E-mail address: jpf@upenn.edu

Dent Clin N Am 65 (2021) 447–473
https://doi.org/10.1016/j.cden.2021.02.003
0011-8532/21/© 2021 Elsevier Inc. All rights reserved.

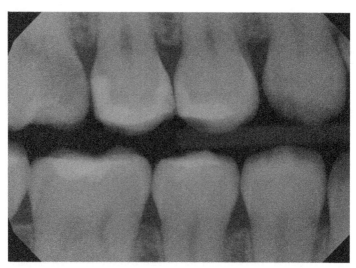

Fig. 1. Health (mandibular + maxillary right posterior) bitewing radiograph: Alveolar crest levels appear radiopaque, flat, and smooth and are appropriately correlated 1–2 mm from the CEJ. Image provided by authors.

clinical examinations. Through radiographs, calcified tissue changes can be visualized. Although they cannot detail cellular activity, they can show the effects of previous cellular experiences with the bone and roots. Radiographs provide crucial diagnostic and treatment planning information to serve as baseline information from which an assessment of treatment outcomes can be prognosticated. An understanding of the advantages and disadvantages of diagnostic imaging, however, as well as the cost and benefits is needed. This involves an appropriate prescription for radiograph

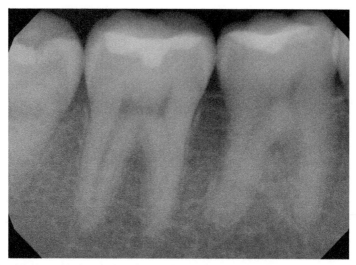

Fig. 2. Health (mandibular right posterior) periapical radiograph: Alveolar crest levels appear radiopaque, flat, and smooth. PDL spaces appear as a thin continuous radiolucent line. Image provided by authors.

type and quantity in order to optimize the effects of radiographs on treatment outcomes. The adaption of digital imaging as a type of radiographic assessment has the ability to change the way periodontal tissues are visualized.

PERIODONTAL RADIOGRAPH TECHNIQUES

Currently, periapical and bitewing radiographs have been used widely to form the basis of radiographic diagnostic information. This combination is used for the evaluation of periodontal diseases in conjunction with a clinical examination.[1] Using these images, clinicians can assess the status of the periodontal bone and predict prognosis and diagnosis accurately.[2] Features, such as the relative alveolar bone height, PDL space around teeth, and bone destruction pattern, can be observed from radiographic images. Alveolar trabecular pattern, radiodensity, and contours of interdental bone can vary, however, depending on x-ray angulation and type of film. The bisection-of-angle technique distorts an anatomic structure's true appearance because it elongates the radiographic image.[3] As a result, the level of the facial bone becomes distorted compared with the lingual, and alveolar bone margin may appear closer to the anatomic crown of the tooth. Horizontal angulation errors that occur result in overlapping tooth images, changes in radiographic PDL space width, and distortion of furcation involvement.[4] In an attempt to avoid these errors, Prichard proposed four criteria for adequate angulation of periapical graphs. These include the following: (1) periapical radiograph should show cusps of molars with occlusal surface, (2) enamel and pulp chambers should be seen and distinct, (3) interproximal spaces should be open, and (4) contacts between adjacent teeth should not overlap unless teeth are out of line. Following these guidelines will help reproduce and standardize reliable radiographs for treatment.

NORMAL INTERDENTAL BONE

The basis of bone change evaluation in periodontal disease is based mainly on the appearance of the interdental alveolar bone. Radiographically, this is the main

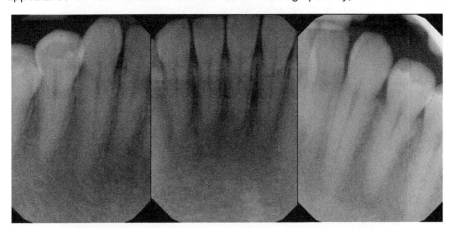

Fig. 3. Health (mandibular anterior sextant) periapical radiograph: Alveolar crest levels appear radiopaque, pointed, and sharp and are appropriately correlated 1–2 mm apical from the CEJ. The PDL appears as a thin uniform and continuous radiolucent line around the entire root structure. Image provided by authors.

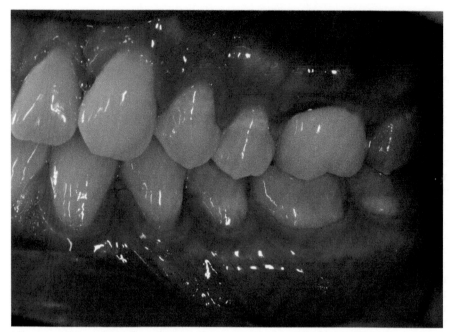

Fig. 4. Health (mandibular + maxillary left posterior sextants) photographic image: Clinical presentation of healthy periodontium. Image provided by authors.

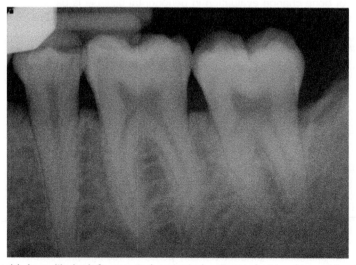

Fig. 5. Health (mandibular left posterior) periapical radiograph: Alveolar crest levels appear radiopaque, flat, and smooth. PDL spaces appear as a thin continuous radiolucent line. Image provided by authors.

observation because the root structure overlaps and obscures both the facial and lingual alveolar bone structure. Interdental bone normally is represented by a radiopaque line, which is located at the alveolar bone margin and adjacent to the PDL.[5] A change in the angulation of an x-ray beam, however, produces changes in appearance.[6] The interdental alveolar crest varies due to the convex anatomy of tooth surfaces and the location of the CEJ. The horizontal width of the bone relative to the width of the proximal root surface also is a factor that causes variation. It is more common for the angulation of the interdental crest to form a parallel line similar to that formed by the CEJs of adjacent teeth (**Figs. 1–5**). In some radiographs, this may result in an angulated appearance of the interdental bone.[7] In certain periodontal conditions, such as medication-induced gingival hyperplasia, radiographic bone presentation appears normal or abnormal. The clinical presentation, however, demonstrates pathology (**Figs. 6 and 7**).

RADIOGRAPHIC APPEARANCE OF PERIODONTAL DISEASE

The destruction of alveolar bone in periodontitis has some generalizable characteristics. These features may be present alone or in combinations. Typically, there is disruption of lamina dura. Fuzziness of crestal aspect of the alveolar bone may be present. This appearance is a result of resorption due to the advancement of gingival inflammation to the periodontal bone.[8] The presence of crestal lamina dura also may indicate periodontal health.[9] The radiographic feature of periodontitis recognized most commonly is the reduction in height of bone due to increasing osteoclastic activity. The interdental septum height is reduced due to the resorption of bone. The

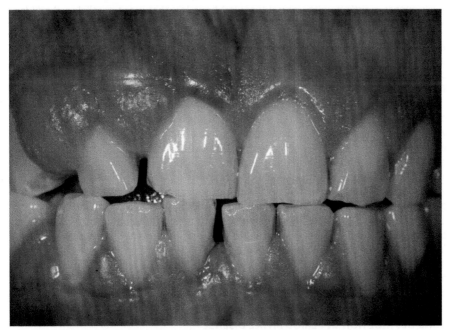

Fig. 6. Periodontal Disease (mandibular + maxillary anterior sextants) photographic image: Clinical presentation of calcium channel blocker plaque-induced hyperplasia. Image provided by authors.

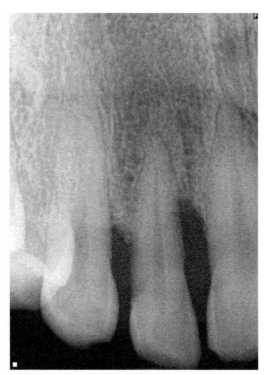

Fig. 7. Periodontal Disease (maxillary right anterior) periapical radiograph: Alveolar crest levels appear indistinct, with vertical (angular) bone loss that is not parallel to the CEJs of adjacent teeth. Image provided by authors.

wedge shape at the interproximal aspects of the crest is created via the widening of the periodontal space, which is apically pointed toward the root. Lastly, a widening of periodontal space creating a wedge shape at the interproximal aspects of the crest. The apex of the wedge pointed apically toward the root.

The surface architecture of the alveolar bone in periodontal disease that was once thought to be of a linear pattern now has been described as "complex" with the advancement of imaging and diagnostic modalities. The visualization of this topology is crucial for both diagnostic and treatment planning. For example, certain areas, such as interradicular areas, are more prone to loss of bone with increasing likelihood during disease progression. As a result, the treatment options vary accordingly. The clinician decides whether or not periodontal osteoplasty surgery with or without ostectomy is appropriate. As a result, bone regeneration would be beneficial and prove to have a positive and predictable outcome. Although the decision for bone regeneration is determined once a surgical flap has been raised for clinical visualization, the advancements of radiological imaging modalities have proved useful in this regard. Two-dimensional imaging has its limitations; portraying a 2-dimensional structure in a planar perspective, visualization of the architecture cannot be predicted as accurately as three-dimensional imagery.

BONE DESTRUCTION IN PERIODONTAL DISEASE

The earliest signs of periodontal disease can be detected only clinically due to specific features of early periodontal disease and the limitations of radiographic imaging.[10]

Radiographs are unable to capture the initial destructive alveolar bone changes. Once there is evidence of some structure changes, however, this is an indication that the disease may have progressed beyond the initial stages of periodontal disease. According to Thomas,[11] radiographic imaging underestimates bone loss severity. The range of variation may be up to 1.6 mm of difference when observing alveolar crest height. This is apparent especially during angulation of radiographs.[7] Radiographs aid the clinician's determination of the remaining bone amount rather than bone loss, indirectly determining the amount of bone loss in periodontal disease. The clinician estimates the amount of bone from the height of the remaining bone to the approximated original physiologic level of the alveolar crest.[11] In some cases of periodontal disease, the location and distribution of periodontal disease may result in a particular diagnosis.[12] To reach a particular diagnosis, radiographic evidence of bone loss around similar locations in different areas of the mouth and at particular surfaces of teeth.[13] This has been included localized periodontal disease, such as Stage III, grade C, localized periodontitis in an adolescent patient where there is an incisal-molar pattern of bone loss (**Fig. 8**).

FURCATION INVOLVEMENT

A complex aspect of periodontal radiograph is the diagnosis of disease of teeth with furcation involvement (**Figs. 9** and **10**). The extent of periodontal disease involvement with furcated teeth is important in determining therapy. Decisions related to the extent and morphology of bone loss can change a potential treatment from a regenerative therapy to tooth extraction, followed by implant placement. The combination of clinical evaluation and radiographic imaging often provides the clinical with information to make the proper diagnosis and plan. Clinical examination with a specific furcation detection probe, such as the Nabers, is used to definitively diagnose furcation involvement.[14] Radiographs may aid this diagnosis; however, due to some limitations, such as improper positioning, anatomic variations, and root superimposition, a furcation may not be visible on a radiograph image. A tooth may appear bifurcated at one angle; however, when adjusted, it may not appear; therefore, it is recommended that radiographs should be taken at different angles to increase the chances of observing a furcation involvement.[15] Walter and colleagues[16] recommend the guideline for assisting furcation detection with radiographs. First, a radiographic observation of furcation

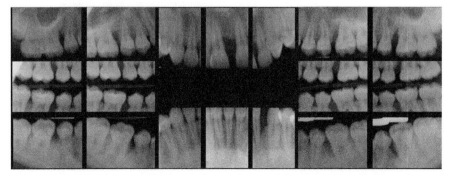

Fig. 8. Stage III, Grade C, Localized Periodontitis in an Adolescent Patient (full-mouth series) FMX radiographic series: Vertical bone loss pattern in anterior sextants and mandibular first molar regions. Image provided by authors.

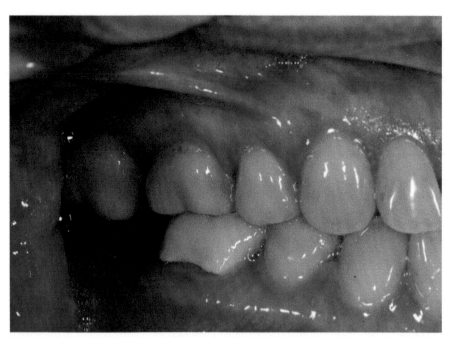

Fig. 9. Periodontal Disease (mandibular + maxillary right posterior sextants) photographic image: Clinical presentation of mandibular molar furcation involvement. Nabors probe instrumentation is needed to determine severity as an adjunctive diagnosis to radiographic assessment. Image provided by authors.

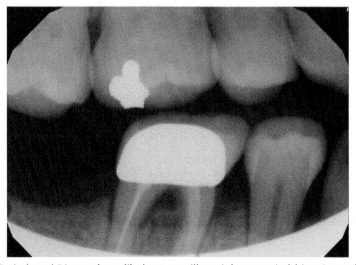

Fig. 10. Periodontal Disease (mandibular + maxillary right posterior) bitewing radiograph: Mandibular alveolar crest levels appear indistinct, with horizontal bone loss beyond the buccal and lingual furcation entrances of the mandibular molar. Image provided by authors.

should be evident clinically, using a probe, especially if there is no evidence of adjacent root bone loss. The reduction in radiodensity of a proposed furcation area may suggest a furcation involvement of the teeth. Lastly, the investigators noted that a marked bone resorption at the site of a single molar root suggests that there may be a furcation involvement.

PATTERN OF BONE DESTRUCTION

The progression of periodontal disease results in physiologic changes of interproximal bone. Such physiologic changes include the different height and contour of the alveolar bone, size and shape of the alveolar medullary space, and the radiodensity of alveolar crest.[17] The height of interdental bone inevitably reduces as disease progresses.[8] The patterns of interdental bone loss could be horizontal, angular, or vertical.[18] There are limitations of radiographic imaging, however, which cannot determine the depth of crater defects as well as the buccal and lingual surface bone destruction.[19] Additionally, if superimposed, mesial and distal bone destruction of a tooth may not be observed. Bone loss, however, interdentally tends to continue on buccal and lingual surfaces.[20] This interdental bone loss forms a trough-like defect that can be difficult to observe in radiographs. Deep craterlike defects may not be observed in radiographs if there are dense plates of interdental bone on buccal and lingual plates. According to Svärdström and Wennström,[21] to allow for sufficient visualization of inner cancellous trabecular bone, a 0.5-mm to 1.0-mm thickness of cortical plate is

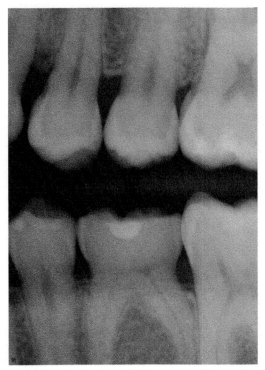

Fig. 11. Stage 1 Periodontal Disease (mandibular + maxillary right posterior) bitewing radiograph: Radiographic bone loss limited to the coronal third (<15%). Image provided by authors.

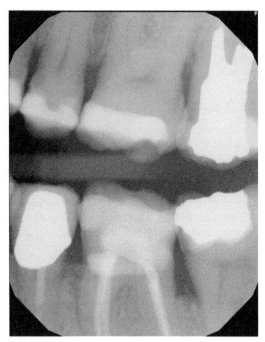

Fig. 12. Stage 2 Periodontal Disease (mandibular + maxillary left posterior) bitewing radiograph: Radiographic bone loss limited to the coronal third (15%–33%). Image provided by authors.

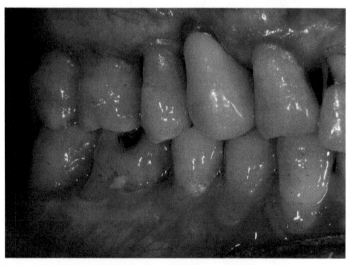

Fig. 13. Stage 3 Periodontal Disease (mandibular + maxillary right posterior sextants) photographic image: Clinical presentation of stage 3 periodontal disease. Image provided by authors.

needed. The classification of periodontal diseases recently has been revised to follow criteria related to progression, complexity, extent of disease, time, tooth loss, and systemic modifiers. According to the American Academy of Periodontology/European Federation of Periodontology 2017 classification, periodontal diseases and condition have been modified to a multidimensional staging and grading system.[17] The staging and grading of periodontitis begin with mild bone attachment of loss (stage 1) before progressing to a more severe form with attachment loss equal to or greater than 5 mm and to loss of 5 or more teeth (stage IV) (**Figs. 11–16**). Health and gingivitis are not included as classification categories.

OCCLUSAL TRAUMA

The clinical signs of trauma from occlusion are clinically evident by worn dentition, temporomandibular joint pain, headaches, and muscular pain. Often, the occlusal trauma affects the tooth-supporting structures. The hard tissue alterations are a result of the wound healing process that aims to strengthen the periodontal structures to allow for increased occlusal loading. These changes in structures can be visualized with radiography (**Fig. 17**). Traumatic occlusion injury results in evident loss of bone density, thickening of the lamina dura, a widening of PDL space, and furcation involvement.

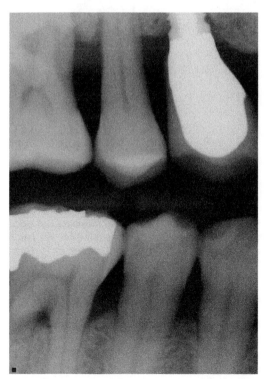

Fig. 14. Stage 3 Periodontal Disease (mandibular + maxillary right posterior) bitewing radiograph: Radiographic bone loss extending to the middle third of root and beyond. Furcation involvement class II and class III. Image provided by authors.

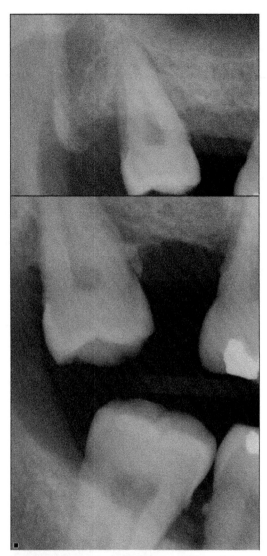

Fig. 15. Stage 4 Periodontal Disease (mandibular + maxillary right posterior) periapical + bitewing radiographs: Radiographic bone loss extending to the middle third of root and beyond. Secondary occlusal trauma (tooth mobility degree 2). Furcation involvement class II/III. Image provided by authors.

CONE BEAM COMPUTED TOMOGRAPHY FOR THE DETECTION OF PERIODONTITIS

Over the past several years, use of cone beam computed tomography (CBCT) for dental applications has become commonplace. CBCT provides high-contrast images of dental structures and, with relevance to periodontology, of osseous structures. The use of this technology provides the clinician and practice with several advantages. The 3-dimensional radiographic imaging helps the clinician visualize the architecture, which, in turn, allows for a more accurate diagnosis and treatment plan. Similar to a panoramic radiograph, the CBCT obtains all images during a single rotation,

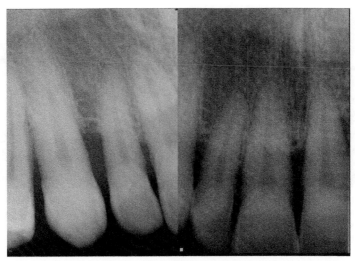

Fig. 16. Stage 4 Periodontal Disease (maxillary anterior) periapical radiographs: Radiographic bone loss extending to the middle third of root and beyond. Secondary occlusal trauma (tooth mobility degree 2). Image provided by authors

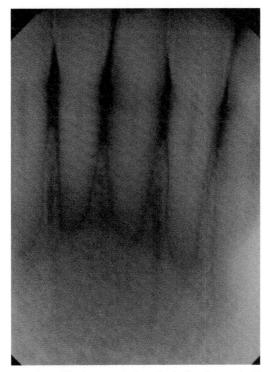

Fig. 17. Occlusal Trauma (mandibular anterior) periapical radiograph: Wear facet at occlusal aspect of central incisor. PDL spaces appear widened with reduced alveolar bone support. Image provided by authors.

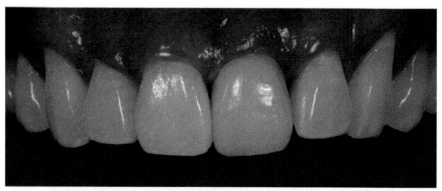

Fig. 18. Health (maxillary anterior sextant) clinical photograph: Clinical presentation of healthy implant periodontium. Marginal tissue presents with a flat shape and a generalized firm consistency. Free gingival tissue generally is smooth, attached gingiva is stippled. Image provided by authors.

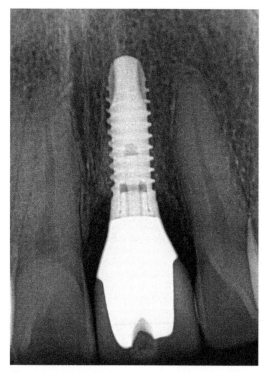

Fig. 19. Health (maxillary anterior incisor) periapical radiograph: Alveolar crest levels appear radiopaque, noting corticated texture. Normal implant bone levels are at first thread. Image provided by authors.

decreasing the time for a scan. Although the reconstruction of imaging data onto a computer increases, the amount of time spent during the scan for both patient and operator has decreased.[22] Limitation of the beam due to the collimation allows for radiation to the specific site of interest after the selection of the optimal field of view.[15] This limitation prevents unnecessary irradiation of other areas. The CBCT produces high-quality images with isotropic voxel resolution that ranges from 0.4 mm to 0.08 mm.[23] This accuracy and precision of all dimensions of the alveolar and tooth structure aid in periodontal-orthodontics analysis as well as implant site evaluation.[24] The most frequent use for CBCT has been in the diagnostic planning for dental implant placement. CBCT, however, does have diagnostic applications in the field of periodontology, in particular with the evaluation of the periodontium. The advantages compared with traditional radiographs include the 3-dimensional imaging of the periodontium and teeth.[25] CBCTs avoid the superimposition that otherwise would have been an obstruction during the traditional radiograph imaging.[26] For example, a 3-wall defect with intact buccal and lingual plates may have been obscured with bitewing and periapical radiographs; however, with CBCT imaging, visualization of the defect size and shape becomes more evident.[23,25]

ULTRASONOGRAPHY

Imaging using ultrasonography can aid in detection of soft tissue–related diseases.[26] There have been various applications of ultrasound usage in periodontology. An

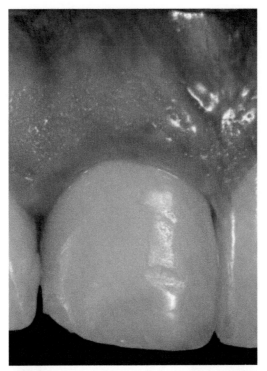

Fig. 20. Health (maxillary anterior incisor) clinical photograph: Clinical presentation of healthy implant site in the maxillary anterior sextant. Periodontal tissue maintains consistent size that is not enlarged, and marginal tissues have a flat shape that follows the contours of the underlying periodontium. Image provided by authors.

ultrasonography probe helps the clinician record measurements of a patient's PDL in relation to the CEJ.[27] An ultrasonic scanner can be used to detect hard and soft periodontium structures to assess dimensional relationship. The scanner also can assess gingival thickness before and after mucogingival surgery as well as the masticatory mucosa.[28,29] Ultrasonic instruments have been used to not only detect large supragingival and subgingival calculus accumulations but also remove bacterial plaque using acoustic microstreaming and the cavitation effects of ultrasound.

PERI-IMPLANT HEALTH AND DISEASE

The dental implant has become a necessary component of daily treatments in the fully or partially edentulous patients. The long-term survival of an osseointegrated implant is dependent on maintaining proper bone levels. Unfortunately, dental implants can suffer from the same diseases as natural teeth. There is a continuum for health to peri-implant mucositis to peri-implantitis with peri-implant bone levels influenced by many pathologic and nonpathologic conditions.[30] Understanding of peri-implant disease has evolved and is currently more than just presence or absence of the implant. As the field has developed, the classification of peri-implantitis has been limited to descriptions of disease progression or those involving soft tissues and/or hard tissues (peri-implant mucositis or peri-implantitis). The American Academy of Periodontology/European Federation of

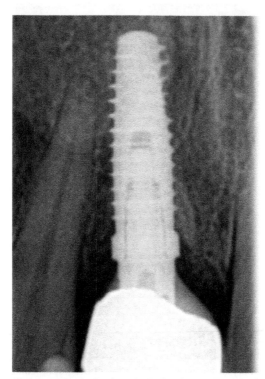

Fig. 21. Health (maxillary anterior incisor) periapical radiograph: Alveolar crest levels appear radiopaque, noting corticated texture. Normal implant bone levels are at first thread. Image provided by authors.

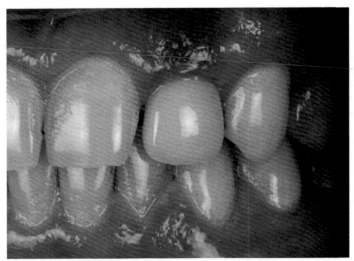

Fig. 22. Mucositis (maxillary anterior incisor) clinical photograph: Clinical presentation of peri-implant mucositis in the maxillary anterior incisor region. Periodontal tissue maintain size that is enlarged and appears edematous. Free gingival surface texture does not appear smooth. Tissue consistency appears boggy. Image provided by authors.

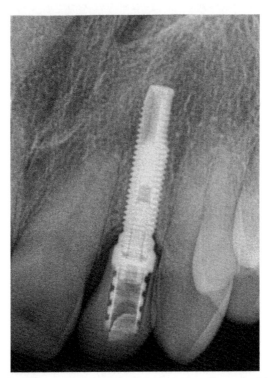

Fig. 23. Mucositis (maxillary anterior incisor) periapical radiograph: Alveolar crest levels appear radiopaque. Bone level appears normal at level of implant platform. Image provided by authors.

Periodontology 2017 classification also included peri-implant diseases.[31] Peri-implant health was defined as the absence of any signs of inflammation and further additional bone loss after the initial healing. When there is the presence of inflammation without further additional bone loss after the initial healing, the disease is termed peri-implantitis mucositis. Lastly, when there is soft tissue inflammation, evidence of bone loss and increasing probing depth after the implant restoration placement, the term is peri-implantitis. These definitions, from health to peri-implantitis, have a range of probing depths.. Therefore, it is recommended that the clinician obtain both radiographic and probing measurements. As discussed, classifications of peri-implantitis have been limited to extent of disease (early, moderate, or advanced) or those involving soft tissues and/or hard tissues (peri-implant mucositis or peri-implantitis).[32–34] There are developing classification systems established, however, based on etiology. The majority of bone loss has been related to bacterial biofilm followed, exogenous trauma, exogenous irritants, absence of keratinized tissue, and extrinsic pathology.[35]

NORMAL PERI-IMPLANT HEALTH

The normal radiographic architecture for dental implants has been governed by surgical placement. Radiographic follow-up studies of initially submerged dental

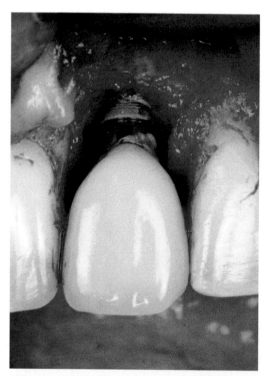

Fig. 24. Peri-implantitis, Cement Retention Etiology (maxillary anterior incisor) clinical photograph: Clinical presentation of peri-implantitis diseased implant in the maxillary anterior incisor region. Residual cement located clinically at the buccal and distal aspects. Image provided by authors.

implants have documented a period of healing and remodeling of approximately 1 year with significant changes in crestal bone levels and relatively small changes thereafter. Albrektsson and colleagues[36] have reported that within the first year after placement, peri-implant bone loss ranged from 0.9 mm to 1.6 mm. Following the first year of service, bone loss should be less than 0.2 mm annually. Bone level alternation during this nonpathologic period has been dependent on the macrodesign of the coronal portion of the implant and restorative protocol. Bone resorption can be maintained at the implant platform, first screw thread, or junction between the smooth and rough surfaces.[37] Contemporary dental implants have surface modification, which can improve the maintenance of bone height, especially during the early healing period. Therefore, bone loss around a rougher surface implant is significantly less (**Figs. 18–21**).

PERI-IMPLANT MUCOSITIS

The onset and response to the mucosal inflammation around implants are similar to those around the natural teeth. The classic signs of inflammation increase, such as probing depth, gingival index, bleeding on probing, and plaque index.[38–41] Microflora and inflammatory response studies for peri-implant diseases have followed those for gingivitis. Often, with local therapy, such as improvement of oral hygiene measures, nonsurgical therapy, and peri-implant supportive protocols, signs of mucositis

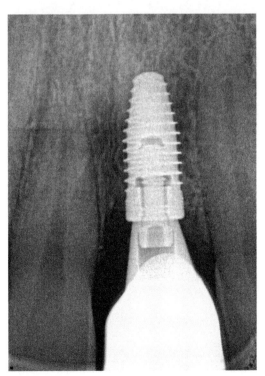

Fig. 25. Peri-implantitis, Cement Retention Etiology (maxillary anterior incisor) periapical radiograph: Alveolar crest levels appear radiopaque. Slightly reduced bone level. Image provided by authors.

decrease.[42] Because peri-implant mucositis is as a soft tissue disease entity, radiographic structures are similar to the healthy implant (**Figs. 22** and **23**).

PERI-IMPLANTITIS INDUCED BY PATHOGENIC BACTERIA

Over the past several years, clinical research has documented not only similarities of periodontitis and dental implant diseases but also periodontitis as a risk for peri-implantitis. History of prior periodontitis, loss of a majority of the natural dentition, insufficient oral hygiene, and residual probing pocket depths have been found as cofactors for implant failure. Overall, the majority of evidence demonstrates that there is a shift of the biofilm from health to disease regarding the biofilm. The biofilm conversion from peri-implant mucositis to peri-implantitis described in the characteristics of peri-implantitis.[43] The species of healthy and/or diseased implant have been

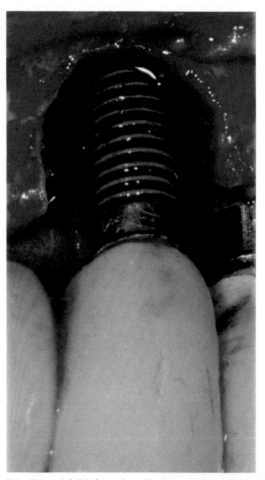

Fig. 26. Peri-implantitis, Bacterial Etiology (maxillary anterior incisor) clinical photograph: Clinical presentation of peri-implantitis diseased implant in the maxillary anterior incisor region. Bacterial in origin. Severe bone loss noted at time of clinical therapy. Image provided by authors.

compared. Sanz-Martin and colleagues[44] studied healthy and diseased implants. The investigation found that both states had a core grouping of pathogens, whereas health had a taxa consistent with periodontal health, and peri-implantitis a taxa consistent with periodontitis. As detected around the natural dentition, species of the red complex, such as *Porphyromonas gingivalis* and *Tannerella forsythia*, some of the most virulent pathogens are found in peri-implantitis. In addition, the bacteria associated with the diseased dental implant seem to be more pathogenic than those in periodontitis. The loss of supporting bone around a dental implant also seems to resemble loss around the natural tooth. Bone loss patterns indicate a horizontal resorption. The

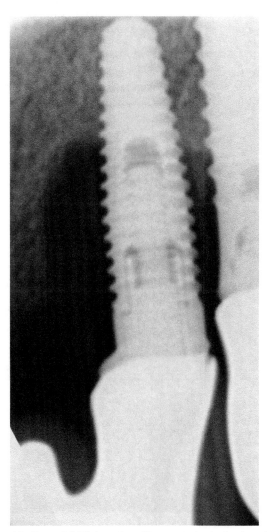

Fig. 27. Peri-implantitis, Bacterial Etiology (maxillary anterior incisor) periapical radiograph: Alveolar crest levels appear radiopaque. Severely reduced abrupt vertical bone loss noted at mesial and distal aspect of implant housing. Image provided by authors.

resorption tends to be around the entire implant unlike with the tooth, which can have a single defect (**Figs. 24** and **25**).

PERI-IMPLANTITIS INDUCED BY EXOGENOUS IRRITANTS RESIDUAL CEMENT

Cemented restorations commonly are used to restore dental implants. It has been shown that excess cement that remains in the sulcus after insertion of the implant-supported restorations can cause inflammation. Several studies have documented the frequency of residual cement and bone loss, which ultimately leads to peri-implant disease. In addition, the issue is complicated by older cementation products that lack radiopacity. Linkevicius and colleagues[45] documented in a patient center investigation that dental radiographs should not be considered a reliable method for cement excess evaluation. The results revealed that cement remnants were detected up to 11.5%, depending on the location. Unfortunately, even radiopaque cements may evade detection. Wadhwani and colleagues[46] found that radiographically dense implant restorative cements may be poor, and, depending on the thickness of the cement, smaller pieces could be undetected. As a result, avoiding cement-retained restorations in difficult-to-access areas has been recommended for practitioners with less experience. The soft tissues related with excess cement typically are inflamed and

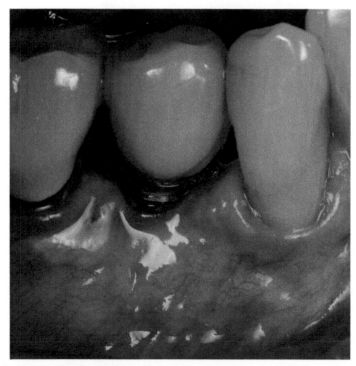

Fig. 28. Peri-implantitis, Lack of Keratinized Tissue Etiology (mandibular right premolar) clinical photograph: clinical presentation of peri-implantitis diseased implant in the mandibular premolar region. Absence of clinical attached mucosa, recession noted. Image provided by authors.

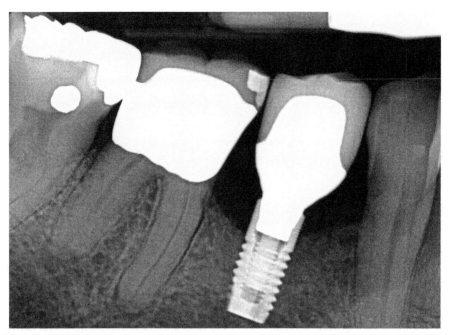

Fig. 29. Peri-implantitis, Lack of Keratinized Tissue Etiology (mandibular right premolar) periapical radiograph: Alveolar crest levels appear diffuse. Horizontal bone loss pattern noted. Image provided by authors.

bleed readily upon probing. The radiographic appearance of bone loss demonstrates a pattern of vertical and/or horizontal resorption (**Figs. 26** and **27**).

PERI-IMPLANTITIS INDUCED BY ABSENCE OF KERATINIZED TISSUE

The tissues that surround an osseointegrated dental implant can be categorized as hard and soft tissues. Both of these components are known as the peri-implant tissues. The importance of the peri-implant tissues is to protect the bone that supports the implant. With the absence of healthy peri-implant tissues, long-term implant success and survival become compromised and less predictable.[47] The dimensions of peri-implant keratinized mucosa may be a risk indicator for peri-implant mucositis. The need for a minimum amount of keratinized tissue in order to maintain peri-implant tissue health has been a controversial issue.[48–52] Some studies suggest that plaque accumulation that resulted in marginal inflammation was more frequent at implant sites with less than 2 mm of keratinized tissue.[53–57] The bone loss patterns in cases of an absence of keratinized tissue generally involve only the buccal aspect of the implant. The loss of bone may extend toward the opposite bone palate. In many cases, the initial bone loss due to inadequate soft tissue can expose the implant surface and lead to plaque accumulation and secondary loss of bone (**Figs. 28** and **29**).

CLINICS CARE POINTS

- Dental radiography is an adjunctive clinical tool that can differentiate between a diagnosis of health/ non-health in periodontal and peri-implant structures.

- Radiographic evaluation of periodontal and peri-implant structures can assess changes on the appearance of the interdental bone.
- Characteristics of periodontal disease and peri-implant disease (peri-implantitis) can present alone or in combinations.

DISCLOSURE

None of the authors has any relevant financial relationships with any commercial interests.

REFERENCES

1. American Dental Association Council on Scientific Affairs. The use of cone-beam computed tomography in dentistry: an advisory statement from the American Dental Association Council on Scientific Affairs. J Am Dent Assoc 2012;143:899–902.
2. Suphanantachat S, Tantikul K, Tamsailom S, et al. Comparison of clinical values between cone beam computed tomography and conventional intraoral radiography in periodontal and infrabony defect assessment. Dentomaxillofac Radiol 2017;46:20160461.
3. Monsour PA. A modification of the bisecting-angle technique for anterior periapical dental radiographs. Oral Surg Oral Med Oral Pathol 1986;62:468–70.
4. Güneri P, Göğüş S, Tuğsel Z, et al. Efficacy of a new software in eliminating the angulation errors in digital subtraction radiography. Dentomaxillofac Radiol 2007;36:484–9.
5. Mckee IW, Glover KE, Williamson PC, et al. The effect of vertical and horizontal head positioning in panoramic radiography on mesiodistal tooth angulations. Angle Orthod 2010;71:442–51.
6. Mauriello SM, Tang Q, Johnson KB, et al. A comparison of technique errors using two radiographic intra-oral receptor-holding devices. J Dent Hyg 2015;89:384–9. Available at: https://pubmed.ncbi.nlm.nih.gov/26684996/. Accessed September 30, 2020.
7. Peker I, Alkurt MT. Evaluation of radiographic errors made by undergraduate dental students in periapical radiography. N Y State Dent J 2016;75:45–8. Available at: https://pubmed.ncbi.nlm.nih.gov/19882842/. Accessed September 30, 2020.
8. Needleman I, Garcia R, Gkranias N, et al. Mean annual attachment, bone level, and tooth loss: a systematic review. J Periodontol 2018;89:S120–39.
9. Lang NP, Bartold PM. Periodontal health. J Periodontol 2018;89:S9–16.
10. Dietrich T, Ower P, Tank M, et al. Periodontal diagnosis in the context of the 2017 classification system of periodontal diseases and conditions – implementation in clinical practice. Br Dent J 2019;226:16–22.
11. Thomas SL. Application of Cone-beam CT in the Office Setting. Dent Clin North Am 2008;52:753–9.
12. Fine DH, Patil AG, Loos BG. Classification and diagnosis of aggressive periodontitis. J Periodontol 2018;89:S103–19.
13. Billings M, Holtfreter B, Papapanou PN, et al. Age-dependent distribution of periodontitis in two countries: Findings from NHANES 2009 to 2014 and SHIP-TREND 2008 to 2012. J Periodontol 2018;89:S140–58.
14. Müller H-P, Eger T. Furcation diagnosis. J Clin Periodontol 1999;26:485–98.

15. Woelber J, Fleiner J, Rau J, et al. Accuracy and usefulness of CBCT in periodontology: a systematic review of the literature. Int J Periodontics Restorative Dent 2018;38:289–97.
16. Walter C, Schmidt JC, Dula K, et al. Cone beam computed tomography (CBCT) for diagnosis and treatment planning in periodontology: A systematic review. Quintessence Int 2016;47:25–37.
17. Papapanou PN, Sanz M, Buduneli N, et al. Periodontitis: consensus report of workgroup 2 of the 2017 world workshop on the classification of periodontal and peri-implant diseases and conditions. J Periodontol 2018;89(Suppl 1): S173–82.
18. Van der Velden U. Diagnosis of periodontitis. J Clin Periodontol 2000;27:960–1.
19. Baelum V, Luan WM, Chen X, et al. A 10-year study of the progression of destructive periodontal disease in adult and elderly Chinese. J Periodontol 1997;68: 1033–42.
20. Schatzle M, Loe H, Lang NP, et al. Clinical course of chronic periodontitis: III. Patterns, variations and risks of attachment loss. J Clin Periodontol 2003;30:909–18.
21. Svärdström G, Wennström JL. Periodontal treatment decisions for molars: an analysis of influencing factors and long-term outcome. J Periodontol 2000;71: 579–85.
22. Walter C, Schmidt JC, Rinne CA, et al. Cone beam computed tomography (CBCT) for diagnosis and treatment planning in periodontology: systematic review update. Clin Oral Investig 2020;24:2943–58.
23. Kim DM, Bassir SH. When is cone-beam computed tomography imaging appropriate for diagnostic inquiry in the management of inflammatory periodontitis? an american academy of periodontology best evidence review. J Periodontol 2017; 88:978–98.
24. Tischler M. CBCT for full-arch implant dental treatment. Dent Today 2016;35(66, 68):70–1.
25. Yeung AWK, Jacobs R, Bornstein MM. Novel low-dose protocols using cone beam computed tomography in dental medicine: a review focusing on indications, limitations, and future possibilities. Clin Oral Investig 2019;23:2573–81.
26. Nasseh I, Al-Rawi W. Cone beam computed tomography. Dent Clin North Am 2018;62:361–91.
27. Lynch JE, Hinders MK. Ultrasonic device for measuring periodontal attachment levels. Rev Sci Instrum 2002;73:2686–93.
28. Tattan M, Sinjab K, Lee E, et al. Ultrasonography for chairside evaluation of periodontal structures: A pilot study. J Periodontol 2020;91:890–9.
29. Muller HP, Kononen E. Variance components of gingival thickness. J Periodontal Res 2005;40:239–44.
30. Fiorellini JP, Luan KW, Chang YC, et al. Peri-implant mucosal tissues and inflammation: clinical implications. Int J Oral Maxillofac Implants 2019;34:s25–33.
31. Jepsen S, Caton JG, Albandar JM, et al. Periodontal manifestations of systemic diseases and developmental and acquired conditions: Consensus report of workgroup 3 of the 2017 World Workshop on the Classification of Periodontal and Peri-Implant Diseases and Conditions. J Periodontol 2018;89(Suppl 1):S237–48.
32. Saaby M, Karring E, Schou S, et al. Factors influencing severity of peri-implantitis. Clin Oral Implants Res 2016;27(1):7–12.
33. Froum SJ, Rosen PS. A proposed classification for peri-implantitis. Int J Periodontics Restorative Dent 2012;32:533–40.
34. Misch CE. The implant quality scale: a clinical assessment of the health–disease continuum. Oral Health 1998;88:15–26.

35. Sarmiento HL, Norton MR, Fiorellini JP. A classification system for peri-implant diseases and conditions. Int J Periodontics Restorative Dent 2016;36:699–705.

36. Albrektsson T, Zarb G, Worthington P, et al. Long- term efficacy of currently used dental implants: A review and proposed criteria of success. Int J Oral Maxillofac Implants 1986;1:11–25.

37. Weber HP, Buser D, Fiorellini J, et al. Radiographic evaluation of crestal bone levels adjacent to nonsubmerged titanium implants. Clin Oral Lmplants Res 1992;3:181–8.

38. Salvi GE, Aglietta M, Eick S, et al. Reversibility of experimental peri-implant mucositis compared with experimental gingivitis in humans. Clin Oral Implants Res 2012;23:182–90.

39. Zitzmann NU, Berglundh T, Marinello CP, et al. Experimental peri-implant mucositis in man. J Clin Periodontol 2001;28:517–23.

40. Schierano G, Pejrone G, Brusco P, et al. TNF-alpha TGF-beta2 and IL-1beta levels in gingival and peri-implant crevicular fluid before and after de novo plaque accumulation. J Clin Periodontol 2008;35:532–8.

41. Gualini F, Berglundh T. Immunohistochemical characteristics of inflammatory lesions at implants. J Clin Periodontol 2003;30:14–8.

42. Carcuac O, Derks J, Charalampakis G, et al. Adjunctive systemic and local antimicrobial therapy in the surgical treatment of peri-implantitis: a randomized controlled clinical trial. J Dent Res 2016;95:50–7.

43. Mombelli A, Décaillet F. The characteristics of biofilms in peri-implant disease. J Clin Periodontol 2011;38(Suppl 11):203–13.

44. Sanz-Martin I, Doolittle-Hall J, Teles RP, et al. Exploring the microbiome of healthy and diseased peri-implant sites using Illumina sequencing. J Clin Periodontol 2017;44:1274–84.

45. Linkevicius T1, Vindasiute E, Puisys A, et al. The influence of the cementation margin position on the amount of undetected cement. A prospective clinical study. Clin Oral Implants Res 2013;24:71–6.

46. Wadhwani C, Hess T, Faber T, et al. A descriptive study of the radiographic density of implant restorative cements. J Prosthet Dent 2010;103:295–302.

47. Costa FO, Takenaka-Martinez S, Cota LO, et al. Peri-implant disease in subjects with and without preventive maintenance: a 5-year follow-up. J Clin Periodontol 2012;39:173–81.

48. Wennström JL, Derks J. Is there a need for keratinized mucosa around implants to maintain health and tissue stability? Clin Oral Implants Res 2012;23(Suppl 6): 136–46.

49. Gobbato L, Avila-ortiz G, Sohrabi K, et al. The effect of keratinized mucosa width on peri-implant health: a systematic review. Int J Oral Maxillofac Implants 2013; 28:1536–45.

50. Lin GH, Chan HL, Wang HL. The significance of keratinized mucosa on implant health: a systematic review. J Periodontol 2013;84:1755–67.

51. Brito C, Tenenbaum HC, Wong BK, et al. Is keratinized mucosa indispensable to maintain peri-implant health? A systematic review of the literature. J Biomed Mater Res B Appl Biomater 2014;102:643–50.

52. Thoma DS, Mühlemann S, Jung RE. Critical soft-tissue dimensions with dental implants and treatment concepts. Periodontol 2000 2014;66:106–18.

53. Chung DM, Oh TJ, Shotwell JL, et al. Significance of keratinized mucosa in maintenance of dental implants with different surfaces. J Periodontol 2006;77: 1410–20.

54. Bouri A, Bissada N, Al-Zahrani MS, et al. Width of keratinized gingiva and the health status of the supporting tissues around dental implants. Int J Oral Maxillofac Implants 2008;23:323–6.
55. Adibrad M, Shahabuei M, Sahabi M. Significance of the width of keratinized mucosa on the health status of the supporting tissue around implants supporting overdentures. J Oral Implantol 2009;35:232–7.
56. Roccuzzo M, Grasso G, Dalmasso P. Keratinized mucosa around implants in partially edentulous posterior mandible: 10-year results of a prospective comparative study. Clin Oral Implants Res 2016;27:491–6.
57. Boynueğri D, Nemli SK, Kasko YA. Significance of keratinized mucosa around dental implants: a prospective comparative study. Clin Oral Implants Res 2013; 24:928–33.

Radiology in Endodontics

Frank C. Setzer, DMD, PhD, MS*, Su-Min Lee, DDS, MSD, DScD

KEYWORDS

- Endodontic radiology • Root canal treatment • Periapical radiograph
- Cone-beam computed tomography • CBCT

KEY POINTS

- Periapical radiographs are the most commonly used modality in Endodontics. The paralleling technique is preferred.
- Angulated radiographs are frequently used to identify superimposed objects or fractures. The SLOB rule (same lingual opposite buccal) is a standard technique.
- Cone-beam computed tomography is increasingly used in Endodontics. Its benefit derives from the ability to provide 3-dimensional image volumes.

INTRODUCTION

Radiography is an integral part of Endodontics. Radiographs are used for prevention, diagnostics, therapy, and follow-up. Shortly after Dr Otto Walkhoff took the first dental radiograph of his teeth in 1895, Dr Edmund Kells first determined endodontic working length by using dental x-rays in 1899, and in 1900, Dr Weston Price first suggested the use of radiographs to evaluate the adequacy of root canal fillings.

Periapical radiographs are the most frequently used type of radiographs for endodontic treatment. Bitewing radiographs are often taken to evaluate restorability before initiating treatment or to check for coronal leakage and decay. Occlusal and lateral cephalometric radiographs are used after dental and facial trauma to identify root or alveolar fractures by providing additional views compared with periapical or panoramic radiographs. The introduction of cone-beam computed tomography (CBCT) provides a 3-dimensional (3D) assessment of oral structures. It is now widely used in addition to periapical radiographs or instead of some traditional imaging techniques, such as occlusal radiographs.

This article provides a practical guide for the most common clinical applications for radiology in Endodontics, focusing on digital periapical radiographs and CBCT imaging.

Department of Endodontics, School of Dental Medicine, University of Pennsylvania, 240 South 40th Street, Philadelphia, PA 19104, USA
* Corresponding author.
E-mail address: fsetzer@upenn.edu

Dent Clin N Am 65 (2021) 475–486
https://doi.org/10.1016/j.cden.2021.02.004
0011-8532/21/© 2021 Elsevier Inc. All rights reserved.

PERIAPICAL RADIOGRAPHS

Periapical radiographs are a type of 2-dimensional (2D) radiograph imaging, arguably the most important and widely used radiographic technique in Endodontics. For decades, conventional films had been used until the modern digital era in dental radiography started with the introduction of the RadioVisioGraphy system in 1989.[1] The digital systems rely on electronic detection of an radiograph-generated image processed and then reproduced on a computer screen. Various digital imaging modalities are currently available.

Digital radiography is firmly established as an indispensable diagnostic tool in endodontic practice. It demonstrated to be an excellent asset for Endodontics because of the number of radiographs indicated before, during, and after an endodontic procedure. Its benefits include a significant reduction in overall radiation dosage, increased speed of obtaining high-resolution digital images, the possibility of digital enhancement and ease of transmissibility, the elimination of manual processing steps and chemical waste, as well as digital data storage. The introduction of digital radiography allowed for a variety of image enhancements and modifications, including inversion, contrast, flashlight, magnification, pseudo colors, and digital measurements of root lengths and curvature angles.[2]

However, periapical radiographs have limitations because of the 2D nature of the images produced, geometric distortions, and anatomic noise. A 2D projection of a 3D object can only provide suggestive and not final evidence in judging a clinical problem.[3] The most common clinical problem is the difficulty of assessing any buccolingual dimensions, which can only be indirectly assessed by periapical radiographs through eccentric radiographs. Also, the bacterial status of hard and soft tissues cannot be determined, and inflammatory tissues cannot be differentiated from healed fibrous scar tissue. Last, radiographs do not provide information about the true nature of the tissue that replaced the bone. Abscesses, granulomas, or cysts resemble radiographically identical osteolytic lesions in a great majority of situations.[4] Lesions in the medullary bone are undetected in the radiographs until there are substantial bone loss and cortical bone involvement. For a hard tissue lesion to be evident on a radiograph, there should be at least a mineral bone loss of 6.6%.[5]

Paralleling and Bisecting Techniques

The paralleling technique (**Fig.1A**) is primarily recommended for endodontic periapical radiographs. It allows for projections with minimal geometric distortions[6] and has a

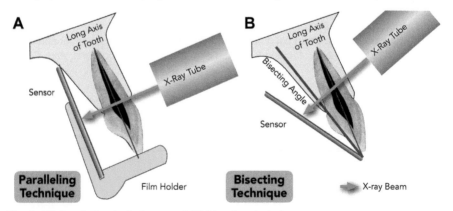

Fig. 1. (*A*) Paralleling technique, and (*B*) bisecting technique.

high level of reproducibility, which is beneficial for comparison with other radiographs throughout a procedure.[7] Briefly, a sensor is placed parallel to the long axis of the tooth undergoing treatment and exposed using radiographs perpendicular to the sensor surface. Special sensor holding devices, such as radiograph holders or hemostats, are required to align the sensor precisely with the radiograph tube. In the maxilla, the sensor may have to be placed at the palatal vault's height in the midline and in the mandible must displace the tongue toward the midline. Compromises may be necessary for patients with limited mouth opening, a severe gag reflex, or poor tolerance to the sensor.[6]

The bisecting angle technique (**Fig.1B**) lets radiographs pass perpendicular to the angle bisector of the angle formed by the tooth's long axis and the radiograph sensor. No holding devices are required. For conventional periapical and bitewing radiography, this technique is unreliable to achieve geometric accuracy, and distortions of anatomy are common. It is difficult to use rectangular collimation with this technique, as extension cone paralleling techniques are used with rectangular collimation to achieve maximum geometric sharpness and increased contrast of the resultant image. Although, when done with proper technique, it produces an only minimal distortion of the tooth length on the resultant images, the superimposition of adjacent anatomic landmarks or pathologic features may lead to difficulties in interpretation.[7] For example, the superimposition of the maxilla's zygomatic process over the root apices of molar teeth will often occur, which results in a characteristic radiopacity that renders interpretation difficult.[7]

Although similar diagnostic results are achievable with either technique, more studies favor the paralleling technique for effectiveness and superior diagnostic quality.[8,9] Whether a radiograph with good quality can be obtained will depend on the proper sensor placement in the patient's mouth and the correct angulation of the radiograph cone in relation to the sensor and oral structures. Proper exposure time and intensity of the radiograph beam must be chosen.

Adjustments in Vertical and Horizontal Angulation

Changes in horizontal radiograph angulation are employed by using the same lingual opposite buccal rule (SLOB), a technique helpful in identifying the relative spatial or buccal-lingual location of an object within the tooth or alveolus (**Fig. 2**). It combines an orthoradial periapical radiograph taken at zero horizontal angulation with additional mesial and/or distal eccentric radiographs. The orthoradial radiograph may lead to the superimposition of buccal and palatal objects on the sensor (**Fig. 3**A). In Endodontics,

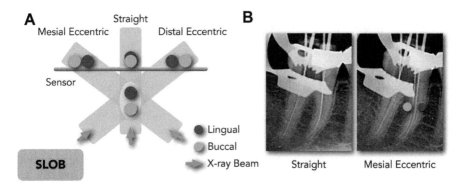

Fig. 2. (*A*) The SLOB rule. (*B*) Clinical example for comparison.

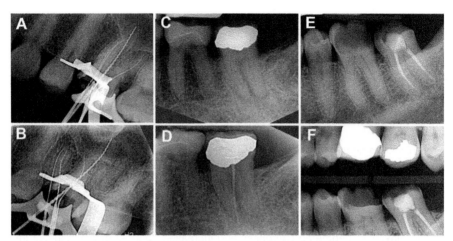

Fig. 3. (*A*) Orthoradial working length radiograph. Note superimposition of files in the mesiobuccal canals. (*B*) Eccentric working length radiograph. Note the visual separation of files in the mesiobuccal canals, allowing precise assessment. (*C*) Mandibular left second molar. Clinically, a sinus tract was present midroot below the furcation area. (*D*) Radiographic sinus tract tracing with a gutta-percha point. The gutta-percha traces to the periapical area, allowing to aid in the diagnosis of periapical, endodontic disease versus periodontal disease deriving from the furcation. (*E*) Periapical radiograph of mandibular left first molar showing deep distal decay with questionable restorability. (*F*) Bitewing radiograph demonstrates amount of sound supracrestal tooth structure. Tooth was deemed restorable.

these objects include roots, canals, instruments, or foreign objects. A secondary radiograph is then acquired with a slightly altered horizontal angulation of the radiograph beam (**Fig. 3**B). An object closest to buccal will appear to move in the opposite direction of the movement of the radiograph tube head, when compared with the orthoradial image. In turn, an object closest to lingual will appear to move in the direction of the movement of the radiograph tube head. For example, in the case of a working length film, if the eccentric direction of the radiograph beam is directed from mesial, a lingual canal will appear mesially on the image. In contrast, if the radiograph beam is directed from distal, the lingual will appear distally. Other than its utilization during root canal treatment, the SLOB rule can be applied to verify the presence or absence of foreign bodies or periapical lesion if radiopaque or radiolucent shadows are superimposed on an orthoradial radiograph.

In trauma, both vertical and horizontal angulations are of importance. Angulation changes may reveal a fracture line that otherwise could be concealed by hard tissue structures if the radiograph beam hits the fracture line within a ±3° angle. Horizontal angulation changes of 10° to 15° from the orthoradial direction should be used to identify a vertical crown, root, or alveolar fracture. Similarly, changes in vertical radiograph beam angulation are used for horizontal fractures. However, it must be appreciated that increases in vertical angulation will lead to a shortening of a tooth's length. Buccal roots will appear shorter than lingual roots in multirooted teeth, as they are at a greater distance from the sensor. A more accurate visualization of lingual roots and their apices is possible by increasing the vertical angulation. Increasing the vertical angulation also alters the vertical relationship of anatomic landmarks and root apices. This effect can determine whether anatomic landmarks lie buccally or lingually, an assessment that has benefit during endodontic surgery.[7] Last, identifying a "double periodontal ligament" by using a 20° horizontal angulation may hint at additional canals in a root with an hourglass cross-section.[10]

Sequence of Periapical Radiographs in Root Canal Therapy

Periapical radiographs are essential for endodontic therapy. They are used for diagnosis, preoperative assessment and patient communication, interpretation of root and root canal system morphology, verification of procedural steps, postoperative assessment of the root filling (obturation), as well as the long-term evaluation of the treatment outcome (follow-up).[5]

Diagnostic and preoperative radiographs

Periapical radiographs intended for endodontic therapy must include the complete area of interest with the full length of the root and at least 3 mm of periapical bone (**Fig. 4**A, B).[11] Ideally, these radiographs should be taken using the paralleling technique, which provides a consistently high quality without shortening or elongation.[6] One radiograph may be sufficient for a single-rooted tooth. For a multirooted tooth, roots and the root canal system may become superimposed (see **Fig. 4**A). A second radiograph with the radiograph beam shifted mesially or distally following the SLOB rule should be taken. A bitewing image may be necessary to assess restorability (see **Fig. 4**B).

Periapical radiographs allow both description of anatomic features and structures and detection of other conditions of the teeth and jaws related or not related to Endodontics. As an overview, **Table 1** lists the most common normal anatomic landmarks and relevant findings related to Endodontics. Because of the 2D imaging of 3D structures, periapical radiographs may see the projection of radiolucent or radiopaque anatomic shadows superimposed on the periapical tissues. Examples of radiolucent

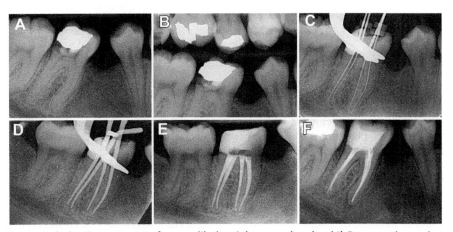

Fig. 4. Endodontic treatment of a mandibular right second molar. (*A*) Preoperative periapical radiograph. Note the radiolucent line representing the periodontal ligament space, depicted by the thin continuous dark line around the root outline. The radiopaque area close to the periodontal ligament of the premolar represents the lamina dura. The trabecular pattern and density the mandibular bone are relatively denser than in the maxilla. (*B*) Corresponding bitewing radiograph to assess restorability. (*C*) Working length radiograph. (*D*) Masterpoint radiograph before root filling. (*E*) Postoperative radiograph. Note temporary filling with radiolucent space indicative of a space holder such as a Teflon band or a cotton pellet. (*F*) Six-month follow-up radiograph. Note that the temporary filling has been replace by a build-up before permanent full-coverage restoration.

Table 1
Normal anatomic landmarks and relevant findings for endodontics

Normal Anatomic Landmarks	Relevant Findings for Endodontics
• Enamel, dentin, cementum, and alveolar bone • Pulp chamber, root canal system, and apical foramen • Periodontal ligament space • Lamina dura • Zygomatic process • Inferior border of the maxillary sinus • Neurovascular canals in the walls of the maxillary sinus • Intermaxillary suture • Incisive foramen • Nasolacrimal duct • Coronoid process of the mandible • Mandibular canal • Mylohyoid ridge • Mental foramen • Lingual foramen • Nutrient canal • Genial tubercles	• Number, course, shape, and length of root canals • Calcification or obliteration of pulp cavity and/or canals • Presence of caries that may threaten to affect the pulp • Widening of periodontal ligament • Nature and extent of periapical and alveolar bone destruction • Internal and external resorptions • Crown and root fractures • Abnormalities like dilaceration and taurodontism • Luxation and intrusion due to trauma • Foreign bodies following trauma • Iatrogenic errors (perforations, fractured instruments, and so forth) • Dens invaginatus with radicular lesion • Apical condensing osteitis • Enostosis (sclerotic bone) • Periradicular cemental dysplasia • Circumferential dentigerous cyst • Hereditary hypophosphatemia • Radicular lingual groove • Estimation and confirmation of root canals before instrumentation (working length determination) • Confirmation of position and adaptation of master cone • Evaluation of outcome of root canal therapy (postoperative radiograph)

shadows include superimposition of the mental foramina, the nasopalatine foramen, or the maxillary sinus, including its recesses. From an endodontic perspective, the effect of bone density reduction by these intrabony cavities may increase the radiolucent effect of the periodontal ligament, making it appear widened, yet still well demarcated and continuous. On the other hand, the effect on the lamina dura's radiopaque line may be the opposite, making it less discernible. Radiopaque shadows may derive from the body of the zygomatic arch, the mylohyoid ridge, and sclerotic bone areas, complicating the assessment of periradicular radiolucencies.

Clinicians must be trained to identify the normal anatomic landmarks and variations owing to pathologic condition.[7] Much of radiographic interpretation is based on the differentiation of normal versus abnormal conditions. Radiographs aid in making an endodontic diagnosis; however, clinical tests and examination, and the patient's medical and dental history must be considered. Endodontics aims to prevent or eliminate apical periodontitis. Diagnostic radiographs allow identifying periapical lesions. Although there is significant variation in jaw lesions, the majority, in particular, proximal to root apices, are odontogenic and inflammatory in nature.[12] Osteolytic processes owing to endodontic disease result from the irritants within a necrotic and infected root canal system. Changes in mineralization and structure of the periapical bone, visualized by radiographic techniques, are the primary indicators of the presence of apical periodontitis and its healing after endodontic treatment.[5,13] If pathologic condition is evident on the radiograph, the complete rarefaction plus normal bone should be recorded on the image. In cases with extensive lesions, a panoramic radiograph or larger-volume CBCT may be indicated.

If a sinus tract is present, it should be traced by inserting a gutta-percha cone into the tract up to the point of resistance and a radiograph taken with it in place. This radiograph will allow determining the path and termination of the sinus tract, revealing its origin, and thus identifying the affected tooth during diagnostic examination (**Fig. 3**C, D). This procedure may be of great benefit if pulpal sensibility tests cannot be adequately performed or multiple teeth present with periapical radiolucencies. Additional exposures with 10° to 15° changes in horizontal and/or vertical angulation need to be considered for diagnosing traumatic dental injuries, including root fractures, luxation, and avulsion injuries.[14]

Working length radiographs

Endodontic working length is an important concept to allow root canal instrumentation and root filling to reach as close to the cemento-dentinal junction as possible (**Fig. 4**C). Working length films are taken with root canal instruments inserted into the canals 0.5 to 1 mm short of the root length estimated on the preoperative radiograph or based on the reading of an electronic apex locator. Working length radiographs must always be taken with the rubber dam in place, to avoid contamination from the oral cavity or accidental swallowing or aspiration of an endodontic instrument. Any file inserted should be equipped with a rubber stop as a length indicator measured from a reproducible reference point. To allow for a correct reading of the instrument tip, a minimum size 15 is indicated (see **Fig. 4**C). The use of smaller file sizes may mislead and result in a wrong length determination. Besides length verification, radiographic imaging at this stage of root canal treatment gives additional information about the root canals' course, shape, and length.

A bisecting angle technique can be used but bears the risk of shortening or elongating individual roots. To avoid having a patient use a finger to support the sensor and expose it to unnecessary radiation, a hemostat or a sensor-holding device (eg, Rinn film holder system) should be used. Film holders will also allow for greater accuracy by applying the paralleling technique if the sensor and radiograph tube are correctly aligned. The sensor should be placed perpendicularly to the radiograph beam. This placement will also allow for greater accuracy and less likelihood of obtaining a partial radiograph if the radiograph beam misses a part of the sensor (cone out). However, sensor placement may still be difficult because of the patient's restricted opening with the rubber dam and sometimes also a frame in place. In the mandibular posterior area, the mouth's closing may relax the mylohyoid muscle, permitting the sensor to be placed further apically. In areas with increased difficulty, such as anterior maxillary teeth with a shallow palate, the placement of a cotton roll between sensor and crowns may be advised to obtain a better angulation.

Following the SLOB rule, for multirooted teeth or roots with more than 1 canal, at least 2 radiographs, one at the direct, standard angle, and the other with an eccentric angulation should be taken. The clinician should place different types of instruments, such as K- and Hedström files, in buccal and lingual canals, respectively, to allow for proper identification of the individual canals.

Masterpoint/master apical file

Before root filling, canal instrumentation and working length should be verified by taking a radiograph with either the final root canal instrument (master apical file [MAF]) or gutta-percha masterpoints selected for obturation (**Fig. 4**D), inserted to the full working length (see **Fig. 4**D). This step will allow for identifying potential iatrogenic errors, such as transportations or perforations before root filling and helps avoid short filling or overfilling. The master point size typically corresponds to the MAF but may require individual adjustment. Certain endodontic filling techniques may require 1 additional radiographic step to verify progression of the obturation. This step includes the lateral compaction (condensation) technique, which incorporates a midobturation image, verifying the placement of the masterpoints with sealer and 2 to 3 accessory cones, as well as warm techniques, such as vertical compaction (condensation) or continuous wave, verifying the apical fill at a downpack stage before the backfill of the canals. The technique for all masterpoint/MAF and midfilling films follows the recommendations for working length radiographs.

Postoperative radiographs

The evaluation of a root filling is mainly based on its radiographic appearance, including proper length, the absence of voids, or extruded filling materials. A postoperative radiograph must only be taken after the placement of a temporary or permanent restoration to ensure an excellent coronal seal (**Fig. 4**E). The rubber dam will be removed before taking postoperative radiographs. The paralleling technique should be used to allow reproducibility and a comparison with preoperative and follow-up radiographs. The importance of these images extends beyond the evaluation of treatment and includes medicolegal documentation.

Follow-up radiographs

Follow-up (recall) radiographs are taken to evaluate the prognosis of an endodontically treated tooth (**Fig. 4**F). Radiographs exposed at different points in time should be compared (see **Fig. 4**F).[15] The follow-up radiograph assesses periapical health or status of healing and may aid in identifying treatment failures. Preoperative, postoperative, and follow-up radiographs should be standardized with respect to their radiation geometry, density, and contrast to allow reliable interpretation of any changes that may have occurred in the periapical tissues owing to treatment.[5] Poorly standardized radiographs may lead to underestimating or overestimating the degree of healing or failure.[16] It has been recommended to use customized stents in order to maximize reproducibility. Elastomeric impression materials may be placed onto the paralleling device's bite block, which is then positioned in the most favorable position, and the patient is asked to bite on it until it sets.[17] The bite block with the patient's impression should be kept for later evaluations. A 1-year follow-up may be sufficient for most endodontic treatments. However, additional radiographs may be necessary if the tooth had presented with a large periapical lesion.

BITEWING RADIOGRAPHS

Bitewing radiographs are a type of 2D radiograph depicting crowns of teeth in either left or right maxillary and mandibular sextants. In Endodontics, they provide useful information regarding the proximal surfaces of the teeth, allow for the detection of interproximal caries, and aid in identifying coronal leakage and restorability, otherwise not visible on a periapical radiograph (**Fig. 3**E, F).

CONE-BEAM COMPUTED TOMOGRAPHY

CBCT is similar in many ways to multidetector computed tomography for the 3D imaging of hard tissue structures. CBCT allows for faster image processing and reduced radiation in comparison to conventional CT, because of its radiograph distribution in a cone shape.[18] In Endodontics, the most common format is a limited field-of-view (FOV) volume in the form of a cylinder with approximately 40 to 50 mm in diameter

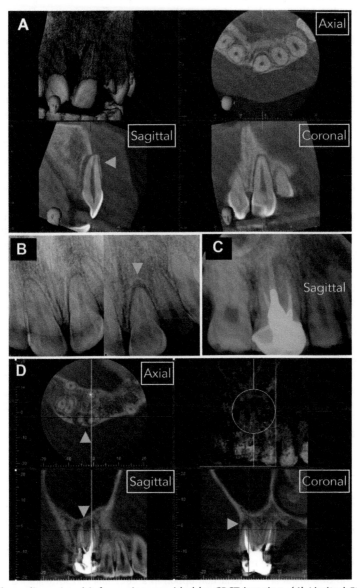

Fig. 5. Three-dimensional information provided by CBCT imaging. (*A*) Limited FOV CBCT. Note luxation of maxillary left central incisor with fracture of alveolar buccal plate and buccal displacement of the root apex (*arrowhead*). (*B*) Corresponding periapical radiographs in 2 vertical angulations, indicative of vertical luxation. No indication of horizontal displacement. (*C*) Periapical radiograph of maxillary right first molar with history of previous endodontic treatment. No indication of periapical lesions. (*D*) Corresponding limited FOV CBCT. Note apical radiolucencies on both buccal roots in axial, sagittal, and coronal views (*arrowheads*).

(**Fig. 5**A, D), depending on the manufacturer. This format provides for the imaging of approximately 4 teeth in the posterior and 6 teeth in the anterior area, ideal for most endodontic diagnostic, treatment planning, and problem-solving tasks. Limited FOV volumes allow for high-resolution scans with minimal distortion, an important aspect considering the minute details necessary to assess in Endodontics. Besides these benefits, a radiation dose up to 15 times lower than conventional CT scans[19] increased the ability to use CBCT imaging in private practice. A 2017 survey of 1083 endodontists found that 80.3% of the practitioners had access to either an on-site or an off-site CBCT machine.[20]

In Endodontics, CBCT is used to aid in the diagnosis of endodontic or nonodontogenic diseases; to identify root and root canal anatomy,[21] external, internal, and apical resorptions[22]; to detect missed canals,[23] intracanal foreign body materials (eg, separated instruments); to evaluate dental trauma[24] (**Fig. 5**A, B); to identify and assess the extent of apical periodontitis[25] (**Fig. 5**C, D); for healing assessment and follow-up of previous endodontic treatments with unclear clinical signs or symptoms[26]; and for surgical treatment planning.[27] CBCT imaging has been shown to demonstrate greater sensitivity and specificity to detect periapical lesions compared with conventional periapical or panoramic radiographs.[28]

For large periapical lesions, where apex locator measurements may be compromised, preoperative CBCT measurements were suggested for working length determination, demonstrating great accuracy.[29] CBCT "guided" techniques were proposed for nonsurgical endodontic treatment, for example, to minimize overall tooth structure loss detecting calcified canals,[30] and for surgical endodontics in close proximity to vulnerable anatomic structures.[31] Most recent applications saw the combination of CBCT imaging with artificial intelligence algorithms for the automated detection of periapical lesions[32] or crown and root fractures.[33]

For many patients and practitioners, the biggest concern regarding CBCT imaging remains radiation exposure. About 48% of the average annual radiation dose per person in the United States (6.2 mSv) derives from diagnostic tests and medical treatments, with 24% of the total radiation dose from any medical CT.[34] The overall guiding principle for practitioners to minimize exposure to radiation remains ALARA ("as low as reasonably achievable"), as stated in Title 10, Section 20.1003 of the Code of Federal Regulations.[35] Clinicians should be aware of and avoid any unnecessary radiation exposure of the patient.

CLINICS CARE POINTS

- Sitting a patient upright for periapical and bitewing radiographs will allow for better visualization of the x-ray beam direction.
- Changing horizontal or vertical angulations of a periapical radiographs for maxillary molars may allow to avoid superimposition of the zygomatic arch.
- Utilization of a metal artifact reduction option in a CBCT imaging software may greatly reduce scatter in the three-dimensional volume.

DISCLOSURE

The authors have nothing to disclose.

REFERENCES

1. Benz C, Mouyen F. Evaluation of the new RadioVisioGraphy system image quality. Oral Surg Oral Med Oral Pathol 1991;72:627–31.
2. Parks ET, Williamson GF. Digital radiography: an overview. J Contemp Dent Pract 2002;15:23–39.
3. Bender IB, Seltzer S. Roentgenographic and direct observation of experimental lesions in bone: I. 1961. J Endod 2003;29:702–6 [discussion 701].
4. Nair PN. New perspectives on radicular cysts: do they heal? Int Endod J 1998;31: 155–60.
5. Gröndahl HG, Huumonen S. Radiographic manifestations of periapical inflammatory lesions. Endod Top 2004;8:55–67.
6. Forsberg J. A comparison of the paralleling and bisecting-angle radiographic techniques in endodontics. Int Endod J 1987;20:177–82.
7. Fava LR, Dummer PM. Periapical radiographic techniques during endodontic diagnosis and treatment. Int Endod J 1997;30:250–61.
8. Hoe KH, Lee SS, Jeon IS, et al. Quantitative analysis of errors in alveolar crest level caused by discrepant projection geometry in digital subtraction radiography: an in vivo study. Oral Surg Oral Med Oral Pathol Oral Radiol Endod 2005;100:750–5.
9. Forsberg J, Halse A. Radiographic simulation of a periapical lesion comparing the paralleling and the bisecting-angle techniques. Int Endod J 1994;27:133–8.
10. Kaffe I, Gratt BM. Variations in the radiographic interpretation of the periapical dental region. J Endod 1988;14:330-5.
11. Van Aken J, Verhoeven JW. Factors influencing the design of aiming devices for intraoral radiography and their practical application. Oral Surg Oral Med Oral Pathol 1979;47:378–88.
12. Becconsall-Ryan K, Tong D, Love RM. Radiolucent inflammatory jaw lesions: a twenty-year analysis. Int Endod J 2010;43:859–65.
13. Cotti E, Campisi G. Advanced radiographic techniques for the detection of lesions in bone. Endod Top 2004;7:52–72.
14. Flores MT, Andersson L, Andreasen JO, et al, International Association of Dental Traumatology. Guidelines for the management of traumatic dental injuries. I. Fractures and luxations of permanent teeth. Dent Traumatol 2007;23:66–71.
15. Friedman S. Prognosis of initial endodontic therapy. Endod Top 2002;2:59–98.
16. Patel S, Dawood A, Whaites E, et al. New dimensions in endodontic imaging: part 1. Conventional and alternative radiographic systems. Int Endod J 2009;42: 447–62.
17. Rudolph DJ, White SC. Film-holding instruments for intraoral subtraction radiography. Oral Surg Oral Med Oral Pathol 1988;65:767–72.
18. Patel S, Durack C, Abella F, et al. Cone beam computed tomography in Endodontics - a review. Int Endod J 2015;48:3–15.
19. Scarfe WC, Farman AG, Sukovic P. Clinical applications of cone-beam computed tomography in dental practice. J Can Dent Assoc 2006;72:75–80.
20. Setzer FC, Hinckley N, Kohli MR, et al. A survey of CBCT use amongst endodontic practitioners in the United States. J Endod 2017;43:699–704.
21. Caputo BV, Noro Filho GA, de Andrade Salgado DM, et al. Evaluation of the root canal morphology of molars by using cone-beam computed tomography in a Brazilian population: part I. J Endod 2016;42:1604–7.

22. Creanga AG, Geha H, Sankar V, et al. Accuracy of digital periapical radiography and cone-beam computed tomography in detecting external root resorption. Imaging Sci Dent 2015;45:153–8.
23. Karabucak B, Bunes A, Chehoud C, et al. Prevalence of apical periodontitis in endodontically treated premolars and molars with untreated canal: a cone-beam computed tomography study. J Endod 2016;42:538–41.
24. Venskutonis T, Plotino G, Juodzbalys G, et al. The importance of cone-beam computed tomography in the management of endodontic problems: a review of the literature. J Endod 2014;40:1895–901.
25. Uraba S, Ebihara A, Komatsu K, et al. Ability of cone-beam computed tomography to detect periapical lesions that were not detected by periapical radiography: a retrospective assessment according to tooth group. J Endod 2016;42:1186–90.
26. Schloss T, Sonntag D, Kohli MR, et al. A comparison of two- and three-dimensional healing assessment after endodontic surgery using CBCT volumes or periapical radiographs. J Endod 2017;43:1072–9.
27. Low KM, Dula K, Burgin W, et al. Comparison of periapical radiography and limited cone-beam tomography in posterior maxillary teeth referred for apical surgery. J Endod 2008;34:557–62.
28. Leonardi Dutra K, Haas L, Porporatti AL, et al. Diagnostic accuracy of cone-beam computed tomography and conventional radiography on apical periodontitis: a systematic review and meta-analysis. J Endod 2016;42:356–64.
29. Üstün Y, Aslan T, Şekerci AE, et al. Evaluation of the reliability of cone-beam computed tomography scanning and electronic apex locator measurements in working length determination of teeth with large periapical lesions. J Endod 2016;42:1334–7.
30. Zehnder MS, Connert T, Weiger R, et al. Guided endodontics: accuracy of a novel method for guided access cavity preparation and root canal location. Int Endod J 2016;49:966–72.
31. Hawkins TK, Wealleans JA, Pratt AM, et al. Targeted endodontic microsurgery and endodontic microsurgery: a surgical simulation comparison. Int Endod J 2020;53:715–22.
32. Setzer FC, Shi KJ, Zhang Z, et al. Artificial intelligence for the computer-aided detection of periapical lesions in CBCT images. J Endod 2020;46:987–93.
33. Shah H, Hernandez P, Budin F, et al. Automatic quantification framework to detect cracks in teeth. Proc SPIE Int Soc Opt Eng 2018;10578:105781K. https://doi.org/10.1117/12.2293603.
34. National Council on Radiation Protection and Measurements. Ionizing radiation exposure of the population of the United States. Bethesda, MD: NCRP; 2009. Report No. 160.
35. Code of federal regulations: 10 CFR 20.1003. Washington, DC, US government printing office. Available at: https://www.nrc.gov/reading-rm/doc-collections/cfr/part020/part020-1003.html. Accessed September 25, 2020.

Imaging in Oral and Maxillofacial Surgery

Steven Wang, DMD, MD, MPH*, Brian Ford, DMD, MD

KEYWORDS

- Oral surgery imaging • CBCT • Panoramic imaging • Panorex • Surgery planning

KEY POINTS

- There are many types of imaging modalities commonly used in oral and maxillofacial surgery.
- The more ubiquitous use of three-dimensional (3D) imaging has allowed for advances in the field of oral and maxillofacial surgery.
- The advances in 3D imaging and surgical software programs have allowed for improved surgical planning and the creation of patient-specific surgical guides and implants.

INTRODUCTION

The scope of oral and maxillofacial surgery treatment and care is very broad, from dentoalveolar surgery, to pathology and reconstruction, to treatment of craniofacial deformities. The effective surgical treatment of patients requires appropriate and accurate diagnostic imaging. The various imaging modalities used in oral and maxillofacial surgery are typically for diagnostic and treatment planning purposes. With the improvements of three-dimensional (3D) imaging and software programs, surgical treatment and care have been enhanced with patient-specific guides, hardware, and implants. This article discusses the various imaging modalities used for a variety of typical oral and maxillofacial surgery procedures.

IMAGING FOR DENTOALVEOLAR SURGERY AND IMPLANTS

The most common procedures for oral and maxillofacial surgeons are dentoalveolar surgery and dental extractions. Imaging with periapical radiography can be used for diagnosis of single-tooth issues such as caries, or for evaluation of single-tooth dental implants with angulation and postoperative documentation. However, panoramic imaging is the typical first-line imaging modality for most dentoalveolar needs and diagnosis in the oral surgery setting.

Department of Oral and Maxillofacial Surgery and Pharmacology, University of Pennsylvania School of Dental Medicine, 240 South 40th Street, 1st Floor Schattner Building, Philadelphia, PA 19104, USA
* Corresponding author.
E-mail address: steven.wang@pennmedicine.upenn.edu

Dent Clin N Am 65 (2021) 487–507
https://doi.org/10.1016/j.cden.2021.02.012
0011-8532/21/© 2021 Elsevier Inc. All rights reserved.

Panoramic imaging allows evaluation of a broad area of the dentofacial complex. With panoramic imaging, oral surgeons are able to evaluate multiple teeth, impactions, relation of teeth to other relevant structures, the bony architecture, generalized periodontal bone health, and other pathologic conditions such as cysts or masses.

Cone-beam computed tomography (CBCT) imaging is particularly useful for dentoalveolar surgery to allow 3D analysis of anatomy and structures. CBCT can be used for evaluation of proximity of teeth to vital structures, or to measure distances and evaluate bone for dental implant placement.

Clinical Applications

Third molars

The panoramic radiograph is the standard radiographic image taken to evaluate third molars for extraction. The approximation of the teeth to the maxillary sinus and inferior alveolar nerves, as well as angulation and depth of impaction, is easily determined with a panoramic image. When evaluating mandibular third molars in close proximity to the inferior alveolar nerve (IAN), findings such as root darkening, root deflection, root narrowing, bifid apex, overlap of the canal, as well as loss of cortical lines of the IAN canal, deflection of the canal, or narrowing of the canal could indicate potential for increased risk of paresthesia or nerve injury if the teeth were to be extracted.[1,2] **Fig. 1** shows a pantomogram where tooth 17 overlaps the IAN, with root darkening, and nerve canal deflection.

CBCT imaging may be beneficial to better understand the proximity of teeth to the IAN when the signs mentioned earlier on pantomogram are present. Although CBCT imaging typically does not change the surgical approach or technique of extracting teeth, the added information may be beneficial in deciding between extraction versus coronectomy to prevent nerve injury.[3–5] An example of this is **Fig. 2**, which shows the CBCT of tooth 17 for the patient in **Fig. 1**. This CBCT image shows the IAN traveling through the roots of tooth 17, thus making coronectomy the procedure of choice if surgery is indicated. 3D imaging with CBCT may be a useful diagnostic tool to aid in surgical planning for procedures on mandibular third molar teeth.

Exposure of Impacted Teeth

A common procedure for oral and maxillofacial surgeons is the exposure and bonding of impacted teeth for orthodontic treatment. Panoramic imaging is useful to visualize these impacted teeth and their general locations, such as in **Figs. 3** and **4**. If these impacted teeth cannot be palpated on clinical examination, intraoral imaging with the commonly known SLOB (same-lingual, opposite-buccal) rule can be performed

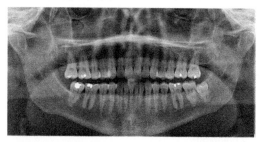

Fig. 1. A panoramic radiograph with tooth 17 showing classic signs of close proximity to the IAN (overlap with the IAN, root darkening, deflection of the canal).

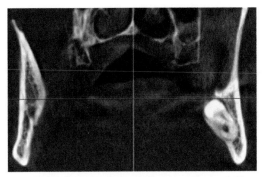

Fig. 2. CBCT of tooth from **Fig. 1** showing IAN traversing through the roots of tooth 17.

for localization of the tooth, but the increased use of CBCT imaging allows 3D localization of these teeth and more anatomic information.[6] This ability is clinically relevant because the location of the teeth in question determines whether the surgical approach should be accomplished from the buccal or the palatal or lingual, leading to decreased morbidity from the procedure.[7] **Figs. 5** and **6** also show the CBCT of the same patients in **Figs. 3** and **4**, respectively, allowing the surgeon to have a better understanding of the surgical access.

Implants

As described elsewhere in this article, imaging for dental implant placement has progressed to 3D analysis via CBCT imaging. Plain film radiography such as periapical radiographs can be used for specific situations where no vital anatomy (IAN, maxillary sinus, bony concavities) is nearby, and clinically sufficient bone width and height are present. If these criteria are not met, then panoramic or CBCT imaging are recommended to allow more precise measurements to relevant anatomy. Panoramic imaging is useful for evaluation of bone height in the posterior maxilla and mandible, to see general distance to the maxillary sinus and IAN, respectively. CBCT imaging can evaluate distances more accurately to vital structures and allow 3D visualization of edentulous spaces. Technological advances with CBCT imaging, planning software, and 3D printing and milling have allowed the creation of surgical guides and guided implant surgery.[8] **Figs. 7–10** show a patient that had an ameloblastoma surgically resected, and bone continuity restored with a free fibula flap, using 3D imaging and dental software programs to surgically plan dental implant placement and subsequent dental rehabilitation.

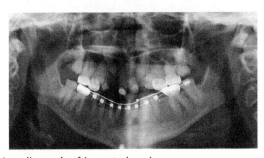

Fig. 3. A panoramic radiograph of impacted canines.

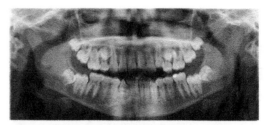

Fig. 4. A panoramic radiograph of impacted premolars.

IMAGING FOR DENTOALVEOLAR AND MAXILLOFACIAL TRAUMA

Dental and maxillofacial injuries range from fractured teeth to complex fractures involving the entire osseous facial skeleton. Diagnostic imaging plays a critical role in the initial diagnosis, treatment planning, and intraoperative and postoperative management of these patients. Until the 1980s, diagnostic imaging consisted of plain films and panoramic radiographs. A major advancement in imaging for facial trauma occurred with the introduction of computed tomography (CT) imaging.[9,10] CT allowed the visualization of injuries in multiple planes. With advances in software, 3D reformatted images became widespread. Continued advancement in CT hardware and software have now changed the way patients with facial trauma are managed.

Dentoalveolar Trauma

Evaluating dental and dentoalveolar trauma begins with a detailed physical examination. Mobile teeth moving in a segment suggest an alveolar fracture, whereas nonmobile fractured teeth suggest an isolated dental trauma. Changes in occlusion could

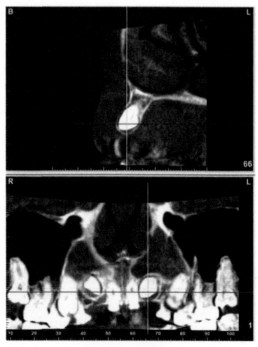

Fig. 5. Cross-sectional and panoramic views of CBCT of impacted canines from **Fig. 3.**

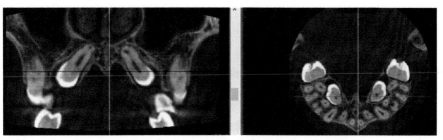

Fig. 6. Coronal and axial views of CBCT of impacted premolars from **Fig. 4**.

arise from a maxillary or mandibular fracture. The imaging technique selected varies based on the physical examination findings. Isolated dental trauma is best evaluated with periapical films because they provide the highest-resolution image. With changes in occlusion or mobile segments of dentition, additional imaging is necessary. Panoramic radiographs may be used to detect mandibular fractures and alveolar fractures. Midface fractures often require 3D imaging to detect.

Dental Luxation Injuries

The diagnosis and management of dental luxation requires careful physical examination and radiographic evaluation. Depending on the type of injury, the treatment and

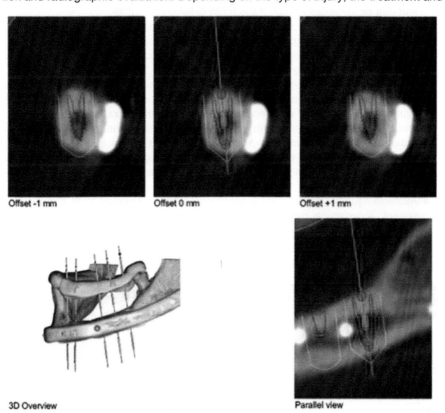

Fig. 7. 3D surgical plan for surgically guided implant placement in a mandible reconstructed with a fibula free flap.

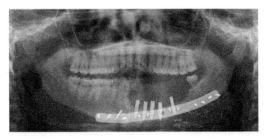

Fig. 8. A panoramic radiograph of implant placement in fibula reconstruction of mandible.

overall prognosis varies.[11,12] Primary teeth are generally managed conservatively, so the following discussion relates to management of permanent tooth luxation injuries.[13]

- *Concussion injuries* present with pain with percussion without loosening or displacement of the tooth. The injury cannot be detected with radiographs and is generally managed conservatively with a soft diet for 1 to 2 weeks.
- *Subluxation injuries* present with a loose tooth in the appropriate position. A periapical radiograph may show widening of the periodontal ligament (PDL) space. A CT scan appears normal. This injury is generally managed conservatively with a soft diet or semirigid fixation if the tooth is severely mobile.
- *Lateral luxation injuries* present with eccentric displacement of a tooth. A periapical radiograph may show widening of the PDL space and can identify a tooth root fracture. A CT scan may identify a comminuted alveolar socket. The injury is treated with repositioning and semirigid fixation.
- *Extrusive luxation* presents with coronal displacement of the tooth. A periapical radiograph confirms partial displacement of the tooth out of the socket. This injury can be managed with repositioning and semirigid fixation.
- *Intrusive luxation* presents with apical displacement of the tooth. A periapical radiograph often confirms the apical displacement and is able to identify any tooth root fractures. A CT scan may identify the comminuted alveolar socket. This injury can be managed with repositioning and splinting or orthodontic extrusion.
- *Avulsion injuries* present with a tooth completely displaced from the alveolar socket. A periapical radiograph shows an empty socket and confirms there is no retained root fragment. This injury is managed with timely reimplantation and semirigid fixation.

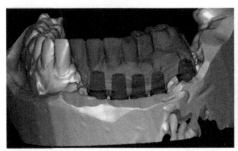
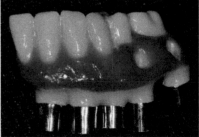

Fig. 9. Software design and lab processed final implant-supported prosthesis.

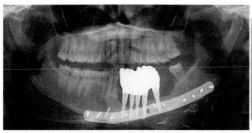
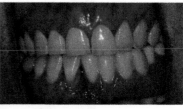

Fig. 10. (*Left*) Pantomogram of final prosthesis. (*Right*) Clinical photograph of final prosthesis.

Alveolar Fractures

An alveolar fracture presents with multiple mobile teeth moving as a single unit. A periapical radiograph may be able to identify a fracture line in the alveolar bone. Panoramic radiograph often appears normal. CT scan is the best modality to radiographically confirm the fracture as well as to ensure there is not a more significant skeletal fracture such as a mandible fracture or a maxillary (Le Fort) fracture. These injuries in both the adult and pediatric population are managed with repositioning and splinting.

Mandibular Fractures

Imaging modalities for mandibular fractures consist of plain films, panoramic radiographs, or CT scans. Given the complex anatomy and various treatment options, CT has become the gold standard for mandibular fractures. Plain films have an overall sensitivity of 62% in identifying mandibular fractures; however, they may be useful in identifying certain fractures, especially in the pediatric population, where there is a concern for the amount of radiation a patient is receiving.[14] In the outpatient dental setting, a pantomogram is able to evaluate the mandible and has a sensitivity of 92% in identifying mandibular fractures.[14] **Fig. 11** shows a 3D rendering from a CT scan that shows a mandibular symphysis and left mandibular subcondylar fracture in detail.

Midface Fractures

The midface includes the maxilla and the paired zygomas. Fractures in this region are best evaluated with a CT scan.[15] Plain film and panoramic radiographs are not often sensitive enough to identify midface fractures. Given the complex and overlapping anatomy of the facial skeleton, CT is the most useful imaging modality. **Fig. 12** shows a bilateral zygomaticomaxillary complex fracture and maxillary fractures.

Intraoperative Computed Tomography

Intraoperative imaging has changed the management of facial trauma. A portable CT scanner is brought into the operating room and a CT scan can be taken while the patient is still under general anesthesia, such as in **Fig. 13**. This approach allows the surgeon to evaluate the repair and make changes if necessary, before leaving the operating room. This technology has reduced the need for so-called take-back surgeries and improved surgical outcomes.[16] In addition to the evaluation of treatment, intraoperative CT has changed treatment algorithms.[17] Before intraoperative CT scans, surgeons often had to expose all aspects of a fracture to assess the reduction of the fracture. With intraoperative CT, surgeons can assess aspects of the fracture without full exposure. This ability reduces the surgical morbidity associated with additional exposure and fixation.[18,19]

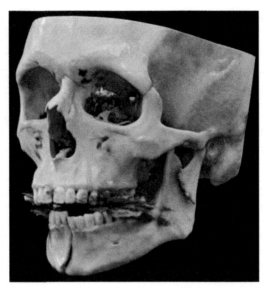

Fig. 11. 3D reconstruction from a CT scan showing mandibular symphysis and left subcondylar fractures.

Virtual Surgical Planning

Virtual surgical planning uses CT images and biomedical engineering software to perform computer-assisted surgical simulation. In addition to allowing surgeons to plan surgery virtually before entering the operating room, osteotomy cutting guides,

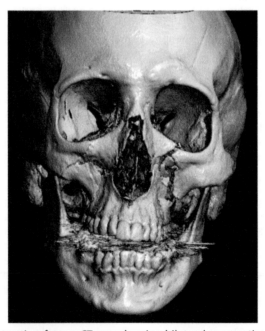

Fig. 12. 3D reconstruction from a CT scan showing bilateral zygomaticomaxillary complex fractures and maxillary sinus fractures.

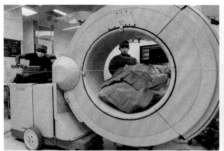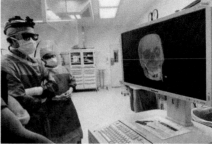

Fig. 13. (*Left*) Intraoperative CT scanner during trauma repair. (Right) Evaluation of intraoperative CT scan to determine further surgical plan.

custom reconstruction plates, and other custom implants can be fabricated.[20–22] The technology has improved patient outcomes and can reduce surgical time.

IMAGING FOR MAXILLOFACIAL PATHOLOGY AND RECONSTRUCTION

Many pathologic conditions in the orofacial region are identified by imaging. Numerous benign and malignant conditions can be clinically asymptomatic and may only be discovered after radiographic evaluation.[23] The radiologic characteristics and findings of all pathologic conditions of the dentofacial structures is beyond the scope of this article, but few pathologic conditions are able to be definitely diagnosed with imaging alone. Surgical biopsy of tissue and diagnosis by histologic analysis is typically required to determine the diagnosis and subsequent definitive management of disorders of the dentofacial structures.

Intraoral radiographs are the typical imaging modality when patients see the dentist with complaints of dental pain and swelling. The patient in **Fig. 14** had a periapical radiograph taken to evaluate teeth associated with an anterior maxillary swelling. A full-mouth series is also the mainstay for evaluation for comprehensive dental care. Pathologic lesions may be found on asymptomatic patients, such as in **Fig. 15**, a periapical radiograph from a full-mouth series taken for comprehensive evaluation. This lesion was biopsied and diagnosed as an ameloblastoma.

Although panoramic imaging should be taken when clinically relevant, and not necessarily as a screening tool to look for disorder in asymptomatic patients, panoramic imaging can be considered to evaluate when teeth have not erupted into the dental arch in the expected time frame or age.[24] Pathologic lesions such as in **Fig. 16** can occasionally be found displacing teeth or impeding their eruption. When reviewing panoramic imaging, careful examination of the entire dentofacial structures is necessary, because lesions may be present in regions of the bone that are not the primary area of interest. **Fig. 17** shows a small lesion in the left mandibular ramus, and, 3 years later, the lesion grew in size, as shown in **Fig. 18**. This lesion was biopsied and excised and was noted to be an odontogenic keratocyst.

When pathologic lesions are found on intraoral or panoramic imaging, 3D characterization of these lesions is often beneficial. CBCT imaging allows the understanding of the extent of intrabony lesions in 3 dimensions, as well as the proximity of lesions to vital structures such as adjacent dentition, the IAN, the extent of protrusion into the maxillary sinus, or perforation of the lesion outside of the bony cortex and invasion into the soft tissue. **Fig. 19** is a CBCT scan of the odontogenic keratocyst in **Fig. 18**, showing proximity of the lesion abutting the IAN. The understanding of the

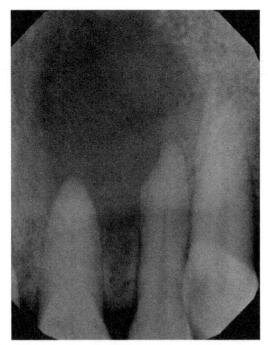

Fig. 14. Periapical radiograph taken of anterior maxillary swelling. Excisional biopsy showed a radicular cyst.

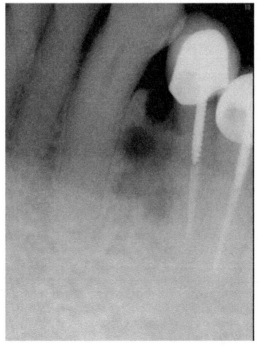

Fig. 15. Periapical radiograph taken during routine visit. Biopsy showed ameloblastoma.

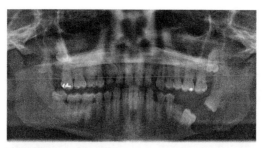

Fig. 16. A panoramic radiograph of radiolucency associated with unerupted teeth 31 and 32. A second radiolucency was associated with impacted tooth 1. These radiolucencies were excised and biopsy showed them to be dentigerous cysts.

location of lesions in proximity to these types of structures is beneficial when planning the surgical management of these lesions.

Clinical Application

With advancements in 3D imaging and CBCT use, as well as surgical planning software, oral and maxillofacial surgery treatment of certain pathologic conditions is enhanced. **Figs. 20** and **21** show a panoramic radiograph and CBCT of a compound odontoma. With the ability to analyze pathologic lesions in 3 dimensions, CBCT of the odontoma allows surgeons to know how many toothlike structures are present, as well as their location, to allow for removal of the entire lesion, resulting in the successful removal shown in **Fig. 22**.

Another clinical application of current imaging technology is to use 3D imaging and software programs to create patient-specific surgical guides and treatment.[25–27] **Fig. 23** shows a radiolucency found on panoramic radiograph taken for the evaluation of swelling associated with a previously placed dental implant. A biopsy confirmed the lesion to be an ameloblastoma, for which the treatment is surgical resection. CT imaging was taken to evaluate the extent of the intrabony lesion. With 3D imaging and

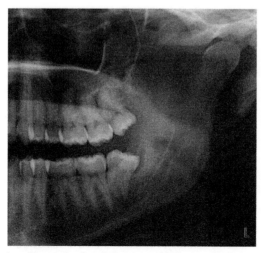

Fig. 17. A panoramic radiograph of radiolucency of left mandibular ramus.

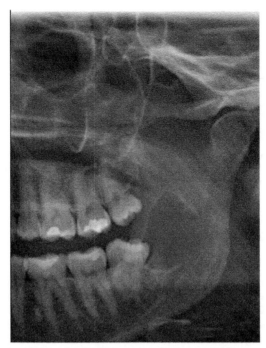

Fig. 18. A panoramic radiograph of radiolucency of left mandibular ramus, 3 years after image from **Fig. 17**. It was biopsied and found to be an odontogenic keratocyst.

surgical planning software, plans such as in **Fig. 24** allow confirmation of the surgical margins of 1 to 1.5 cm, and creation of surgical cutting guides to use during surgery. The patient was subsequently treated with resection with the cutting guides, followed by bone grafting (**Fig. 25**).

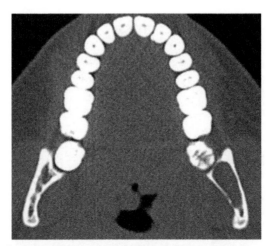

Fig. 19. CBCT of odontogenic keratocyst of left mandibular ramus from patient in **Figs. 17** and **18**.

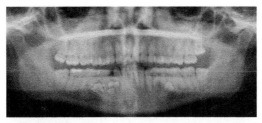

Fig. 20. A panoramic radiograph of a compound odontoma preventing eruption of the right mandibular premolars 28 and 29.

Head and Neck Cancer

The diagnosis of oral cancer depends on obtaining a tissue sample from the lesion. This tissue then undergoes histopathologic analysis by a pathologist who makes the diagnosis. Once the diagnosis of oral cancer has been established, the treating surgeon obtains advanced radiologic imaging. The imaging to evaluates the primary tumor, adjacent structures, and cervical lymph nodes, and assesses for distant metastases. The imaging modalities used in oral cancer evaluation include MRI with intravenous contrast, ultrasonography, CT with intravenous contrast, and PET to help stage the cancer.[28]

A panoramic radiograph and periapical films are useful for evaluating the dentition before definitive treatment. CT scans of the head, neck, and chest are used to assess for potential metastases. MRI of the neck is used to evaluate the soft tissue extent of the tumor and to assess for perineural involvement. Ultrasonography can be used to assess the cervical lymph nodes and to help guide fine-needle aspiration for cytologic evaluation. PET is often combined with the aforementioned studies. PET is a nuclear medicine study where a radiotracer is administered intravenously. The radiotracer is preferentially taken up by cells with a high metabolic rate, such as cancer, and can be useful in identifying metastatic disease.[29,30]

Treatment of head and neck cancer depends not only on the type of cancer but on the stage of that cancer as well. The TNM (tumor, node, metastasis) classification for cancer staging relies not only on detailed physical examination and histopathologic evaluation but also on the radiologic studies presented earlier.[31]

IMAGING FOR TEMPOROMANDIBULAR JOINT DYSFUNCTION AND SURGERY

The temporomandibular joint (TMJ) is an anatomically and biomechanically complex structure. There are many clinical entities that affect the TMJ. Temporomandibular

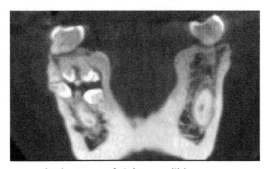

Fig. 21. CBCT of compound odontoma of right mandible.

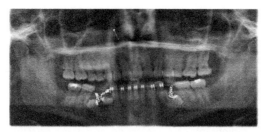

Fig. 22. Postoperative pantomogram after removal of odontoma and exposure and bonding of impacted teeth.

disorder (TMD) is an umbrella term for disorders that affect the TMJ, the muscles of mastication, or both.[32] The clinical evaluation of patients with TMD can be challenging because many signs and symptoms overlap with multiple disorders. In order to correctly diagnose and treat patients with TMD, advanced imaging is often required.

Pantomogram

A panoramic radiograph or pantomogram is often the first radiologic study obtained to evaluate the condyle in patients with TMD. Degenerative joint disease can be diagnosed by identifying surface erosion, osteophyte formation, subcortical cysts, or sclerosis. Conditions that affect the length of the condyle, such as condylar hyperplasia, may be identified. Neoplastic processes such as osteochondroma or synovial chondromatosis may also be identified. Given the limited diagnostic accuracy of the orthopantomogram, more advanced imaging is frequently obtained.[33,34]

MRI

MRI is the gold standard for evaluating the articular disc and soft tissue structures of the TMJ.[35] The imagining technique involves obtaining sagittal, oblique, and coronal plane images of the joint in both the open-mouth and closed-mouth positions. Evaluating the images in both the closed-mouth and open-mouth positions allows an assessment of the biomechanics of the joint. By comparing disc position relative to the condylar head in the open-mouth and closed-mouth views, the diagnosis of disc displacement with or without reduction can be identified. Pathologic entities such as disc perforation, joint effusions, and other neoplastic processes can also be evaluated with MRI.

Computed Tomography/Cone-beam Computed Tomography

Evaluating the TMJ with CT provides a more detailed examination of the osseous component of the joint. It allows evaluation in multiple planes and allows detailed

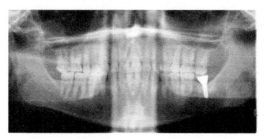

Fig. 23. Ameloblastoma in area of swelling below a dental implant.

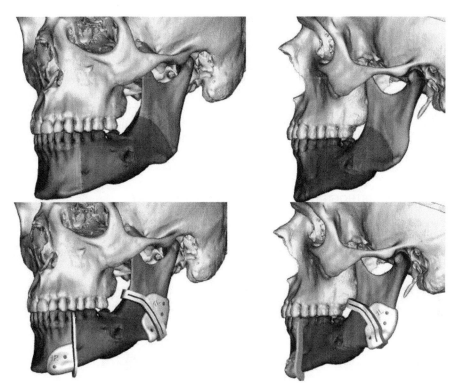

Fig. 24. 3D reconstructions from CBCT, with virtual surgical plan with appropriate resection margins, and creation of surgical cutting guides. Courtesy of Materialise.

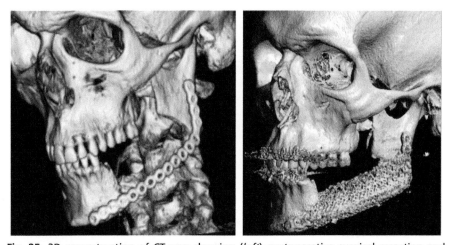

Fig. 25. 3D reconstruction of CT scan showing (*left*) postoperative surgical resection and (*right*) subsequent bone grafting for reconstruction.

accurate measurements.[32] CBCT has been found to be an acceptable alternative to medical-grade CT scans at diagnosing osseous TMJ abnormalities.[36]

Advances in Oral and Maxillofacial Surgery

Operating on the TMJ is challenging because of the complex anatomy of the area. Recent advances have made operating on the TMJ more successful and safer. Virtual surgical planning and patient-specific implants have revolutionized TMJ surgery with custom TMJ alloplastic replacements. CT angiograms can evaluate the proximity of vasculature to the joint, and interventional radiology techniques such as the embolization of blood vessels in close proximity to the TMJ have reduced the bleeding risk for high-risk patients.[37]

IMAGING FOR ORTHOGNATHIC AND CRANIOFACIAL SURGERY

Classic imaging for orthognathic surgery evaluation and treatment includes the panoramic radiograph and posteroanterior and lateral cephalograms (the evaluation of these images for diagnosis is reviewed in the Nipul K. Tanna and colleagues' article,

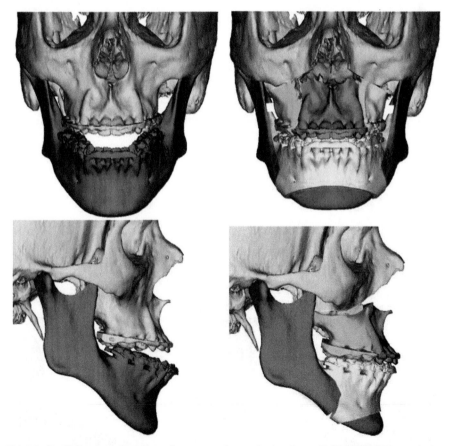

Fig. 26. (*Left*) 3D reconstruction of preoperative occlusion from CBCT. (*Right*) 3D rendering of virtual surgical plan of 3-piece Le Fort, mandibular bilateral sagittal split osteotomy, and genioplasty. Courtesy of Materialise.

"Imaging in Orthodontics," in this issue). These 3 types of images combined can allow some semblance of 3D analysis of maxillary and mandibular growth and pathologic circumstances that may need to be corrected with joint orthodontic and oral surgical care, or orthognathic surgery. The use of lateral cephalograms for diagnostic purposes allows surgeons and orthodontists to identify jaws that are deficient or excessive, and whether to perform surgery on the maxilla, mandible, or both.

CBCT imaging provides the ability to evaluate and analyze the maxillofacial anatomy more accurately.[38–40] With current virtual surgical planning software using CBCT imaging, 3D models and renderings can be used for surgical planning. With these technologies, surgeons are able to perform virtual osteotomies, move jaws in 3 dimensions, and better visualize the impact of these movements in all dimensions. **Fig. 26** shows a 3D preoperative rendering, as well as the proposed surgical plan of a 3-piece maxillary Le Fort advancement and mandibular bilateral sagittal split osteotomy setback with reduction genioplasty. **Fig. 27** also shows the ability of the 3D software from a CBCT scan to allow visualization of bony interferences or gaps in bone that could affect the positioning or stability of the proposed surgical movements.

In addition to better visualization, surgical planning, and understanding of surgical movements, using CBCT imaging along with advancements in surgical planning software and with milling and printing of titanium plates, custom computer-aided design and computer-aided manufacturing surgical cutting guides and plates can be fabricated to allow accurate patient-specific implants. Custom, patient-specific cutting guides and custom plates, such as those shown in **Fig. 28**, allow accurate surgical outcomes and decreased surgical time, which can lead to improved patient outcomes and decreased operative morbidity.[41–44] The use of 3D CBCT imaging and advances in surgical planning software has revolutionized orthognathic surgery diagnosis, planning, and treatment.

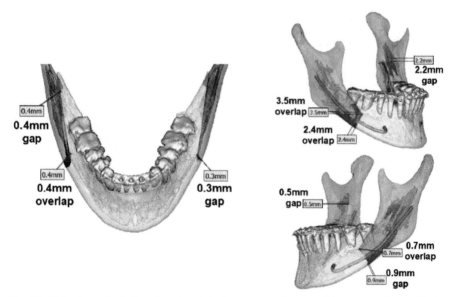

Fig. 27. Virtual surgical plan showing interferences and gaps with proposed mandibular movements. Courtesy of Materialise.

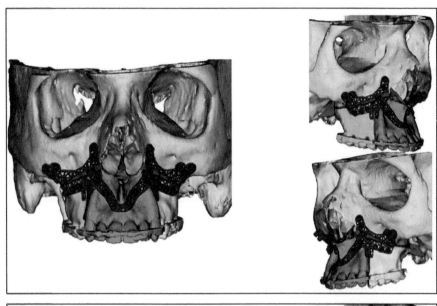

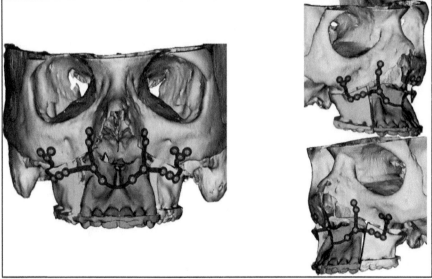

Fig. 28. 3D printed cutting guide (*above*), and 3D printed surgical plate (*below*). Courtesy of Materialise.

CLINICS CARE POINTS

- Panoramic imaging is the mainstay for evaluation of third molars, but CBCT imaging may be useful for evaluation of teeth overlapping or abutting the IAN to avoid permanent nerve injury.
- CBCT imaging is useful for dental implant placement to evaluate bone volume and distance from relevant anatomic structures, and for the creation of surgical guides.

- CT imaging is most useful for evaluation of maxillofacial trauma.
- MRI is most useful for the evaluation of soft tissue, such as the position of the TMJ disk and other soft tissue structures.
- CBCT imaging and surgical planning software have revolutionized the orthognathic surgery planning process.

DISCLOSURE

The authors have nothing to disclose.

REFERENCES

1. Rood J, Shehab B. The radiological prediction of inferior alveolar nerve injury during third molar surgery. Br J Oral Maxillofac Surg 1990;28:20–5.
2. Su N, Wijk A, Berkhout E, et al. Predictive value of panoramic radiography for injury of inferior alveolar nerve after mandibular third molar surgery. J Oral Maxillofac Surg 2017;75:663–79.
3. Araujo G, Peralta-Mamani M, Silva A, et al. Influence of cone beam computed tomography versus panoramic radiography on the surgical technique of third molar removal: a systematic review. Int J Oral Maxillofac Surg 2019;48:1340–7.
4. Matzen L, Christensen J, Hintze H, et al. Influence of cone beam CT on treatment plan before surgical intervention of mandibular third molars and impact of radiographic factors on deciding on coronectomy vs surgical removal. Dentomaxillofac Radiol 2013;42:98870341.
5. Guerrero M, Botetano R, Beltran J, et al. Can preoperative imaging help to predict postoperative outcome after wisdom tooth removal? A randomized controlled trial using panoramic radiography versus cone-beam CT. Clin Oral Investig 2014;18: 335–42.
6. Mozzo P, Procacci C, Tacconi A, et al. A new volumetric CT machine for dental imaging based on the cone-beam technique: preliminary results. Eur Radiol 1998;8:1558–64.
7. Majumdar S, Hossain M, De N, et al. Effect of diagnosis by two-dimensional radiography versus CBCT on surgical aspects of transmigrated impacted mandibular canines. J Maxillofac Oral Surg 2020;19:461–7.
8. Bell C, Sahl E, Kim Y, et al. Accuracy of implants placed with surgical guides: thermoplastic versus 3D printed. Int J Periodontics Restorative Dent 2018;38: 113–9.
9. Johnson D. CT of maxillofacial trauma. Radiol Clin North Am 1984;22:131–43.
10. Daffner R, Gehweiler J, Osborne D, et al. Computed tomography in the evaluation of severe facial trauma. Comput Radiol 1983;7(2):91–102.
11. Diangelis A, Andreasen J, Ebeleseder K. Guidelines for the management of traumatic dental injuries: 1. fractures and luxations of permanent teeth. Pediatr Dent 2017;39(6):401–11.
12. Andersson L, Andreasen J, Day P, et al. Guidelines for the management of traumatic dental injuries: 2. avulsion of permanent teeth. Pediatr Dent 2017;39(6): 412–9.
13. Malmgren B, Andreasen J, Flores M, et al. Guidelines for the management of traumatic dental injuries: 3. Injuries in the primary dentition. Pediatr Dent 2017;39(6): 420–8.

14. Chayra G, Meador L, Laskin D. Comparison of panoramic and standard radiographs for the diagnosis of mandibular fractures. J Oral Maxillofac Surg 1986; 44(9):677–9.
15. Louis M, Agrawal N, Truong T. Midface Fractures II. Semin Plast Surg 2017; 31(2):94–9.
16. Cuddy K, Khatib B, Bell R, et al. Use of intraoperative computed tomography in craniomaxillofacial trauma surgery. J Oral Maxillofac Surg 2018;76(5):1016–25.
17. Ellis E, Perez D. An algorithm for the treatment of isolated zygomatico-orbital fractures. J Oral Maxillofac Surg 2014;72(10):1975–83.
18. Borad V, Lacey M, Hamlar D, et al. Intraoperative imaging changes management in orbital fracture repair. J Oral Maxillofac Surg 2017;75(9):1932–40.
19. Higgins A, Hurrell M, Harris R, et al. A study protocol for a randomised controlled trial evaluating the effects of intraoperative computed tomography on the outcomes of zygomatic fractures. Trials 2019;201(1):514.
20. Herford A, Miller M, Lauritano F, et al. The use of virtual surgical planning and navigation in the treatment of orbital trauma. Chin J Traumatol 2017;20(1):9–13.
21. Tarsitano A, Badiali G, Pizzigallo A, et al. Orbital reconstruction: patient-specific orbital floor reconstruction using a mirroring technique and a customized titanium mesh. J Craniofac Surg 2016;27(7):1822–5.
22. Maloney K, Rutner T. Virtual Surgical Planning and Hardware Fabrication Prior to Open Reduction and Internal Fixation of Atrophic Edentulous Mandible Fractures. Craniomaxillofac Trauma Reconstr 2019;12(2):156–62.
23. Macanovic M, Gangidi S, Porter G, et al. Incidental bony pathology when reporting trauma orthopantomograms. Clin Radiol 2010;10:842–9.
24. Rushton V, Horner K. The use of panoramic radiology in dental practice. J Dent 1996;24(3):185–201.
25. Shenaq D, Matros E. Virtual planning and navigational technology in reconstructive surgery. J Surg Oncol 2018;118(5):845–52.
26. Hua J, Aziz S, Shum J. Virtual surgical planning in oral and maxillofacial surgery. Oral Maxillofac Surg Clin North Am 2019;31(4):519–30.
27. Steinbacher D. Three-dimensional analysis and surgical planning in craniomaxillofacial surgery. J Oral Maxillofac Surg 2015;73(12):S40–56.
28. Mukherji S, Castelijns J, Castillo M. Squamous cell carcinoma of the oropharynx and oral cavity: how imaging makes a difference. Semin Ultrasound CT MR 1998; 19(6):463–75.
29. Rohde M, Nielsen A, Johansen J, et al. Head-to-head comparison of chest X-Ray/Head and Neck MRI, Chest CT/Head and Neck MRI, and 18F-FDG PET/CT for detection of distant metastases and synchronous cancer in oral, pharyngeal, and laryngeal cancer. J Nucl Med 2017;58(12):1919–24.
30. Senft A, de Bree R, Hoekstra O, et al. Screening for distant metastases in head and neck cancer patients by chest CT or whole body FDG-PET: a prospective multicenter trial. Radiother Oncol 2008;87(2):221–9.
31. Lydiatt W, Patel S, O'Sullivan B, et al. Head and Neck cancers-major changes in the American Joint Committee on cancer eighth edition cancer staging manual. CA Cancer J Clin 2017;67(2):122–37.
32. Sommer O, Aigner F, Rudisch A, et al. Cross-sectional and functional imaging of the temporomandibular joint: radiology, pathology, and basic biomechanics of the jaw. Radiographics 2003;23(6):e14.
33. Kaimal S, Ahmad M, Kang W, et al. Diagnostic accuracy of panoramic radiography and MRI for detecting signs of TMJ degenerative joint disease. Gen Dent 2018;66(4):34–40.

34. Talmaceanu D, Lenghel L, Bolog N, et al. Imaging modalities for temporomandibular joint disorders: an update. Clujul Med 2018;91(3):280–7.
35. Roth C, Ward R, Rsai S, et al. MR imaging of the TNJ: a pictorial essay. Appl Radiol 2005;34:9–16.
36. Larheim T, Abrahamsson A, Kristensen M, et al. Temporomandibular joint diagnostics using CBCT. Dentomaxillofac Radiol 2015;44(1):20140235.
37. Santillan A, Hee Sur M, Schwarz J, et al. Endovascular preoperative embolization for temporomandibular joint replacement surgery. Interv Neuroradiol 2020;26(1):99–104.
38. Caloss R, Atkins K, Stella JP. Three-dimensional imaging for virtual assessment and treatment simulation in orthognathic surgery. Oral Maxillfac Surg Clin North Am 2007;19(3):287–309.
39. Naran S, Steinbacher D, Taylor J. Current concepts in orthognathic surgery. Plast Reconstr Surg 2018;141(6):925–36.
40. De Riu G, Virdis P, Meloni S, et al. Accuracy of computer-assisted orthognathic surgery. J Craniomaxillofac Surg 2018;46(2):293–8.
41. Mazzoni S, Bianchi A, Schiariti G, et al. Computer-aided design and computer-aided manufacturing cutting guides and customized titanium plates are useful in upper maxilla waferless repositioning. J Oral Maxillofac Surg 2015;73(4):701–7.
42. Wong A, Goonewardene M, Allan B, et al. Accuracy of maxillary repositioning surgery using CAD/CAM customized surgical guides and fixation plates. Int J Oral Maxillofac Surg 2020;5027(20):30325–3028.
43. Brunso J, Franco M, Constantinescu T, et al. Custom-machined miniplates and bone-supported guides for orthognathic surgery: a new surgical procedure. J Oral Maxillofac Surg 2016;74(5):1–12.
44. Schneider D, Kämmerer P, Hennig M, et al. Customized virtual surgical planning in bimaxillary orthognathic surgery: a prospective randomized trial. Clin Oral Investig 2019;23(7):3115–22.

Radiographic Interpretation in Oral Medicine and Hospital Dental Practice

Katherine France, DMD, MBE[a],*,
Anwar A.A.Y. AlMuzaini, DDS, MS, BDM, MSOB[b,1],
Mel Mupparapu, DMD, MDS, DABOMR[a]

KEYWORDS

- Hospital dentistry • Oral medicine • Temporomandibular disorders • Facial pain
- Salivary gland disease • Cone beam computed tomography (CBCT)
- Magnetic resonance imaging (MRI) • Positron emission computed tomography (PET)

KEY POINTS

- A wide variety of basic and advanced imaging modalities in dentistry and medicine are employed in oral medicine practice regardless of setting.
- Several oral medicine conditions, in particular facial pain, require imaging for appropriate diagnosis and treatment, and may require a variety of imaging modalities in their assessment.
- Salivary gland disease also presents a diagnostic conundrum, and imaging in diagnosis and treatment may be prescribed according to findings and suspected etiologies.
- Before hospital procedures and during hospital admissions, plain radiography and occasionally advanced imaging are essential to reach diagnosis and treat patients.
- Many patients undergoing surgical procedures are referred for dental evaluation and determination of teeth that require intervention, commonly assessed using plain radiography.

INDICATIONS AND GENERAL GUIDELINES

Oral medicine is the eleventh dental specialty recognized by the American Dental Association (ADA).[1] The scope of oral medicine practice is wide and includes management of patients with a variety of orofacial concerns and local manifestations of systemic conditions.

[a] University of Pennsylvania School of Dental Medicine, 240 South 40th Street, Philadelphia, PA 19104, USA; [b] Ministry of Health, Kuwait City, Kuwait
[1] Present address: Saud Bin Abdulaziz Street, PO Box 2156, Kuwait City, Kuwait.
* Corresponding author.
E-mail address: kfrance@upenn.edu

Dent Clin N Am 65 (2021) 509–528
https://doi.org/10.1016/j.cden.2021.02.010
0011-8532/21/© 2021 Elsevier Inc. All rights reserved.

dental.theclinics.com

Most of the plain images obtained in a dental practice are digital, captured via either solid state (charge-coupled device/complementary metal–oxide–semiconductor) or storage phosphor–based (photostimulable phosphor sensors) using intraoral x-ray machines. Digital panoramic radiographs commonly are obtained as a first-line radiographic examination if patients are unable to open their mouth or otherwise cannot tolerate intraoral imaging. The resolution of panoramic radiographs is 4 line pairs per millimeter (lppm) to 5 lppm,[2] far less than intraoral digital radiographs (7–24 lppm).[3]

Digital skull views (extraoral) also can be obtained in any practice setting provided there is a dedicated cephalostat unit attached to the x-ray machine. The extraoral unit can be either a panoramic x-ray machine or a cone beam computed tomography (CBCT) machine with a cephalostat arm extension. Lateral oblique views are obtained at the hospital to view the body of the mandible and the condyles bilaterally if a panoramic radiograph machine is not available, although, in general, they are considered obsolete.

CBCT machines are an integral part of dental practice. In oral medicine practice, CBCT is used for evaluation of craniofacial anomalies; pathology extending beyond the teeth; soft tissue calcifications of head and neck; and anatomic structures, including the TMJs, external auditory meati, foramina and fossae, inferior alveolar nerve canals, incisive foramen and nasopalatine canals, paranasal sinuses, nasal fossa, and ostiomeatal complex, to name a few. CBCT can be obtained for a focused area (small field of view [FOV]), single jaw (medium FOV) or the entire skull (large FOV) based on the area being investigated. Interpretation can be performed either in house or by sending to an oral and maxillofacial radiologist for formal interpretation and reporting. CBCTs obtained at the dental office can be coded using the ADA code on dental procedures and nomenclature.[4] There are 3 medical codes (Current Procedural Terminology) available for CBCT-related image capture, interpretation, and 3-dimensional (3-D) rendering.[5]

IMAGING FOR FACIAL PAIN

After a thorough history and physical examination, the oral medicine specialist examining a patient with facial pain may use several imaging techniques to identify the source. These include digital radiographs of the teeth and jaws, cervical spine series, selected FOV CBCT, magnetic resonance imaging (MRI) with and without contrast, and magnetic resonance angiography. A brain MRI can be acquired to identify any definitive vascular, neural, or bony pathology that would give rise to the facial pain. Magnetic resonance neurography is emerging as a useful diagnostic test for detection of abnormalities of craniospinal nerves below the skull base.[6]

Imaging for Trigeminal Neuralgia and Atypical Facial Pain

Trigeminal neuralgia, also known as tic douloureux, is a chronic pain condition affecting the trigeminal nerve (fifth cranial nerve).[7] MRI is the diagnostic test of choice to rule out a tumor, multiple sclerosis, or an impinging blood vessel. In some cases, imaging is not possible for reasons including presence of cardiac pacemakers or metal implants, and, in such cases, recording of trigeminal reflexes to assess trigeminal nerve function is an established alternative assessment method.[8]

Atypical facial pain, also known as persistent idiopathic facial pain and atypical odontalgia, is a nonspecific pain where no organic cause can be identified.[9] The pain does not follow the anatomic pathways of cranial or peripheral nerves.[10] Patients must be investigated thoroughly before a diagnosis of atypical facial pain is reached. Investigations may include intraoral periapical radiographs, panoramic radiography, CBCT, CT head with and without contrast, and brain MRI. The choice of imaging is selected by the oral medicine practitioner, depending on the clinical findings and characterization of facial pain.[11]

Imaging for Temporomandibular Joint Disorders

Temporomandibular disorders (TMDs) may affect the joint, joint-associated structures, or muscles of mastication and can manifest as impaired jaw function, pain, or joint sounds.[12] The oral medicine specialist has primary responsibility for several TMDs and should be familiar with the radiographic appearance of the temporomandibular joint (TMJ) and TMJ-related disorders. A thorough clinical examination of the TMJ and orofacial region is essential prior to determining the need for diagnostic TMJ imaging. A necessary first step in evaluating possible TMDs is to rule out any odontogenic or orofacial source that could be causing a patient's complaint. Indications for TMJ imaging vary with each patient. The following imaging modalities frequently are used in assessing the TMJ: panoramic radiography, MRI, computed tomography (CT), CBCT, ultrasound (US), and scintigraphy.

Panoramic imaging

Panoramic radiography is a readily available modality used to evaluate the joints bilaterally and assess the jaws and orofacial structures for any abnormalities that would necessitate further diagnostic imaging (**Fig. 1**). Indications for panoramic imaging of the TMJ can include assessment of suspected joint tumors, condylar hypoplasia/hyperplasia, or degenerative bone disease.[13] The oral medicine specialist should be cautious in interpreting condylar morphology using only a panoramic image because the beam orientation allows examination of only the central and lateral parts of the condyle.[14,15] The superimposition of structures of the skull and zygomatic arch also limits the diagnostic value in assessing the glenoid fossa and articular eminence. This is supported by the American Academy of Oral and Maxillofacial Radiology position statement on imaging of the TMJ, which states that panoramic imaging is an ideal modality for TMD patients only in assessing the teeth and jaw structures to rule out any gross osseous or odontogenic sources of the patient's complaint.[14]

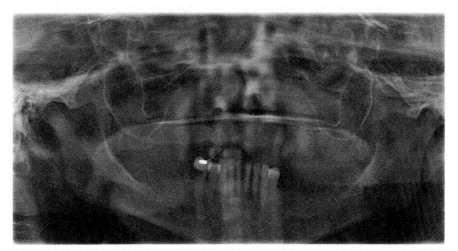

Fig. 1. Panoramic radiograph in which the patient position is not centered, resulting in differing appearances of the left and right mandibular condyles. In addition, this radiograph shows multiple areas of gross dental decay, which may account for or complicate a presentation of facial pain.

Magnetic resonance imaging

MRI is the recommended imaging modality to assess the TMJ, including the articular disk, due to its ability to visualize both bone and soft tissues.[16] On a T1-weighted image, the bone marrow and posterior attachment have a high signal due to fat content whereas the disk and bone display a low signal. A T2-weighted image again reveals a low signal of the disk and bone with an occasional high signal seen in the intermediate zone of the disk.[17] Fluid-attenuated inversion recovery (FLAIR) sequence from T2-weighted images has been investigated for join effusions and found to have a strong correlation with decreased signal intensity, suggesting variable protein content in effusions.[18] FLAIR signal intensity was found to be higher in painful joints compared with joints without pain, which may be due to increased protein.[19] It also has been suggested that FLAIR is useful in detecting bone marrow changes of the condyle, such as edema, in painful joints of patients with TMD.[20] Joint effusion is represented radiographically by a high signal area in a T2-weighted MRI image and there is evidence of an increased frequency of joint effusion in disks that are displaced.[21] An MRI study found patients with disk displacements (both with and without reduction) frequently presented with joint pain and joint effusion, although the causal relationship is not clear.[22]

Ultrasound

There are cases where imaging the TMJ with MRI is not possible, including when cost is prohibitive, claustrophobic patients, or in patients with cardiac pacemakers. Ultrasound (US) represents an acceptable, cost-effective, and noninvasive alternative method for assessing the TMJ in such cases. Joint effusions and disk displacements in the closed mouth and opened mouth positions can be detected by US of the TMJ.[23] Sonography is less sensitive and less specific than an MRI or helical CT in the detection of TMJ internal derangements but may still provide useful information.[24]

Multidetector computed tomography/cone beam computed tomography

CBCT is superior to panoramic radiography in evaluating the TMJ because it allows assessment of bone structures in 3 planes and reconstructs the image utilizing the long axis of the mandibular condyle; this allows visualization of the condylar position relative to the fossa.[25] CBCT also is superior to CT for imaging the TMJs due to its significantly lower radiation exposure to the patient and higher spatial resolution of the image.[16] CBCTs perform equally to multidetector CT (MDCT) in detecting osseous and morphologic changes of the TMJ[13,15,16,26] and are superior to MRI and panoramic radiographs in diagnosing arthritic changes of the TMJ.[27] The same findings and indications for a CT apply to CBCT. The following conditions can be evaluated with MDCT/CBCT.

Osteoarthritis

Osteoarthritis is the most common degenerative joint disease (DJD) that affects the TMJs. Although disk position and shape cannot be assessed by a CT or CBCT, a more posteriorly positioned mandibular condylar head in the glenoid fossa can be a sign of disk displacement and internal derangement. An MRI confirms the diagnosis of internal derangement as the disk is best visualized there.[28]

MDCT or CBCT findings that indicate TMJ osteoarthritis include osteophytes, surface erosions, generalized sclerosis, and subcortical/subchondral cysts. The oral medicine specialist should be cautious in evaluating DJD. Narrowing of the TM joint space is not considered a reliable indicator of DJD because it also can occur in otherwise healthy joints or in joints exhibiting disk displacements only. Likewise, flattening of the condylar head, glenoid fossa, or articular eminence is indicative of DJD only when associated with osteophyte formation because it otherwise could indicate remodeling of the condylar head that occurs with aging or a displaced disk.[29] In addition, osteophytes have been noted as an anatomic variation, and cortical surface irregularities have been found in asymptomatic individuals. Barring significant changes and evidence of bone destruction, it is prudent to consider subtle findings as normal anatomic variations, especially in asymptomatic patients.[30] A promising future direction for CBCTs in assessing osteoarthritis includes utilizing 3-D virtual surface models in assessing condylar morphology, because condylar resorption in TMJ osteoarthritis has been correlated with pain.[31]

Inflammatory Arthritis

Inflammatory arthritis represents a group of conditions causing inflammation of the joints' synovial membrane.[28] Discussion of all inflammatory arthritides is beyond the scope of this article, and only the most common condition likely encountered in the oral medicine clinic, rheumatoid arthritis (RA), is discussed.

RA is the most common inflammatory arthritis. Early osseous changes may be detected on CBCT. The classic CT radiographic finding of RA is cortical erosion without bone proliferation, which can be coupled with osteoarthritic changes, such as flattening of the articular surfaces, subchondral sclerosis, and osteophyte formation. These radiographic findings, however, are nonspecific and may be present in other inflammatory arthritides as well.[27] Correlation with clinical signs and symptoms and serology may be required to assess the patient accurately. Findings of a normal disk position on an MRI with evidence of bone destruction should lead the clinician to suspect trauma or the presence of a rheumatic disease because the articular disk frequently is found in a normal position in inflammatory arthritic cases.[30] In a systematic review conducted by Mupparapu and coworkers,[31] 2-dimensional radiographs, CBCT, MDCT, and MRI were found to be the most common methods employed in the detection of RA. PET-CT was found to be useful for quantifying TMJ involvement in active RA.[31]

IMAGING FOR BONE LESIONS

Imaging for Osteomyelitis

Osteomyelitis is defined as inflammation of the bone marrow spaces and the vessels that leads to either bone loss or necrosis. This process may be acute, subacute, or chronic. Outcomes depend on the severity of the inflammation and blood supply to the area affected. When a necrotic part of the bone becomes isolated, they are termed a *sequestrum*. Sequestra typically are more radiopaque (radiodense) than surrounding bone on plain films due to accelerated deposition of calcium and phosphates. Demonstration of a sequestrum on a radiograph is the hallmark of osteomyelitis. In addition, infected bone gives the classic radiographic moth-eaten appearance (**Figs. 2** and **3**). Intraoral radiographs may not demonstrate these features. A panoramic radiograph may demonstrate some features but due to the 2-dimensional nature of the modality, does not show all the affected areas. MDCT is the best modality to show the osteomyelitic area. MDCT is ideal for this purpose due to its better inherent contrast (higher kilovoltage peak and radiation dose). A CBCT also may be acceptable if an MDCT is not available. Several studies show the utilization of additional advanced imaging modalities for early detection of osteomyelitis. This includes single-photon CT (SPECT) and PET-CT, both of which may be able to visualize early changes before they become apparent on a radiograph, due to the higher sensitivity and specificity of these techniques. This is attributed to the higher sensitivity and specificity of these techniques. SPECT is best utilized in initial diagnosis, and fluorodeoxyglucose F 18 ^{18}F-FDG-PET can be used adjunctively and during follow-up in cases of chronic osteomyelitis.[32]

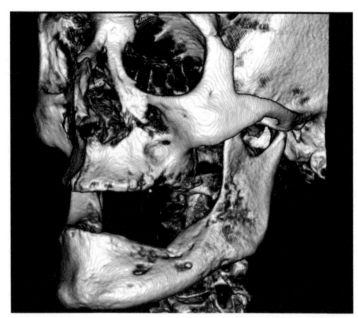

Fig. 2. CBCT 3-D reconstruction of a patient who reported left mandibular pain and swelling. The appearance of left mandibular body demonstrates morphologic bony changes consistent with chronic infection in the area.

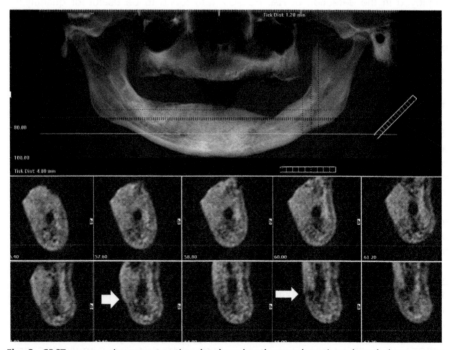

Fig. 3. CBCT panoramic reconstruction (top) and orthogonal sections (rows) demonstrate chronic osteomyelitis of left mandibular body and angle (*arrows*).

Imaging for Osteoradionecrosis of the Jaw and Medication-Related Osteonecrosis of the Jaw

Osteonecrosis of the jaw is bone death due to lack of blood circulation. When infected, the area becomes clinically detectable through mucosal ulceration and bone exposure. Medication-related osteonecrosis of the jaw (MRONJ) is the term for when this condition occurs secondary to use of a medication that interferes with normal physiologic bone turnover (bone resorption and/or bone deposition). The best radiographic modality for visualizing these changes is a high-resolution CBCT (less than 100-μm pixel resolution).[33] Radiographic and histologic appearance of bone necrosis is identical regardless of etiology. Unexplained bone loss and or separation (sequestrum) may be suspected on intraoral or panoramic radiographs and can be confirmed via MDCT or CBCT (**Fig. 4**). MRI is advantageous for evaluation of the nerves.

Oral Cancer

Imaging is an integral part of the investigation for oral cancer, whether a primary malignancy or a metastatic lesion. Occasionally, malignant changes can be recognized in intraoral radiographs, but they generally are more evident when evaluated on extraoral imaging and coupled with clinical presentation. For example, oral squamous cell carcinoma can extend into alveolar bone. Although CBCT shows bone invasion and destruction, due to limitations in contrast, MDCT is preferred. An MRI is indicated when the suspected lesion is of soft tissue origin or if occult or inaccessible for oral examination.[34] More advanced imaging like technetium Tc 99m, SPECT, or PET-CT is preferred when the cancer is suspected to be widespread. These tests generally are done in conjunction with an oncologist. Biopsy and staging are mandatory in all suspected and confirmed cases of cancer.[35]

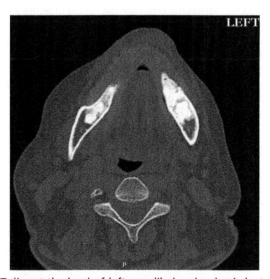

Fig. 4. Axial MDCT slice at the level of left mandibular alveolus (edentulous) in a patient with florid cemento-osseous dysplasia, showing areas suggestive of osteonecrosis and exposure of a small portion of the mucosa. Mucosal dehiscence and bone exposure suggests stage 1 MRONJ. Typically, such a patient has prior history of intake of either bisphosphonates or some form of antiangiogenic medication.

IMAGING FOR SALIVARY GLAND DISEASE

Several pathologies can affect the salivary glands, including inflammatory and infectious diseases, obstructions, neoplasms, and autoimmune disorders. Signs of salivary gland disease include diffuse enlargement or limited enlargement with or without pain. These clinical findings often are nonspecific and require further diagnostic evaluations for a more definitive diagnosis. Several imaging modalities are available for salivary gland diagnosis and management.[36,37]

Plain Radiography

Given the availability of advanced imaging modalities, there is little clinical value in plain radiography of the salivary glands.[38]

Ultrasound

US is a noninvasive, safe, and readily available modality that is useful in initially assessing the salivary glands.[39] US performance is comparable to CT and MRI in detecting superficial salivary gland tumors that are hypoechoic compared with normal salivary glandular tissue.[37] US is the modality of choice in evaluating superficial parotid masses that are palpable.[40] It also has proved successful in confirming clinically suspicious masses and differentiating benign from malignant neoplasms. High-grade malignant neoplasms may appear as nonhomogenous hypoechoic regions with irregular ill-defined borders.[41] In addition, lesions can be biopsied with an US-guided core needle.[42,43] US drawbacks include overlap of adjacent structures, which impairs its ability to detect deeper lesions.[44]

US can successfully detect sialoliths of the salivary glands, where they appear as echogenic foci.[45] The high sensitivity of US in diagnosing sialoliths makes it an acceptable alternative to sialography[46] and the imaging modality of choice in assessing sialoliths due to the lack of radiation exposure and availability.[47]

Sialoliths and microbial organisms often are the cause of acute inflammatory conditions of the salivary glands. US can detect edema and inflammation of the gland and rule out sialoliths or abscesses within the glandular parenchyma that may be causing the acute sialadenitis.[48]

In addition, US is a commonly used modality to assess the extent of salivary gland involvement in Sjögren syndrome.[49] Involvement of the glands is evident via atrophy, fibrosis, and sialectasis.[37] Sialectasis appears as hypoechoic and anechoic regions.[50] A meta-analysis concluded that US of Sjögren syndrome patients may be an acceptable alternative to other imaging modalities in evaluating the salivary glands.[51]

Sialography

Sialography (**Fig. 5**) involves injection of a contrast medium into the glands, allowing visualization of ductal anatomy and parenchyma. Indications include suspected strictures and sialoliths.[52]

Plain film sialography is contraindicated in acute inflammation or infections of the salivary glands, because the contrast medium may cause further spread of the inflammatory mediators. An acceptable alternative is magnetic resonance sialography.[53] Compared with conventional sialography, magnetic resonance sialography utilizes no radiation, is noninvasive, and does not require contrast medium.[54] The following are indications for a magnetic resonance sialography examination: xerostomia, sialolithiasis, ductal stenosis, sialadenitis, and Sjögren syndrome.

Magnetic resonance sialography has been reported to have 100% sensitivity and 93% specificity in detecting ductal stenosis.[45] It is contraindicated in salivary gland

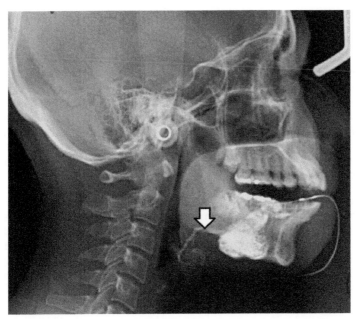

Fig. 5. Lateral skull radiograph showing the filling phase of submandibular sialography. Radiographic water-soluble contrast medium is used for imaging the gland and identifying any changes to normal anatomy (arrow).

hypofunction, because saliva serves as the contrast media. Its low spatial resolution makes it inferior to conventional sialography in that regard.[55] Because it does not utilize contrast media, however, it can be used in acute inflammation or infection of the salivary gland where conventional sialography is contraindicated.[56]

CBCT sialography shows promise for assessing recurrent salivary gland swelling and intraglandular pathologies.[57] When compared with plain film sialography, CBCT sialography detects strictures and sialoliths and can better visualize the salivary gland parenchyma and ductal anatomy.[52]

Cone Beam Computed Tomography

CBCT has been shown to accurately detect sialoliths with results comparable to CT and magnetic resonance sialography and superior to plain radiography and US.[58] This makes CBCT an acceptable first choice of imaging modality in diagnosing sialoliths.

Magnetic Resonance Imaging

MRI utilizes no radiation and allows greater visualization of soft tissues compared with CT scans. Similar to CT scans, it is possible to evaluate the boundaries and extension of a lesion on MRI and determine its location.[56] A standard neck protocol is used. The following conditions are indications for an MRI examination of the salivary glands.

Tumors of the salivary glands

MRI is the imaging modality of choice in assessing tumors of the salivary gland.[46] A majority of salivary gland tumors occur in the parotid gland followed by minor salivary glands, submandibular glands, and sublingual glands.[59] The most common benign parotid gland tumor is the pleomorphic adenoma, which has a high signal on a T2-weighted image, with signal intensity, depending on whether the area is myxoid or cellular. It is not possible, however, to differentiate radiographically between pleomorphic adenoma and basal cell adenoma or myoepithelioma (all variants of pleomorphic adenoma). The higher apparent diffusion coefficient of pleomorphic adenoma makes diffusion-weighted MRI a promising diagnostic modality in assessing this tumor.[60] With MRI, it is possible to evaluate tumors' margins, extent of perineural spread (in malignant tumors), and extension in deep parotid lobes. A T2-weighted image of a malignant tumor reveals hypointense areas and nonhomogenous signals, irregular margins, and invasion into surrounding tissues.[40] The facial nerve also is visualized best on MRI and this is essential to identify prior to parotid gland surgeries.[56]

Sjögren syndrome

MRI has been reported to be useful in detecting Sjögren syndrome. Findings include low homogeneity of the parotid gland on a T1-weighted image and a salt-and-pepper appearance of the glands, caused by lymphocytic infiltration, on T1-weighted and T2-weighted images.[49] Furthermore, patients with Sjögren syndrome are at a higher risk of developing parotid gland lymphomas and thus MRI examination is warranted when these patients present with any mass of the parotid gland.[37]

Computed Tomography

CT has excellent spatial resolution and high sensitivity and thus is the imaging modality of choice in assessing inflammation and calcification of the salivary glands. Drawbacks include beam hardening artifacts caused by dental restorations.[61]

Salivary Gland Scintigraphy

Salivary gland function can be evaluated with nuclear medicine. This is not used routinely, however, in clinical practice. Nuclear scintigraphy involves intravenous injection of technetium Tc 99m sodium pertechnetate, administration of sialagogues to increase salivary secretion, and capturing images to assess salivary gland uptake.[62] It generally is a safe and noninvasive procedure; however, there are no guidelines or consensuses on protocols or interpretation, which in turn leads to great interobserver variability and minimal clinical benefit. Indications include evaluating salivary gland function in Sjögren syndrome patients or following radiotherapy to the head and neck.[46]

Fluorodeoxyglucose F 18 PET

There is limited diagnostic value in ^{18}F-FDG–PET, which is used mainly to stage malignant salivary glands tumors, evaluate nodal metastasis, and assess response to therapy. It is used in combination with a contrast-enhanced CT in order to localize a tumor. ^{18}F-FDG's uptake is increased in cells with high metabolic activity, such as tumor cells; however, there also is increased uptake by salivary glands with benign conditions, such as sialolithiasis, infections, and benign tumors, including Warthin tumors. In addition, some salivary gland malignancies, such as adenoid cystic carcinomas, exhibit low uptake. Due to these discrepancies, in the event an asymmetric ^{18}F-FDG uptake of the salivary glands is noted, an MRI and/or fine-needle aspiration cytology is necessary to confirm diagnosis.[63]

IMAGING FOR THE ADMITTED PATIENT

Patients Seen in the Hospital Setting for Oral Medicine Complaints

Patients present to the hospital for a wide range of complaints, some of which lie within the scope of practice of the oral medicine specialist. These include but are not limited to facial pain, oral lesions, salivary gland disease, and functional limitations of the orofacial complex. Generally, presentation to the hospital occurs due to new-onset or acute exacerbation of these conditions and must be evaluated in that context. Although some of these conditions, such as a variety of oral lesions, can be evaluated clinically by an oral medicine specialist, there are others, including facial pain and salivary gland disease, that may require imaging to reach a final diagnosis.

Specific considerations for imaging of facial pain patients in a hospital setting are discussed below. Additional imaging considerations for facial pain and salivary gland disease are discussed previously. Facial pain includes a wide variety of presentations, causes, and manifestations; a thorough review is beyond the scope of this article. Certain severe and/or intractable pain, however, may particularly precipitate hospital evaluation, including for acute intractable migraine.[64] Other facial pains, due to severity, lack of definitive etiology, or corresponding secondary issues, also may require hospitalization for evaluation.

Plain radiography

For patients admitted for evaluation of facial pain, a variety of imaging methods may be available. Both panoramic radiography and periapical radiography may be accessible, particularly in hospitals with dental services, and both are relatively fast, are easy to interpret, and result in low radiation exposure to patients. Panoramic images are useful particularly in evaluation of TMDs and other facial pains in their immediate visualization of the mandibular condyles together with the teeth and jaw bones, although the condylar appearance varies with the position of the patient within the focal trough (see **Fig. 1**). Panoramic radiography allows for evaluation of any odontogenic cause of the pain and cursory evaluation of other facial structures, including the condyles. Panoramic images also can act as a diagnostic adjunct in patients with limited mouth opening, which may result, among other causes, from TMDs and odontogenic infections.[65]

In addition, patients admitted for unrelated issues may demonstrate exacerbation or onset of oral and facial pain and related problems, both odontogenic and nonodontogenic. Such pains also can be evaluated through plain radiography. Given the difficulties with hygiene, communication, and risk factors in this population, inpatients require speedy and appropriate care for new oral and facial complaints, including appropriate imaging for diagnosis. Assessment of dental pain has been found to be a common need among inpatients, both spurring admission and complicating a hospital stay.[66] With imaging appropriate for the complaint, a definitive diagnosis often can be reached, and the problem addressed.

Computed tomography

Many facial pain patients have an unclear cause of their condition and may require further evaluation. For these purposes, advanced imaging can be helpful in determining any underlying pathology. Medical CT scans provide a relatively accurate view of the hard and soft tissues in 3-D and can be used to evaluate mandibular condyle morphology, assess for osseous pathology, and screen for other underlying causes. Given the speed of acquisition of CT scans, they are useful particularly as preliminary diagnostic tools, including in cases of severe headache or suspicion of trauma.[64]

Magnetic resonance imaging

MRI also can be useful in the evaluation of TMD and facial pain. MRI can provide an intracranial view for evaluation of neuropathic pain and pain of unknown origin. Given its superior soft tissue resolution, MRI also can be used to image the soft tissues of the temporomandibular joint or other affected facial structures. In this way, indications mirror those in outpatient evaluation.[65]

Assessment of the Presurgical Patient and Other Clearance Settings

In addition to patients admitted for evaluation and management, many patients require dental evaluation either before or during an admission. These evaluations generally include both clinical and radiographic components and aim to identify any severe, acute, or active dental infection. Although these evaluations may identify other chronic dental concerns, they primarily are focused on finding and controlling infection that may complicate a patient's immediate course. In this way, rather than clearing the patient, a term often used, the dental or oral medicine specialist is assessing patient status, including risk posed by the proposed medical intervention. In obtaining an understanding of the patient's dental status, providers can advise both the patient and supervising medical team.[67] Pretreatment evaluation requires radiographic evaluation and has been recommended in several situations, as discussed below.

Cardiac surgery

Evaluation of patients before cardiac surgery has been accepted for decades as a standard of care.[68] Generally, patients receive dental evaluation before elective but not emergent procedures in order to control the postsurgical risk of endocarditis.[69] Particularly in patients at high risk of postoperative endocarditis, including those with a previous endocarditis history, patients receiving cardiac valve replacements, intravenous drug users, and others, this evaluation may allow timely management of severe and active dental disease.[70] Despite this recommendation, evidence as to the value of this examination for patient outcomes and endocarditis rates has not been proved definitively, and the benefits and drawbacks to this practice must be considered.[68,69]

Transplantation

Dental examination and control of acute dental disease also are recommended before transplantation, including but not limited to kidney, liver, and hematopoietic stem cell. Control of active or potential acute infection in a hospital setting before transplant allows a decreased patient risk during healing from the procedure and provides a controlled environment for any needed treatment (**Fig. 6**).[71] Dental examination before transplant is a widely accepted practice, with an estimate of 80% of facilities requiring this step before kidney transplant.[72] This dental evaluation also is recommended widely before pediatric transplantations and represents one of the most common inpatient dental needs for children.[73]

Chemotherapy

Given the immunosuppression inherent to chemotherapy and, to a lesser extent, immunotherapy, evaluation and eradication of as much dental disease as possible is generally recommended before treatment commences.[74] Depending on the patient condition and details of the diagnostic process, full control of dental disease may not be practical, but an oral evaluation for acute infection nonetheless is recommended. All nonrestorable teeth, teeth with pericoronitis, and teeth with significant periodontal disease are recommended to be extracted before therapy commences and as early as possible before therapy to allow sufficient time for healing (**Fig. 7**).[75] This

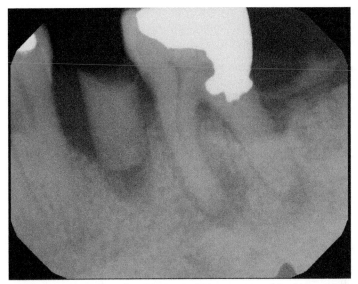

Fig. 6. Mandibular left molar periapical view captures tooth #19 with severe periodontal disease and an apical radiolucency and tooth #20 with minimal remaining bone support and a circumferential apical radiolucency. Both areas represent potential loci of infection in a surgical patient.

recommendation to remove loci of infection, in particular areas that could cause serious infection, has been promoted by the National Cancer Institute since 1990.[76] More recently, studies suggest that dental caries and periodontal inflammation may not have a direct connection to worse treatment outcomes, reinforcing the need to

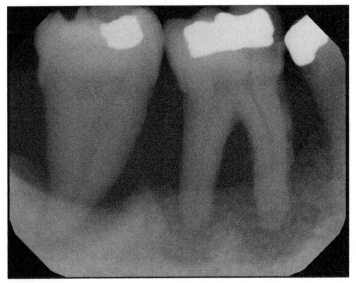

Fig. 7. Mandibular right molar periapical view showing severe periodontal disease involving teeth #31 and #32. Given the extent of disease, extraction would be recommended for these teeth before commencement of chemotherapy or surgical intervention.

focus on major oral risk factors in precancer care.[77] The recommendation applies to pediatric cancer patients as well, particularly resulting in inpatient dental evaluations for children without a dental home.[73]

Recommended radiographs

In evaluating patients before medical procedures and treatments, it is of primary importance to identify and control dental disease. This often can be achieved through panoramic radiographs, selected periapical films, or a combination (**Fig. 8**). Both panoramic radiography and periapical radiography often are available in a hospital setting for evaluation of inpatients and can be used to rule out or determine the extent of dental disease.[73] For patients seen before hospitalization, a full dental evaluation, including selective radiographs, is recommended. Radiographs can estimate risk of infection after procedures and allow the specialist to weigh the risks and benefits to intervening before a procedure.[71] In this way, radiographs are an essential part of a risk stratification for patients undergoing medical treatment.

Patients Requiring Hospital Dentistry

Hospital dentistry refers to the range of dental procedures performed for patients in a hospital setting. These can include both operating room dentistry, where procedures are performed during a session of general anesthesia in either a hospital or surgery center operating room, and procedures performed in a dental clinic that exists as part of a hospital. The latter generally consists of outpatient procedures provided primarily to populations who are admitted for other concerns or whose medical comorbidities prevent their treatment in community settings. In both cases, patients require a full evaluation, including a radiographic examination, in order to provide appropriate treatment.

Patients seen in a hospital as outpatients often receive radiographs according to national guidelines (such as the ADA/Food and Drug Administration guidelines in the United States). Although these patients need to receive care in controlled settings, radiographs often can be captured, including panoramic images, periapical, and bitewing images. That said, for some patients, including those with anatomic

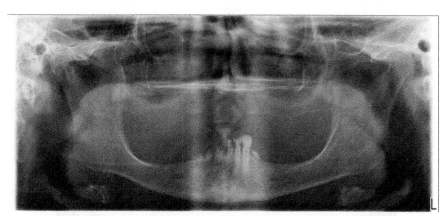

Fig. 8. Panoramic radiograph showing multiple root tips and areas of gross caries and illustrating teeth that would be recommended for extraction before surgical intervention. Given the quality of the image and the resolution of the remaining teeth, periapical views for further evaluation are unnecessary in this case.

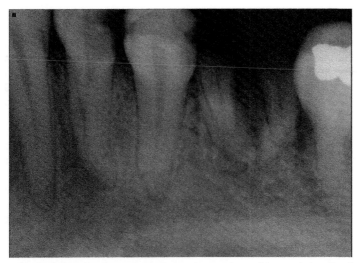

Fig. 9. Mandibular left premolar periapical view in a patient with poorly localized pain illustrates retained root tips of tooth #19 with apical radiolucency and deep caries on tooth #21 distal with an apical radiolucency, likely representing the source of the patient's facial pain.

limitations, such as limited mouth opening, active gag reflexes, and developmental difficulties, some adjustments to radiographs may be needed.

Dentistry may be limited to an operating room, however, for a certain set of patients. These include patients with physical and psychiatric disorders that preclude their treatment in an outpatient setting. For these patients, it often is challenging if not impossible to obtain radiographs prior to the surgical session.[78]

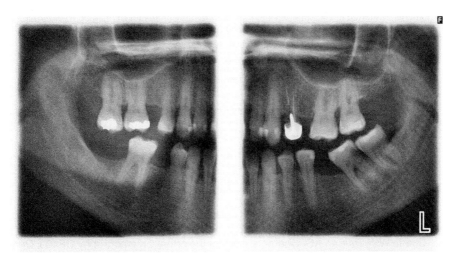

Fig. 10. Panoramic radiograph obtained in the extraoral bitewing mode showing the premolar regions bilaterally. This technique usually is supplemented with maxillary and mandibular central incisor periapical radiographs to make the radiographic examination complete (radiograph courtesy Steven R. Singer, DDS, Rutgers School of Dental Medicine, Newark, NJ).

For patients with anatomic and behavioral limitations seen in both inpatient and outpatient hospital settings, radiographs remain essential to accurate treatment. In patients admitted for ongoing medical issues, in whom the most common complaint is dental pain, followed by possible infections, mobile teeth, and lost fillings, limited and selected periapical radiographs with or without a panoramic radiograph may be sufficient to determine the causative factor and necessary treatment (**Fig. 9**).[66] This is equally true for children admitted for oral pain and possible oral infections, who may be able to tolerate local imaging.[73]

Patients who have special health care needs, however, may need adjustments to radiographic guidelines based on the treatment planned and the patient tolerance.[79] These can include limiting imaging to local views while in the operating room, limiting to panoramic imaging, and employing extraoral bitewing technique (**Fig. 10**) as tolerated.[80] Extraoral bitewing radiographs are more comfortable and can be captured as part of a panoramic radiograph, allowing detailed interproximal views, including third molars, with high accuracy.[81] This technique, as well as panoramic radiography, also provides the benefit of limiting aerosol production via gagging, which is applicable particularly for patients with infectious and contagious diseases.

CLINICS CARE POINTS

- CBCT has become an increasingly prevalent portion of oral medicine practice and often is used in place of several older modalities.
- Facial pain with a suspected neurologic source requires brain imaging before diagnosis and treatment.
- Treatment of TMDs often requires basic and advanced imaging for appropriate diagnosis and treatment.
- Imaging method of choice in salivary gland disease depends on the suspected etiology and the goals of treatment.
- Patients evaluated in a hospital setting may require basic or advanced imaging to determine causes of or contributors to their current complaints.
- Patients with planned surgical procedures often require dental evaluation and risk assessment in order to determine their status.
- For patients who cannot be seen in an outpatient setting, radiographs still play an essential role in treatment.

DISCLOSURE

The authors have nothing to disclose.

REFERENCES

1. Stoopler ET. Oral medicine achieves specialty recognition by the American dental association. J Orofac Sci 2020;12:1–2.
2. Scarfe WC, Farman AG. Characteristics of the orthopantomography OP100. Dentomaxillofac Radiol 1998;27:51–7.
3. Mupparapu M, Nadeau C. Oral and maxillofacial imaging. Dent Clin North Am 2016;60:1–37.
4. Code on dental procedures and nomenclature (CDT code). Available at : https://www.ada.org/en/publications/cdt. Accessed July 23, 2020.

5. American College of Radiology. CPT and ICD-10 coding resources. Available at: https://www.acr.org/Advocacy-and-Economics/Radiology-Economics/Coding-Resources. Accessed August 26, 2020.

6. Chhabra A, Bajaj G, Vadhwa V, et al. MR neurographic evaluation of facial and neck pain: normal and abnormal craniospinal nerves below the skull base. Radio-graphics 2018;38:1498–513.

7. Cruccu G, Finnerup NB, Jensen TS, et al. Trigeminal neuralgia. Neurology 2016; 87:220–8.

8. Gronseth G, Cruccu G, Alksne J, et al. Practice parameter: the diagnostic eval-uation and treatment of trigeminal neuralgia (an evidence-based review): report of the quality standards subcommittee of the American academy of neurology and the european federation of neurological societies. Neurology 2008;71(15): 1183–90.

9. Kawasaki K, Sugawara S, Watanabe K, et al. Differences in the clinical character-istics of persistent idiopathic facial pain (atypical odontalgia) patients with or without neurovascular compression of the trigeminal nerve. Pain Med 2020;21: 814–21.

10. Clarkson E, Jung E. Atypical facial pain. Dent Clin North Am 2020;64:249–53.

11. Shah R, Chauhan N. Somatoform pain disorder presenting as 'atypical facial pain": a rare presentation in a 13-year-old. Indian J Psychol Med 2017;39:500–2.

12. Okeson JP, de Leeuw R. Differential diagnosis of temporomandibular disorders and other orofacial pain disorders. Dent Clin North Am 2011;55:105–20.

13. Talmaceanu D, Lenghel LM, Bolog N, et al. Imaging modalities for temporoman-dibular joint disorders: An update. Clujul Med 2018;91:280–7.

14. Brooks SL, Brand JW, Gibbs SJ, et al. Imaging of the temporomandibular joint: a position paper of the American academy of oral and maxillofacial radiology. Oral Surg Oral Med Oral Pathol Oral Radiol Endod 1997;83:609–18.

15. Petersson A. What you can and cannot see in tmj imaging–an overview related to the rdc/tmd diagnostic system. J Oral Rehabil 2010;37:771–8.

16. Alkhader M, Ohbayashi N, Tetsumura A, et al. Diagnostic performance of mag-netic resonance imaging for detecting osseous abnormalities of the temporoman-dibular joint and its correlation with cone beam computed tomography. Dentomaxillofac Radiol 2010;39:270–6.

17. Bag AK, Gaddikeri S, Singhal A, et al. Imaging of the temporomandibular joint: an update. World J Radiol 2014;6:567–82.

18. Imoto K, Otonari-Yamamoto M, Nishikawa K, et al. Potential of fluid-attenuated inversion recovery (flair) in identification of temporomandibular joint effusion compared with t2-weighted images. Oral Surg Oral Med Oral Pathol Oral Radiol Endod 2011;112:243–8.

19. Kuroda M, Otonari-Yamamoto M, Sano T, et al. Diagnosis of retrodiscal tissue in painful temporomandibular joint (tmj) by fluid-attenuated inversion recovery (flair) signal intensity. Cranio 2015;33:271–5.

20. Kodama S, Otonari-Yamamoto M, Sano T, et al. Signal intensity on fluid-attenuated inversion recovery images of condylar marrow changes correspond with slight pain in patients with temporomandibular joint disorders. Oral Radiol 2014;30:212–8.

21. Khawaja SN, Crow H, Mahmoud RFG, et al. Is there an association between temporomandibular joint effusion and arthralgia? J Oral Maxillofac Surg 2017; 75:268–75.

22. Roh HS, Kim W, Kim YK, et al. Relationships between disk displacement, joint effusion, and degenerative changes of the tmj in tmd patients based on mri findings. J Craniomaxillofac Surg 2012;40:283–6.
23. Marotti J, Heger S, Tinschert J, et al. Recent advances of ultrasound imaging in dentistry–a review of the literature. Oral Surg Oral Med Oral Pathol Oral Radiol 2013;115:819–32.
24. Hayashi T, Ito J, Koyama J-I, et al. The accuracy of sonography for evaluation of internal derangement of the temporomandibular joint in asymptomatic elementary school children: comparison with MR and CT. AJNR Am J Neuroradiol 2001;22:728–34.
25. Librizzi ZT, Tadinada AS, Valiyaparambil JV, et al. Cone-beam computed tomography to detect erosions of the temporomandibular joint: Effect of field of view and voxel size on diagnostic efficacy and effective dose. Am J Orthod Dentofacial Orthop 2011;140:e25–30.
26. Zain-Alabdeen EH, Alsadhan RI. A comparative study of accuracy of detection of surface osseous changes in the temporomandibular joint using multidetector ct and cone beam ct. Dentomaxillofac Radiol 2012;41:185–91.
27. Larheim TA, Abrahamsson AK, Kristensen M, et al. Temporomandibular joint diagnostics using cbct. Dentomaxillofac Radiol 2015;44:20140235.
28. Barghan S, Tetradis S, Mallya S. Application of cone beam computed tomography for assessment of the temporomandibular joints. Aust Dent J 2012;57:109–18.
29. Ahmad M, Hollender L, Anderson Q, et al. Research diagnostic criteria for temporomandibular disorders (rdc/tmd): development of image analysis criteria and examiner reliability for image analysis. Oral Surg Oral Med Oral Pathol Oral Radiol Endod 2009;107:844–60.
30. Larheim TA, Hol C, Ottersen MK, et al. The role of imaging in the diagnosis of temporomandibular joint pathology. Oral Maxillofacial Surg Clin N Am 2018;30:239–49.
31. Mupparapu M, Oak S, Chang YC, et al. Conventional and functional imaging in the evaluation of temporomandibular joint rheumatoid arthritis: a systematic review. Quintessence Int 2019;50(9):742–53.
32. Hakim SG, Bruecker CWR, Jacobsen H Ch, et al. The value of FDG-PET and bone scintigraphy with SPECT in the primary diagnosis and follow-up of patients with chronic osteomyelitis of the mandible. Int J Oral Maxillofac Surg 2006;35:809–16.
33. Mupparapu M. Medication-related osteonecrosis of the jaw (MRONJ): bisphosphonates, antiresorptives, and antiangiogenic agents. What next? Quintessence Int 2016;47:7–8.
34. Heusschen R, Muller J, Duray E, et al. Molecular mechanisms, current management and next generation therapy in myeloma bone disease. Leuk Lymphoma 2018;59:14–28.
35. Mupparapu M, Shanti RM. Evaluation and staging of oral cancer. Dent Clin North Am 2018;62:47–58.
36. Atkinson C, Fuller J 3rd, Huang B. Cross-sectional imaging techniques and normal anatomy of the salivary glands. Neuroimaging Clin N Am 2018;28:137–58.
37. Burke CJ, Thomas RH, Howlett D. Imaging the major salivary glands. Br J Oral Maxillofac Surg 2011;49:261–9.
38. Ogle OE. Salivary gland diseases. Dent Clin North Am 2020;64:87–104.
39. Carotti M, Ciapetti A, Jousse-Joulin S, et al. Ultrasonography of the salivary glands: the role of grey-scale and colour/power doppler. Clin Exp Rheumatol 2014;32:S61–70.

40. Ettl T, Schwarz-Furlan S, Gosau M, et al. Salivary gland carcinomas. Oral Maxillofac Surg 2012;16:267–83.
41. Bhatia KSS, Dai YL. Routine and advanced ultrasound of major salivary glands. Neuroimaging Clin N Am 2018;28:273–93.
42. Novoa E, Gürtler N, Arnoux A, et al. Diagnostic value of core needle biopsy and fine-needle aspiration in salivary gland lesions. Head Neck 2016;38:E346–52.
43. Song IH, Song JS, Sung CO, et al. Accuracy of core needle biopsy versus fine needle aspiration cytology for diagnosing salivary gland tumors. J Pathol Transl Med 2015;49:136–43.
44. Prasad RS. Parotid gland imaging. Otolaryngol Clin North Am 2016;49:285–312.
45. Abdel Razek AAK, Mukherji S. Imaging of sialadenitis. Neuroradiol J 2017;30: 205–15.
46. Afzelius P, Nielsen MY, Ewertsen C, et al. Imaging of the major salivary glands. Clin Physiol Funct Imaging 2016;36:1–10.
47. Ardekian L, Klein HH, Araydy S, et al. The use of sialendoscopy for the treatment of multiple salivary gland stones. J Oral Maxillofac Surg 2014;72:89–95.
48. Orlandi MA, Pistorio V, Guerra PA. Ultrasound in sialadenitis. J Ultrasound 2013; 16:3–9.
49. Fujita A. Imaging of sjogren syndrome and immunoglobulin g4-related disease of the salivary glands. Neuroimaging Clin N Am 2018;28:183–97.
50. Mandel L. Salivary gland disorders. Med Clin North Am 2014;98:1407–49.
51. Delli K, Dijkstra PU, Stel AJ, et al. Diagnostic properties of ultrasound of major salivary glands in sjogren's syndrome: A meta-analysis. Oral Dis 2015;21:792–800.
52. Jadu FM, Lam EWN. A comparative study of the diagnostic capabilities of 2d plain radiograph and 3d cone beam ct sialography. Dentomaxillofac Radiol 2013;42:20110319.
53. Yousem DM, Kraut MA, Chalian AA. Major salivary gland imaging. Radiology 2000;216:19–29.
54. Gadodia A, Seith A, Sharma R, et al. Magnetic resonance sialography using ciss and haste sequences in inflammatory salivary gland diseases: Comparison with digital sialography. Acta Radiol 2010;51:156–63.
55. Rastogi R, Bhargava S, Mallarajapatna GJ, et al. Pictorial essay: salivary gland imaging. Indian J Radiol Imaging 2012;22:325–33.
56. Murdoch-Kinch CA. Salivary gland imaging. J Calif Dent Assoc 2011;39:649–54.
57. Kroll T, May A, Wittekindt C, et al. Cone beam computed tomography (cbct) sialography–an adjunct to salivary gland ultrasonography in the evaluation of recurrent salivary gland swelling. Oral Surg Oral Med Oral Pathol Oral Radiol 2015; 120:771–5.
58. Dreiseidler T, Ritter L, Rothamel D, et al. Salivary calculus diagnosis with 3-dimensional cone-beam computed tomography. Oral Surg Oral Med Oral Pathol Oral Radiol Endod 2010;110:94–100.
59. Wang X, Luo Y, Li M, et al. Management of salivary gland carcinomas - a review. Oncotarget 2017;8:3946–56.
60. Lingam RK, Daghir AA, Nigar E, et al. Pleomorphic adenoma (benign mixed tumour) of the salivary glands: Its diverse clinical, radiological, and histopathological presentation. Br J Oral Maxillofac Surg 2011;49:14–20.
61. Ugga L, Ravanelli M, Pallottino AA, et al. Diagnostic work-up in obstructive and inflammatory salivary gland disorders. Acta Otorhinolaryngol Ital 2017;37:83–93.
62. Wu CB, Xi H, Zhou Q, et al. The diagnostic value of technetium 99m pertechnetate salivary gland scintigraphy in patients with certain salivary gland diseases. J Oral Maxillofac Surg 2015;73:443–50.

63. Purohit BS, Ailianou A, Dulguerov N, et al. Fdg-pet/ct pitfalls in oncological head and neck imaging. Insights Imaging 2014;5:585–602.

64. Ali AS, Stillman M. What inpatient treatments do we have for acute intractable migraine? Cleve Clin J Med 2018;85:514–6.

65. Liang H. Imaging in orofacial pain. Dent Clin North Am 2018;62:553–651.

66. Hashem IW, Gillway D, Doshi M. Dental care pathways for adult inpatients in an acute hospital: a five-year service evaluation. Br Dent J 2020;228:687–92.

67. Patton LL. The fallacy of pre-kidney transplantation "dental clearance." Oral Surg Oral Med Oral Pathol Oral Radiol 2019;128:1–4.

68. Lockhart PB, DeLong HR, Lipman RD, et al. Effect of dental treatment before cardiac valve surgery: systematic review and meta-analysis. J Am Dent Assoc 2019; 150:739–47.

69. Gandhi N, Silvay G. How important is dental clearance for elective open heart operations? Ann Thorac Surg 2015;99:377.

70. Casale MJ, Lurie JM, Khromava M, et al. Dental clearance and postoperative heart infections: observations from a preoperative evaluation clinic for day-admission surgery. J Perioper Pract 2020;30:97–101.

71. Hicks JL. Oral care of the patient with liver failure, pretransplant – a retrospective study. Spec Care Dentist 2015;35:8–14.

72. Segelnick SL, Weinberg MA. The periodontist's role in obtaining clearance prior to patients undergoing a kidney transplant. J Periodontol 2009;80:874–7.

73. Kanuga S, Sheller B, Williams BJ, et al. A one-year survey of inpatient dental consultations at a children's hospital. Spec Care Dentist 2012;32:26–31.

74. Michelet M. Caries and periodontal disease in cancer survivors. Evid Based Dent 2012;13:70–3.

75. Elad S, Raber-Durlacher JE, Brennan MT, et al. Basic oral care for hematology-oncology patients and hematopoietic stem cell transplantation recipients: a position paper from the joint task force of the multinational association of supportive care in cancer/international society of oral oncology (MASCC/ISOO) and the European society for blood and marrow transplantation (EBMT). Support Care Cancer 2015;23:223–36.

76. Elad S, Thierer T, Bitan M, et al. A decision analysis: the dental management of patients prior to hematology cytotoxic therapy or hematopoietic stem cell transplantation. Oral Oncol 2008;44:37–42.

77. Schmalz G, Tulani L, Busjan R, et al. Dental and periodontal treatment need after dental clearance is not associated with the outcome of induction therapy in patients with acute leukemia: Results of a retrospective pilot study. Adv Hematol 2020;6710906. https://doi.org/10.1155/2020/6710906.

78. Schnabl D, Guarda A, Guarda M, et al. Dental treatment under general anesthesia in adults with special needs at the university hospital of dental prosthetics and restorative dentistry of Innsbruck, Austria: a retrospective study of 12 years. Clin Oral Investig 2019;23:4157–62.

79. American Academy of Pediatric Dentistry. Prescribing dental radiographs for infants, children, adolescents, and individuals with special health care needs. Pediatr Dent 2018;40:213–5.

80. Kumar R, Khambete N, Priya E. Extraoral periapical radiography: an alternative approach to intraoral periapical radiography. Imaging Sci Dent 2011;41:161–5.

81. El-Ela WHA, Farid MM, Mostafa MSE. Intraoral versus extraoral bitewing radiography in detection of enamel proximal caries: an ex vivo study. Dentomaxillofac Radiol 2016;45:20150326.

The Digital Clone

Intraoral Scanning, Face Scans and Cone Beam Computed Tomography Integration for Diagnosis and Treatment Planning

Julian Conejo, DDS, MSc[a], Adeyinka F. Dayo, BDS, MS[b],
Ali Z. Syed, BDS, MHA, MS, DABOMR[c],
Mel Mupparapu, DMD, MDS, DABOMR[d],*

KEYWORDS

- Face scanners • Intraoral scanning • Digital impression • Digital wax-up

KEY POINTS

- With the improvement of optical scanning technology, the study of facial morphology using 3-dimensional face scanners has gained importance and reached a new level.
- Intraoral scanners are typically connected to mobile carts as a complete unit with the computer and monitor. More recent versions of scanners are connected wireless to laptop computers.
- The typical printable file format in 3-dimensional imaging is in standard triangulation language and the images are standard triangulation language image files.
- Integrating cone beam computed tomography data with digital impressions and digital wax-ups with the prosthetic plan is the gold standard for prosthetically driven implantology and interdisciplinary treatment planning.

FACIAL SCANNERS AND THEIR ROLE IN THE CREATION OF A VIRTUAL DENTAL PATIENT

The recognition of the facial morphology is necessary for the preoperative, postoperative evaluation, and symmetry assessment. It has significant applications in dentistry. Facial morphology and analysis are very critical in various disciplines of dentistry such

[a] Department of Preventive and Restorative Sciences, University of Pennsylvania School of Dental Medicine, Robert Schattner Center, Suite #350, 240 South 40th Street, Philadelphia, PA 19104, USA; [b] University of Pennsylvania School of Dental Medicine, Robert Schattner Center, 240 S 40th Street, Philadelphia, PA 10104, USA; [c] Admitting & Oral and Maxillofacial Radiology Clinics, Oral and Maxillofacial Radiology, Department of Oral and Maxillofacial Medicine & Diagnostic Sciences, CWRU School of Dental Medicine, Office # 245 C, 9601 Chester Avenue, Cleveland, OH 44106, USA; [d] University of Pennsylvania School of Dental Medicine, 240 S 40th Street, Suite 214, Philadelphia, PA 19104, USA
* Corresponding author.
E-mail address: mmd@upenn.edu

Dent Clin N Am 65 (2021) 529–553
https://doi.org/10.1016/j.cden.2021.02.011
0011-8532/21/© 2021 Elsevier Inc. All rights reserved.

as craniofacial surgery, maxillofacial surgery, orthodontics, craniofacial orthodontics, prosthodontics, and forensics. Facial scan analysis is presently a new highlight area of research. Conventional strategies for assessing facial morphology were based entirely on 2-dimensional (2D) methods.[1,2] In the past, using 2D imaging and photographs, mathematical instruments were used to obtain the facial analysis data.

With the improvement of optical scanning technology, the study of facial morphology using 3-dimensional (3D) face scanners has gained traction and reached to a new level from 2D to 3D.[3,4] One such example is shown in **Fig. 1**, where a facial scan is displayed via a design software(InLab by Dentsply-Sirona).

A facial scanner is a noninvasive measuring tool that can acquire 3D facial models in an open data format with real skin texture color and a scanning process that is typically very short. The literature increasingly reported that 3D facial scanners could be used in the dental clinics, with the 3D facial samples acquired by scanners being used for 3D quantitative diagnostics and treatment assessment.[4–6]

With the advancements in technology, the volumetric data obtained from the CBCT scans, intraoral scans may be superimposed to create a 3D virtual patient. This virtual patient can help in preoperative procedures, treatment planning, and patient outcomes. The data points such as facial landmarks can be obtained using the 3D face scanning using the scanner.

The advancements in technology have not only improved the speed and accuracy of the treatment but also has enhanced outcomes in the facial esthetics, facial profile and in creating the digital smile design. Greater accuracy improves the quality of the data recorded from the face scanner, which ultimately improves the outcome.[7]

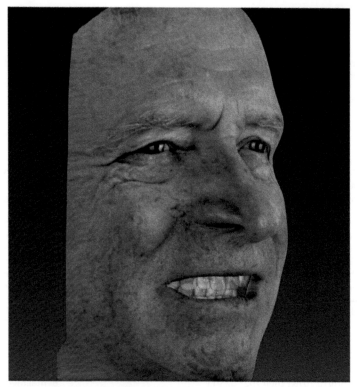

Fig. 1. Facial scan displayed via design software.

There are 2 fundamental types of facial scanners: laser scanners and white light scanners. Although the equipment is different, both types of scanning systems use the principle of triangulation to produce a 3D image of the face. Laser scanners project multiple dots or lines on the patient's face, forming a triangle between the laser (typically 200 FPS infrared class I Laser compliant), light sensor (usually a camera), and the patient. The laser pattern moves over the face to scan the surface area and create a 3D image. The distance of the different surface levels on the patient's face is determined by triangulation. In contrast, white light scanners project light patterns onto the face, forming a triangle between the projector, light sensor (ie, camera), and the patient. In addition, there are different types of scanning systems including fixed and moveable systems.[8] Fixed scanners, such as the OBI Scanner (Viale Lombardia 6, 20133 Milano, Italy) are supported by a tripod placed directly in front of the seated patient. The patient is prompted to make specific head movements (ie, right, left, upward, downward) by the software.[9] Moveable scanners, such as the Artec Evan Scan, are portable and moved around the face to acquire a 3D scan.[10]

Three-dimensional scans are easily obtained using a smartphone with a dedicated application[11] and the corresponding software. Face scans use fast, noncontact scanning and are generally well-tolerated by the patient. Laser stripe is safe for the human eye and unperceived by the patient except when it passes directly over the pupils. However, some face scanners flash a series of bright lights to capture the 3D image, which could cause slight discomfort for some patients.[12] To ensure a constant state of facial expression, the patient is directed to close his or her eyes during the light flashes.[13] Each scanning system has a different range that the patient must stay within for the duration of the scanning process.[14] To ensure that the patient's head is still and in its natural position, support of the head and neck can be used. In addition, hair should be secured away from the face to decrease noise data[13] and facial expressions should be kept unchanged during the scanning process. Moreover, controlled indoor lighting is preferred to avoid image distortion owing to the sensitivity of the light sensors.[14] Some interferences may be seen owing to the reflective surfaces of teeth. However, this could be corrected after image capture.[15]

To obtain a holistic and more accurate 3D image, multiple scans can be taken in different facial positions (rest position, smiling position, and cheek retracted position). The scans are then aligned using the forehead to obtain more information on the patient's smile line, tooth display, and soft tissue. Integrating 3D facial scans with intraoral and extraoral scans provides valuable information for treatment planning.[16] If the operator wishes to scan the teeth separately, facial scanning software allows for the implementation of virtual facebow transfer technique. To use the virtual facebow technique, markers (round opaque stickers) are attached to the margin of the left or right eye orbit and the Beyron points on both sides.[17]

After scanning is complete, the files are saved and imported into the software, which allows for size and lighting adjustments, display from various angles, and merging of 3D images.[9] If the accuracy of the scan is perceived as less than optimal, the scanning software is used for postcapture manipulation including: smoothing skin, improving mesh quality, and filling holes in scan.[12] After the completion of the necessary edits, the 3D scanned image is used for various treatment plans,[18] such as orthodontic treatment and the fabrication of dental prostheses.[15]

ROLE OF INTRAORAL SCANNERS IN THE CREATION OF A VIRTUAL PATIENT

Different technologies are used to obtain a digital impression of teeth and surrounding intraoral tissues.[19] These technologies are constantly updated and refined, so are the actual scanners to make them more user and patient friendly as well as easy to navigate and handle in the oral cavity. A strategic scanning technique that subsequently captures all areas and angles has to be used and become routine for maximum scanning efficiency and quality outcomes. Current intraoral scanners do not require the once-necessary antireflective powder and have to ability to scan. Besides eliminating all the uncomfortable aspects of a conventional impression, one of the great advantages of intraoral scanning is that select areas, which may not have been adequately captured, can simply be rescanned without having to retake the entire impression.[20]

Intraoral scanners function by projecting structured light (white, red, or blue), which is recorded as individual images or video and compiled by the software after recognition of specific points of interest. A 3D model is then generated by matching the points of interest taken under different angles. Extreme points can also be eliminated statistically to decrease noise.[21]

The time needed for taking a digital impression is less than that for a conventional impression.[22] In addition, patients clearly prefer the digital scan. Digital full-arch impressions taken with an intraoral scanner seem to have slight deviations in respect to cross-arch accuracy.[23] Other researchers have found similar accuracy levels between scanners.[24] A recent literature review concluded that, currently, the literature does not support the use of intraoral scanners for long-span restorations on teeth or implants[7] and there remain areas in respect to digital impressions of dental implants that need further investigation.[25] However, new intraoral scanning technologies such as photogrammetric imaging allow for high accuracy even for full-arch implant restorations.[26]

Scanning technique and sequence also play a major role. When properly applied, the digital impression technique seems to be more accurate than a conventional impression.[27,28] A surgical guide in preparation in a proprietary design software is shown in **Fig. 2** (CoDiagnostix, Dental Wings GmbH, Düsseldorfer, Germany).

Traditionally, intraoral scanners were connected to mobile carts as a complete unit with the computer and monitor. More recent versions of scanners are connected wirelessly to laptop computers. Companies that produce scanners as well as dental chairs offer the option of incorporating the scanner into the dental chair.

CAD/CAM Design Software

The ability to visualize and analyze digital impressions immediately after scanning is one of the key advantages of the chairside workflow.[29] Unlike conventional impressions, where errors are often only detected after fabricating the mastercast, an erroneous or deficient digital impression can be analyzed and corrected immediately.

Different software is available for each type of CAD/CAM system: clinical or laboratory. The reason is that restorations and materials for chairside CAD/CAM are more limited owing to time restrictions. The main objective of the chairside workflow is to complete the final ceramic restoration in 1 visit, avoiding the need for a temporary restoration and a second appointment for delivery. With the developments in high-strength ceramic materials and implant prosthetic solutions, the latest chairside CAD/CAM software versions are now able to produce fixed dental prosthesis and implant supported restorations. Dental restoration design software has become increasingly user friendly, with many features like preparation finish line detection and tooth digital "wax up" now automated. The clinician can select from digital libraries of natural tooth shapes and morphologies or create a mirror image of an existing tooth in the patient's mouth. With these features, truly esthetic and natural tooth shapes that are not handmade by a dental technician can be applied based on the

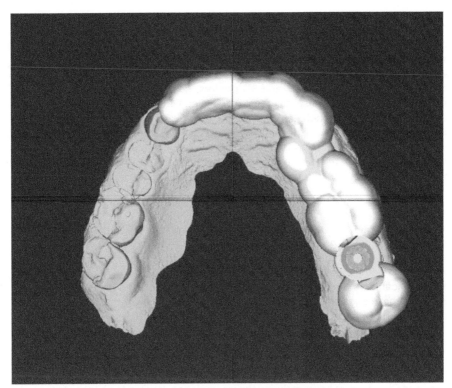

Fig. 2. Surgical guide in preparation in a proprietary design software.

individual esthetic needs and desires of the specific patient. The .STL or other files and tooth libraries can be imported from other sources. Advanced options include digital smile design features and even face scan technology to optimize esthetic outcomes.[29,30]

Several clinicians who want to incorporate digital impressions in their practice but do not want to mill and finish the restorations in house can select a semichairside workflow, which includes the intraoral scan without the design and milling of restorations. After review of the scan images and definition of the preparation margins, the digital impression is sent electronically to the dental laboratory where the restorations are fabricated.[30] System-specific software is available for that feature (eg, Sirona connect, Dentsply Sirona). The laboratory can then use compatible laboratory-specific software for the design and manufacturing (eg, exocad, Exocad GmbH).

Archiving stone study models and mastercasts requires ample digital storage space. Digital scans and datasets can be stored and archived virtually on a designated server. It is important, however, to understand and follow patient data privacy rules and regulations when deciding where to store patient data and scan files. With most systems, CAD data are handled and transmitted in an .STL format, which has become the standard file format in 3D printing and rapid prototyping. Other formats that are currently used are .PLY, .DCM, and .UDX. To communicate with a milling machine, these file formats are "translated" into "millable" data file formats (CNC). The .STL files describe only the surface geometry of a 3D object without any representation of color, texture, or other common CAD model attributes.[30]

The nitty gritty of digital intraoral scanning (optical scanners)
The pixel size, pixel dimension, or pixel resolution all refer to one thing only and that is the number of pixels in the image defined as $X \times Y$, where X represents the number of pixel columns and Y represents the number of pixel rows. To obtain the value on megapixels, the $X \times Y$ value has to be divided by 1 million.[31] Interaction with human–machine interfaces such as 2D and 3D printers, scanners, cameras, and computer monitors bring in a form of spatial resolution called DPI resolution, where DPI stands for dots per inch. It is sometimes referred to PPI or pixels per inch. If the DPI of an image 72, there will be 72×72 pixels in each square inch of the printed image if seen at full zoom, seen on screen and measured using virtual rulers. A change in the DPI can change everything in terms of printing. The following formula has to be kept in mind before any adjustments can be done.

Printed size (inches^2) = Image size (pixel^2) / DPI resolution (DPI)

The pixel size and DPI should maintain a constant relationship if the printed size has to remain constant. If the DPI is changed (and often can be while converting the format of the images), then it affects the printable quality of the image.[31] This factor has applications in both digital radiography and digital photography.

The typical printable file format in 3D imaging is in standard triangulation language (STL) and the images are. STL image files. If a digital radiographic or photographic volume are to be printed, the DICOM (.DCM) image files have to be converted to .STL files. It is also possible now that a DICOM radiographic file and a .STL digital intraoral 3D photographic file can be matched and merged for the creation of a virtual patient.

Digital intraoral scanning generates a point cloud and these points join together and form an unfiltered image. Through interpolation, final image takes shape. Errors, known as Chord errors happen during the interpolation, leading to changes in the point density (resolution) generated by the scanner. The numbers of points generated in a digital intraoral scan would determine the scan resolution; the higher the point number, the higher the resolution. The resolution is obtained by a ratio of the number of points as noted in the .STL file and the surface are of the area examined and it is represented as points per millimeter squared (ppmm).

In a study looking at the various resolutions of intraoral scanners,[32] it was noted that Omnicam from Sirona had the highest resolution (>79 ppmm)followed by True-Definition by 3M (>54 ppmm), Trios by 3Shape (>41 ppmm) and iTero by Cadent (>34 ppmm). Each of the scanners have their own method of image capture from simple light oscillation or continuous 3D video capture to more complicated multiple colored beams forming a single white beam of light capturing single images and measuring out of plane coordinates of object points by sampling with continuous image acquisition.[32]

Digital radiography (cone beam computed tomography imagers)
Resolutions in digital radiographic data can be isotropic or anisotropic depending on the closeness of the voxel to an isotropic cube. The word *isotropic* literally means, "equal direction." The green prefix "an" makes it "imperfect" or "un-equal." Hence, anisotropic means "un-equal directions or dimensions."[33] Digital radiographic data can be interpreted in physical dimensions either in pixel/voxel dimensions (micrometers) or spatial dimensions represented in line pairs per millimeter (lppm).

The spatial resolution of CBCT images is approximately 1 order magnitude lower than that of intraoral radiographs. The actual resolution would be closer to 1 lppm after accounting for the scatter effects, patient movement, and so on.

CONE BEAM COMPUTED TOMOGRAPHY: THE CREATION OF VIRTUAL SKELETAL DATA

CBCT volume acquisition enables the dentist to be able to see the maxillofacial structures 3-dimensionally for not only diagnosis of dentoalveolar pathology, but also to plan the dental treatment including the restorations and prosthodontic care. Since the introduction of root form implants in dentistry, placement of dental implants are enabled by an accurate depiction of the mandibular and maxillary anatomy. The quality of the image depicted depends on the pixel resolution, which can be controlled to a certain extent by the operator. This would be contingent upon the type of CBCT machine and the manufacturer-set pixel resolutions based on the fields of view (FOV) chosen for the patient.

Essentially, there are 3 distinct broad categories that affect the final outcome of the CBCT volume and its diagnostic quality.[34]

Category 1: Machine Properties

FOV chosen, voxel size, focal spot, noise, dynamic range, machine column stability, kV, mA, native acquisition software, and scanner calibration.

Category 2: Patient Related

Patient positioning, stability, density of skeletal structures and amount and density of restorative materials in the teeth.

Category 3: Software for Interpretation

Software design, ease of manipulation of the data, multimodal reformation with ease, 3D reconstruction and ability to read DICOM formatted basis images from several independent CBCT machines.

The Cone Beam Computed Tomography Revolution

CBCT is technology has been introduced to dental practice a little more than 2 decades ago, although conceptually the technology existed even longer. The first CBCT machines approved by the US Food and Drug Administration were commercially available in the United States since 2000.[35] NewTom DVT9000 was the first CBCT unit (Quantitative Radiology srl, Verona, Italy) that was available for clinical use. Other machines were approved by the US Food and Drug Administration in quick succession as many US and foreign manufacturers started manufacturing similar units with various modes of acquisition and with optional FOV settings. Today, there are more than 20 different CBCT machines that are available commercially.

Cone Beam Computed Tomography Scan Acquisition

CBCT acquisition can be done with the patient in 3 possible positions, namely, standing, sitting, or supine. All 3 positions have advantages and disadvantages but in both sitting and standing positions, the patients' head is restrained so that the movement is minimized. The restrain also is pertinent to supine position but the anticipated movement is very minimal if patients are instructed well and have a good neck support within the machine. The scan times vary and in general more than that needed for a panoramic acquisition.

Scan Volumes

CBCT acquisition is task dependent and there are several modes of acquisition (**Fig. 3**).

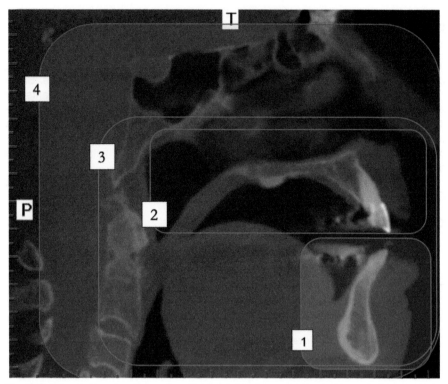

Fig. 3. Schematic showing the various fields of view in a cone beam computed tomography scan acquisition.

Small volumes limited to area within 1 jaw (≤5 cm)
Singe arch (maxilla or mandible) (5–7 cm)
Medium volumes (both maxilla and mandible including skull base) (10–15 cm)
Large volumes (maxilla and mandible, skull base, and most of the cranium) (>15 cm)

The smaller the volume acquired, the higher the spatial resolution of the images. At the same time, if the radiation dose is increased, the quantum noise.

Effective Doses from Cone Beam Computed Tomography Scans

Limited volume
Effective doses for a small volume 4 × 4 cm field of view ranged from 20 to 31 µSv.[35]

Medium and large volumes
In the medium or large FOV mode, the effective doses for some machines reached as high as 1073 µSv in high-resolution modes,[35] although the effective doses are much lower in normal modes. It is known that the effective doses as well as the file sizes become higher as the pixel size is set to be smaller in high-resolution modes.

Cone Beam Computed Tomography Volume Storage

Volumetric data can be stored locally as well as remotely. In a study conducted by Rice and co-workers,[36] it was noted that only 37% of the respondents in their survey used picture archiving and communication system for storage whereas, a large majority of those surveyed used local onsite servers for storing the CBCT data. In the same survey, the authors noted that data were stored either as DICOM volumetric sets by about 53% of users surveys and about 46% of users stored their data in raw or native formats.[36] A typical picture archiving and communication system (MiPACS, Lead Technologies, Charlotte, NC) and its functionality is illustrated in **Fig. 4**.

Cone Beam Computed Tomography Volume Retrieval

CBCT data can be retrieved from its location on a remote server using the functionality of networking. This is called "data transfer" or "data import."

   The DICOM slices (or basis images) are downloaded to a temporary folder within the users terminal and can be opened with a specific software that is, either a native software or a third-party software. One example of a native software is Carestream 3D imaging software if Carestream CBCT machines are used for acquisition. Software programs like Anatomage (Invivo, Santa Clara, CA) are considered third-party because the company does not manufacture or sell a CBCT machine. The software can be used to read the data as long as the data can be retrieved in DICOM format and made available on the terminal.

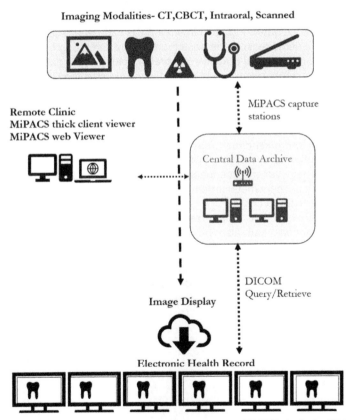

MiPACS ® is a Registered Trademark of Medicor Imaging, LEAD Technologies, USA
Image Created by Mel Mupparapu, DMD

Fig. 4. Schematic showing the workflow using a picture archiving and communication system.

Cone Beam Computed Tomography Image Display

Although 4K monitors are sufficient for majority of the tasks associated with CBCT viewing, many major medical centers use medical grade diagnostic radiology monitors that have specific requirements. In a study comparing the commercial off-the-shelf color monitors to medical grade monitors in radiographic diagnostic tasks, medical grade monitors were found to be superior.[37]

The gold standard of resolutions is used for mammography in the medical imaging. Currently, full field digital mammography is considered a highest spatial image and hence a 5 MP display is required by the US Food and Drug Administration unless the modality of mammogram is not full field digital mammography or if it is a digitized film from full field digital mammography.

Low spatial sources such as CT scan, CBCT, or MRI work well on 2 MP displays or equivalent by pixel pitch in larger formats such as 4 MP, 30″ diagonal monitors. Ultrasound images can be viewed on 1 to 2 MP monitors. In general, 3MP displays are overall suitable for most medical and dental imaging.[38]

Typically most, CBCT data can be displayed in 3 dimensions and also as a composite 3D reconstruction. The displays are sagittal, coronal and axial. Most of the basic displays start with maximum intensity projection (**Fig. 5**) first before the multiplanar reconstructions are looked at. Maximum intensity projection based images are diagnostic for calcifications and a quick assessment of any skeletal asymmetries. The 3D reconstructions as noted **Fig. 6** (Carestream CS 9300 at a resolution of 250 μm) are popular for the same reason; the bone morphology and topography can be easily studied. Because most dental practitioners prefer looking at the data in a panoramic format, a panoramic reconstruction is also achievable using the CBCT data in most software algorithms. The additional advantage of the DICOM dataset is that the volumetric 3DRs can be printed using 3D printers. The printed volumes can be used for mock surgeries, demonstrations, and presurgical planning.

Spatial resolution and pixel dimensions

The spatial resolution of an imaging system is the ability to distinguish and discriminate objects that have varying attenuations separated by small distances. It is represented in line pairs per centimeter (lp/cm). The values that are attainable range from 14 to 16 lp/cm to 22 to 24 lp/cm.[39,40]

In general, pixel resolutions (spatial resolutions) range from 0.40 mm to 0.076 mm. The spatial resolutions can also be represented in micrometers; 1 mm equal

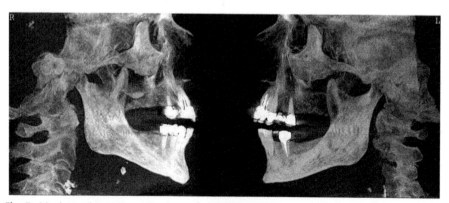

Fig. 5. Maximum intensity projections of a patient showing the right and left sides. Several calcifications were noted in the volume including carotid calcifications bilaterally.

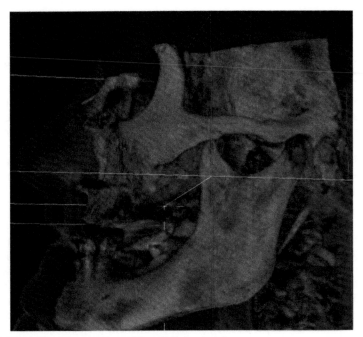

Fig. 6. A CBCT 3D reconstruction with soft tissue overlay.

1000 μm. So, the values range from 400 μm to 76 μm. The larger the pixel value, the smaller the resolution. It is recommended that the optimal resolution for endodontic diagnosis is 200 μm. This would be the average width of the periodontal ligament space.[35] For other diagnostic purposes namely large cystic lesions, tumors, fractures, skull evaluations, temporomandibular joint evaluations, 200 to 400 μm pixel resolutions are used to achieve good diagnostic yield at the same time keeping the file sizes optimal. A typical large volume CBCT will have greater than 500 basis images and a small volume CBCT may have between 200 and 300 basis images. The file size of a small volume may be around 50 to 100 MB, whereas the larger volumes may go up to 200 to 250 MB. If the resolutions are increased, then these sizes can even larger. As the volumes increase, especially in a networked environment, the retrieval of these images becomes an issue and the management of these volumes depend on the speeds of internet connection and the compression algorithms used as well as the characteristics of the remote server. A 1 GB internet connection with good upload as well as download speeds is recommended for a networked CBCT applications.

Merging cone beam computed tomography data with intraoral scan data
Assessment and handling of Digital Radiographic Data and Digital Photographic Data. With the advancements in digital techniques, it is now possible to merge the datasets of both CBCT and IOSD precisely so that the newly merged data can be used for implant-related or orthognathic surgical treatment planning, occlusal rehabilitation and other key functions during a full-mouth reconstruction.[41]

However, there are key differences in the way resolutions are measured between digital images versus digital radiographs. Digital radiographs are a measure of attenuation differences between areas of different densities within human body whereas, digital images of teeth or associated structures are created by reflective photography in 3D format.[42]

INTEGRATING CONE BEAM COMPUTED TOMOGRAPHY SCANS AND INTRAORAL SCANS TO CREATE THE "DIGITAL CLONE"

Integrating the diagnostic and treatment planning benefits of CBCT with digital impressions from intraoral scanners, and digital wax-ups with the prosthetic plan is the gold standard for prosthetically driven implantology and interdisciplinary treatment planning.

The following workflow exemplifies the step by step process on how to predictably obtain the digital clone of patients' initial clinical situation for optimal diagnosis and planning purposes.

1. Preliminary digital impressions (**Figs. 7–9**)

    Full arch maxillary and mandibular intraoral scans are made, assuring that all hard and soft tissue structures are clearly captured with the intraoral scanner (CEREC Omnicam, DentsplySirona). After the maxillary and mandibular files have been reviewed and cleaned by removing any unnecessary data, a third file from the buccal view to capture the maxilla-mandibular relation is made. This buccal scan will correlate the previous scans and recreate the patients existing occlusion. Depending on the specific needs, it can be recorded in maximal intercuspal position (maximum intensity projection) if a limited number of teeth will be restored, or in centric relation if a full mouth rehabilitation approach is required.

    After the buccal scan is correlated, the files are exported as a standard triangulation language (.STL) file.

2. Digital Wax-up (**Figs. 10–13**)

    In the design software (InLab, DentsplySirona), the digital wax-up is made and a file including the new morphology and position of the teeth is also exported in .STL file format. In the example case, a full-mouth wax-up is made. When all teeth are modified, the surrounding soft tissue areas need to be maintained for accurate stitching between the different files.

3. Segmentation of the CBCT scan (**Fig. 14**)

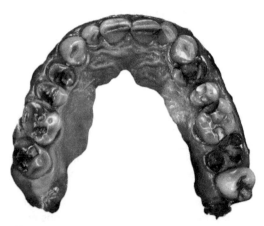

Fig. 7. Full arch maxillary scan.

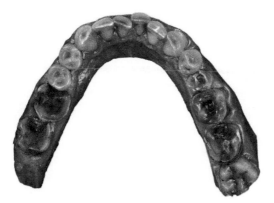

Fig. 8. Full arch mandibular scan.

The DICOM file is uploaded into the planning software (CoDiagnostix, Dental Wings) and the segmentation is made for optimal orientation and visualization. This step provides finer visualization of the areas of interest; in this example, it is the maxilla.

4. Establishing the Panoramic Curve (**Fig. 15**)

The panoramic curve is established by following the arch form, apical to the cemento enamel junction for ideal visualization of single and multiple rooted teeth (CoDiagnostix, Dental Wings).

See **Fig. 9**. for an ideal panoramic curve form occlusal view.

5. Adding Model Scans (**Fig. 16**)

After the segmentation and panoramic steps are completed, additional .STL files can be uploaded into the planning software to create the digital clone.

The 3D position of the dental implants should be planned considering the new tooth arrangement, but the 3D printed surgical guide will be designed over the preoperative .STL file to provide more stability during the surgical procedure to achieve optimal implant positioning. For this reason, it is important to upload both preoperative and wax-up. STL files.

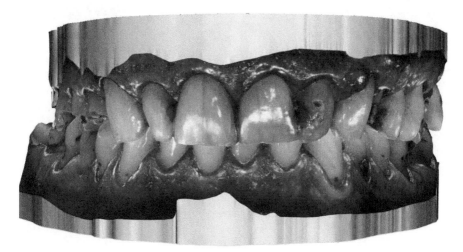

Fig. 9. Full arch buccal scan.

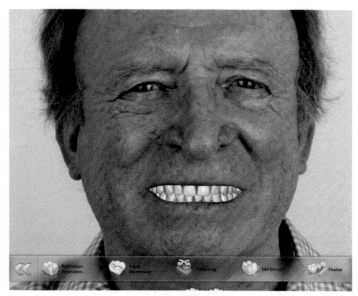

Fig. 10. Extraoral photo for dental–facial integration of the digital wax-up.

Landmarks alignment: In the alignment step, landmarks are placed on the same areas on both files (DICOM and preoperative .STL). The software will notify once the alignment is completed. A minimum of 3 landmarks are needed. This is followed by landmarks alignment between DICOM and preoperative .STL files (**Fig. 17**).

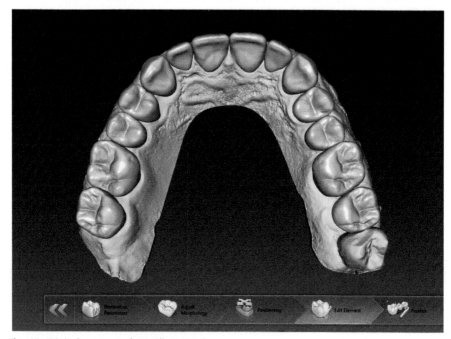

Fig. 11. Digital wax-up of maxillary teeth.

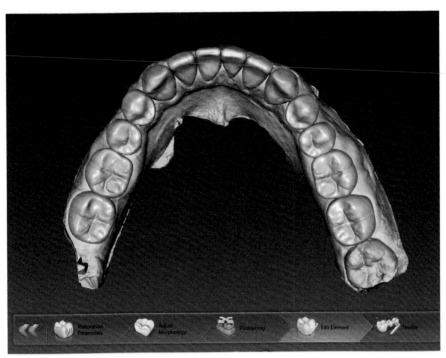

Fig. 12. Digital wax-up of mandibular teeth.

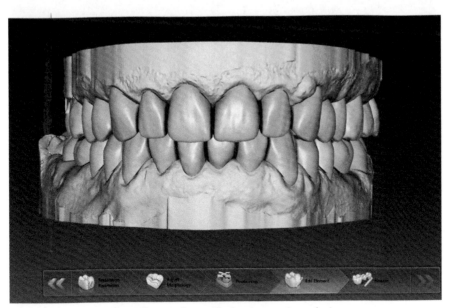

Fig. 13. Buccal view of maxillary and mandibular wax-up in occlusion.

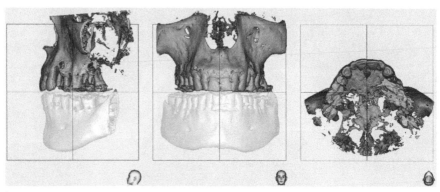

Fig. 14. Segmentation and orientation of the maxilla.

5. Alignment Verification of Layers (**Fig. 18**)

It is of utmost importance that the clinician evaluates the correct alignment of the different files, because this will set the base for the upcoming planning steps. By navigating the DICOM file from the 3 views and assuring that the yellow line that represents the outside surface of the preoperative model matches with the outline of the radiographic image, the correct stitching of the files is confirmed.

6. Wax-up .STL File (**Fig. 19**)

The same process is completed for the addition of the wax-up .STL file.

7. Landmarks Alignments in Soft Tissue (**Fig. 20**)

Because the surfaces of all teeth have been modified, the landmarks need to be placed in soft tissue areas that have not been altered like the tuberosity, palatal rugae, and canine eminence.

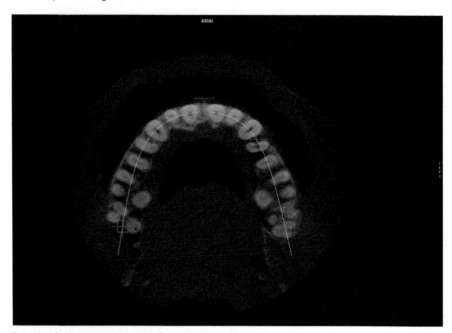

Fig. 15. Ideal panoramic curve form occlusal view.

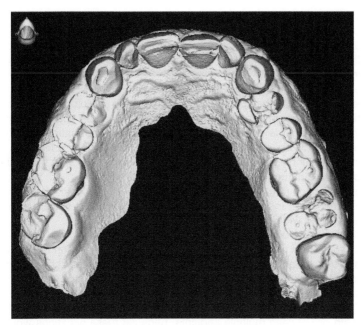

Fig. 16. Occlusal view of. an STL file of preoperative maxillary arch.

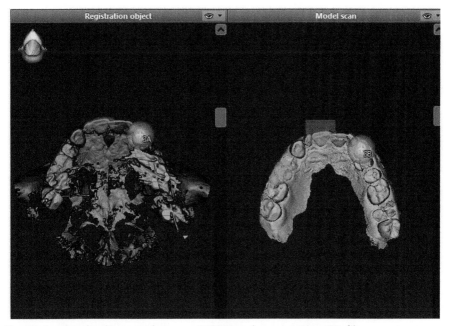

Fig. 17. Landmarks alignment between DICOM and preoperative .STL files.

8. Alignment Verification Between Layers (**Fig. 21**)

   The alignment verification of the 3 layers (DICOM, preoperative .STL and wax-up. STL) is made by navigating the image from the 3 views and confirming that the yellow and orange lines match with the outline of the radiographic image.

9. Three-dimensional View (**Fig. 22**)

   The 3D image with the accurate stitching between all files provides the foundation for the treatment planning step. All 3 files can be activated and deactivated during the diagnosis process. Relevant information regarding soft and hard tissue defects can be visualized in detail. This leads to a better implant planning phase, ensuring that it is in harmony with the final desired prosthetic outcome (CoDiagnostix, Dental Wings).

10. Implant Selection (**Fig. 23**)

   From the library in the software, the determined implant system with specific length and width can be visualized.

11. Prosthetically Driven Implant Planning (**Fig. 24**)

   Previsualization of the contour of the final restoration, the soft tissue thickness, and the available bone and anatomic structures provides the ideal conditions to determine the final implant position.

   A safety area warning for proximity with anatomic structures can be activated. This tool is recommended to avoid implants too proximal to the neighbor teeth or between multiple implants, because these situations would cause future complications.

12. Guided Implant Placement (**Fig. 25**)

   Different approaches for the implant placement can be selected. A surgical guide limited to a pilot drill is the minimum recommended for better accuracy and final 3D implant position (Straumann guided surgery).

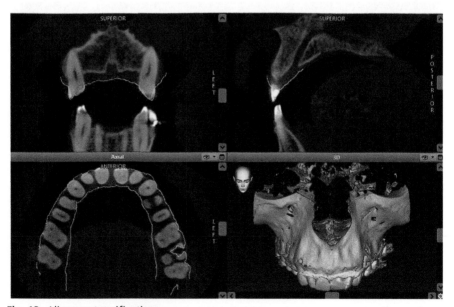

Fig. 18. Alignment verification.

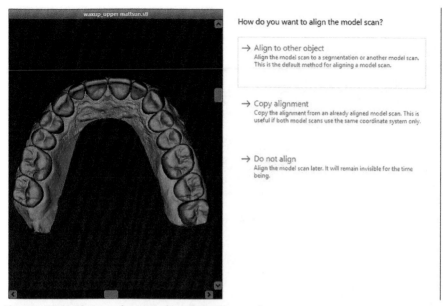

Fig. 19. Occlusal view of an .STL file of maxillary arch wax-up.

A fully guided sequence can also be selected. This protocol has the advantage that a vertical stop between the burs of the surgical kit and the surgical guide can reduce significantly the risk of sinus perforations, nerve collision, or fenestrations.

For both pilot drill or fully guided protocols, determining the correct sleeve is an important final step (**Fig. 26**). Evaluating that the sleeve is not in contact to the

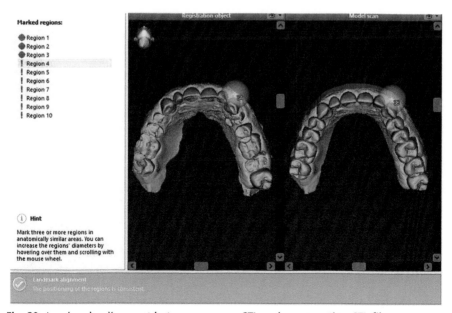

Fig. 20. Landmarks alignment between wax-up .STL and preoperative .STL files.

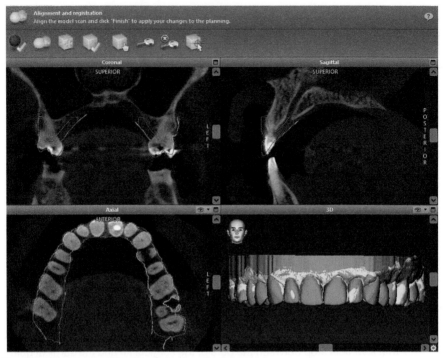

Fig. 21. Alignment verification between the 3 layers.

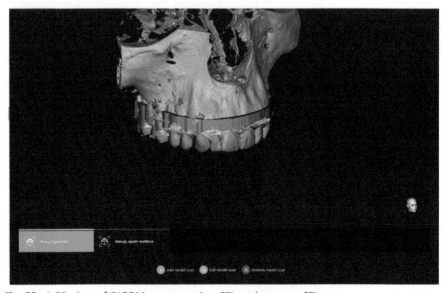

Fig. 22. A 3D view of DICOM, preoperative .STL and wax-up .STL.

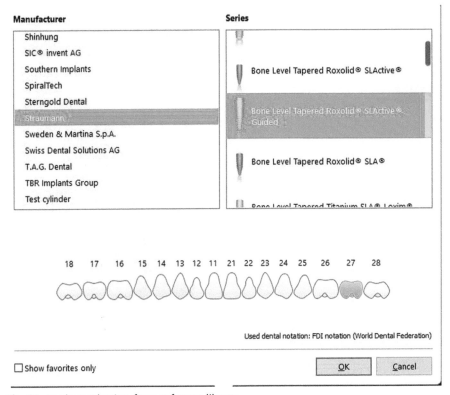

Fig. 23. Implant selection from software library.

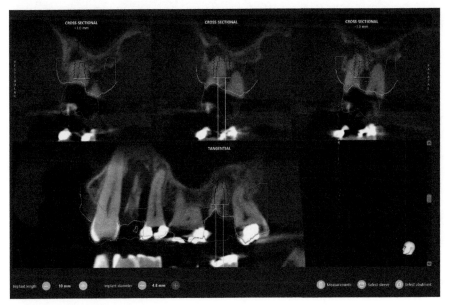

Fig. 24. Virtual implant placement.

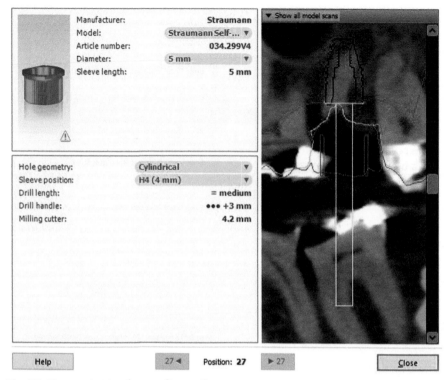

Fig. 25. Sleeve selection from software library.

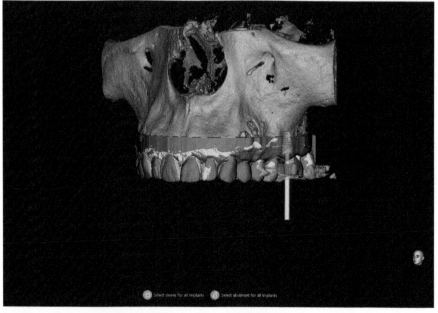

Fig. 26. A 3D view including implant and sleeve placement.

proximal teeth or penetrating in the soft tissue is important before sending the guide for production. Flap or flapless approaches can be selected by the clinicians in a case-by-case specific need.

13. Design of Surgical Guide

After determining the final implant position, surgical approach and respective sleeves, the surgical plan can be sent for production of the surgical stent. The 3D printed resin guides have become a reliable production method.

14. Design of Custom Healing Abutment

With software and hardware advancements, it is also possible to 3D print or mill custom healing abutments of immediate provisional restorations, enhancing the soft tissue conditions for ideal final restorations.

This step-by-step workflow can be implemented with multiple intraoral scanners and implant planning software. Key concepts, steps, and explanations should be implemented independently of the software and hardware available.

CLINICS CARE POINTS

- Facial scans, 3D intraoral photographs and cone beam computed tomography (CBCT) images can be used in the creation of a digital clone of the patient

- The typical file format in 3D imaging is Standard Triangulation Language (STL) and the images are .STL file format

- Integrating Cone Beam Computed Tomography (CBCT) data with digital impressions from intraoral scanners, and digital wax-ups with the prosthetic plan is the "gold standard" for prosthetically driven implantology and interdisciplinary treatment planning

- A surgical guide limited to a pilot drill is recommended at a minimum for better accuracy and final 3D implant position

- With the advancements in digital techniques, it is now possible to merge the datasets of both CBCT and intraoral scanners precisely so that the newly merged data can be used for implant-related or orthognathic surgical treatment planning, occlusal rehabilitation and other key functions during a full-mouth reconstruction.

DISCLOSURE

The authors have nothing to disclose.

REFERENCES

1. Berlin NF, Berssenbrugge P, Runte C, et al. Quantification of facial asymmetry by 2D analysis—A comparison of recent approaches. J Craniomaxillofac Surg 2014; 42(3):265–71.

2. Kim J, Jung H, Jung Y, et al. A simple classification of facial asymmetry by TML system. J Cranio-Maxillofacial Surg 2014;42(4):313–20.

3. Berssenbrugge P, Berlin NF, Kebeck G, et al. 2D and 3D analysis methods of facial asymmetry in comparison. J Craniomaxillofac Surg 2014;42(6):e327–34.

4. Toma AM, Zhurov A, Playle R, et al. Reproducibility of facial soft tissue landmarks on 3D laser-scanned facial images. Orthod Craniofac Res 2009;12(1):33–42.

5. Damstra J, Fourie Z, De Wit M, et al. A three-dimensional comparison of a morphometric and conventional cephalometric midsagittal planes for craniofacial asymmetry. Clin Oral Investig 2012;16(1):285–94.

6. Djordjevic J, Pirttiniemi P, Harila V, et al. Three-dimensional longitudinal assessment of facial symmetry in adolescents. Eur J Orthod 2013;35(2):143–51.

7. Rudolph H, Salmen H, Moldan M, et al. Accuracy of intraoral and extraoral digital data acquisition for dental restorations. J Appl Oral Sci 2016;24:85–94.

8. D'Apuzzo N. Overview of 3D surface digitization technologies in Europe. Proceedings Volume 6056; Three-Dimensional Image Capture and Applications VII. 2006. https://doi.org/10.1117/12.650123.

9. Mangano F, Mangano C, Margiani B, et al. Combining intraoral and face scans for the design and fabrication of computer-assisted design/computer-assisted manufacturing (CAD/CAM) Polyether-Ether-Ketone (PEEK) implant-supported bars for maxillary overdentures. Scanning 2019;2019:4274715.

10. Yamamoto S, Miyachi H, Fujii H, et al. Intuitive facial imaging method for evaluation of postoperative swelling: a combination of 3-dimensional computed tomography and laser surface scanning in orthognathic surgery. J Oral Maxillofac Surg 2016;74(12):2506.e1-10.

11. Lo Russo L, Di Gioia C, Salamini A, et al. Integrating intraoral, perioral, and facial scans into the design of digital dentures. J Prosthet Dent 2020;123(4):584–8.

12. Boehnen C, Flynn P. Accuracy of 3D Scanning Technologies in a Face Scanning Scenario. Fifth International Conference on 3-D Digital Imaging and Modeling (3DIM'05). Ottawa, June 13-16, 2005. https://doi.org/10.1109/3dim.2005.13.

13. Zhao YJ, Xiong YX, Wang Y. Three-dimensional accuracy of facial scan for facial deformities in clinics: a new evaluation method for facial scanner accuracy. PLoS One 2017;12(1):e0169402.

14. Djordjevic J, Toma AM, Zhurov AI, et al. Three-dimensional quantification of facial symmetry in adolescents using laser surface scanning. Eur J Orthod 2014;36(2):125–32.

15. Park JM, Oh KC, Shim JS. Integration of intraoral digital scans with a 3D facial scan for anterior tooth rehabilitation. J Prosthet Dent 2019;121(3):394–7.

16. Hassan B, Greven M, Wismeijer D. Integrating 3D facial scanning in a digital workflow to CAD/CAM design and fabricate complete dentures for immediate total mouth rehabilitation. J Adv Prosthodont 2017;9(5):381–6.

17. Hong SJ, Noh K. Setting the sagittal condylar inclination on a virtual articulator by using a facial and intraoral scan of the protrusive interocclusal position: a dental technique. J Prosthet Dent 2021;125(3):392–5 [published online ahead of print, 2020 Mar 24].

18. Liu H, Bai S, Yu X, et al. Combined use of a facial scanner and an intraoral scanner to acquire a digital scan for the fabrication of an orbital prosthesis. J Prosthet Dent 2019;121(3):531–4.

19. Richert R, Goujat A, Venet L, et al. Intraoral scanner technologies: a review to make a successful impression. J Healthc Eng 2017;2017:8427595.

20. Galhano GÁ, Pellizzer EP, Mazaro JV. Optical impression systems for CAD-CAM restorations. J Craniofac Surg 2012;23(6):e575–9.

21. Seelbach P, Brueckel C, Wöstmann B. Accuracy of digital and conventional impression techniques and workflow. Clin Oral Investig 2013;17(7):1759–64.

22. Yuzbasioglu E, Kurt H, Turunc R, et al. Comparison of digital and conventional impression techniques: evaluation of patients' perception, treatment comfort, effectiveness and clinical outcomes. BMC Oral Health 2014;14:10.

23. Lee SJ, Macarthur RX, 4th, et al. An evaluation of student and clinician perception of digital and conventional implant impressions. J Prosthet Dent 2013;110(5):420–3.

24. Ender A, Mehl A. *In-vitro* evaluation of the accuracy of conventional and digital methods of obtaining full-arch dental impressions. Quintessence Int 2015; 46(1):9–17.
25. Patzelt SB, Emmanouilidi A, Stampf S, et al. Accuracy of full-arch scans using intraoral scanners. Clin Oral Investig 2014;18(6):1687–94.
26. Mangano F, Gandolfi A, Luongo G, et al. Intraoral scanners in dentistry: a review of the current literature. BMC Oral Health 2017;17(1):149.
27. Rutkūnas V, Gečiauskaitė A, Jegelevičius D, et al. Accuracy of digital implant impressions with intraoral scanners. A systematic review. Eur J Oral Implantol 2017; 10(Suppl 1):101–20.
28. Bratos M, Bergin JM, Rubenstein JE, et al. Effect of simulated intraoral variables on the accuracy of a photogrammetric imaging technique for complete-arch implant prostheses. J Prosthet Dent 2018;120(2):232–41.
29. Svanborg P, Skjerven H, Carlsson P, et al. Marginal and internal fit of cobalt-chromium fixed dental prostheses generated from digital and conventional impressions. Int J Dent 2014;2014:534382, 54.
30. Zaruba M, Mehl A. Chairside systems: a current review. Int J Comput Dent 2017; 20(2):123–49.
31. Rakhshan V. Image resolution in the digital era: notion and clinical implications. J Dent (Shiraz) 2014;15:153–5.
32. Medina-Sotomayor P, Pascual-Moscardó A, Camps I. Relationship between resolution and accuracy of four intraoral scanners in complete-arch impressions. J Clin Exp Dent 2018;10:e361–6.
33. Difference between isotropic and anisotropic. Available at: http://www. differencebetween.net/science/chemistry-science/difference-between-isotropic-and-anisotropic/. Accessed September 12, 2020.
34. Bueno MR, Estrela C, Azevedo BC, et al. Development of a new cone-beam computed tomography software for endodontic diagnosis. Braz Dent J 2018; 29:517–29.
35. Scarfe WC, Levin MD, Gane D, et al. Use of cone beam computed tomography in endodontics. Int J Dent 2009;2009:634567.
36. Rice DD, Abramovitch K, Olson GW, et al. Data management practices of cone beam computed tomography volumes: an exploratory user survey. Oral Surg Oral Med Oral Pathol Oral Radiol 2019;128(2):e100–7.
37. Krupinski EA. Medical grade vs off-the-shelf color displays: influence on observer performance and visual search. J Digit Imaging 2009;22:363–8.
38. Requirements for medical imaging monitors-part I. Available at: https://otechimg. com/publications/pdf/wp_medical_image_monitors.pdf. Accessed September 6, 2020.
39. Miracle AC, Mukherji SK. Conebeam CT of the head and neck, part 1: physical principles. AJNR Am J Neuroradiol 2009;30:1088–95.
40. Miracle AC, Mukherji SK. Conebeam CT of the head and neck, part 2: clinical applications. AJNR Am J Neuroradiol 2009;30:1285–92.
41. Carosi P, Ferrigno N, De Renzi G, et al. Digital Workflow to Merge an Intraoral Scan and CBCT of edentulous maxilla: a technical report. J Prosthodont 2020; 29(8):730–2.
42. Brüllmann D, Schulze RK. Spatial resolution in CBCT machines for dental/maxillofacial applications-what do we know today? Dentomaxillofac Radiol 2015;44(1): 20140204.

Physiologic and Pathologic Calcifications of Head and Neck Significant to the Dentist

Steven R. Singer, DDS[a], Irene H. Kim, DMD, MPH[b],
Adriana G. Creanga, BDS, MS, DABOMR[a],
Mel Mupparapu, DMD, MDS, DABOMR[b],*

KEYWORDS

- Radiology • Digital radiography • Cone beam computed tomography • Diagnosis
- Head and neck imaging

KEY POINTS

- A broader range of commonly calcified structures can be viewed in cone beam computed tomography (CBCT) examinations than in other diagnostic dental imaging studies. Head and neck calcifications are within the soft tissue and hence are better attenuated and visible on CBCT.
- Dental practitioners must recognize subtle alterations of normal bony anatomy and not mistake them as pathology.
- A wide range of calcifications includes mostly benign entities as well as age-related calcifications and remodeling of normal anatomic structures and dystrophic calcifications. Often, these changes are incidental findings on dental imaging studies.
- Occasionally, bony or soft tissue changes can alert the clinician to more sinister disease processes, such as a malignancy. Such changes always have other clinical findings before changes appear on radiographs.
- CBCT seldom is the primary method for detecting diseases affecting the soft tissues of the head and neck.

INTRODUCTION

The increased use of advanced imaging in dental practice, in particular, cone beam computed tomography (CBCT), has highlighted the need to recognize head and neck calcifications that are of importance to the dentist. Many of these calcifications are within a soft tissue and hence are better attenuated and visible on CBCT. Alterations of normal bony anatomy are subtle, but the dental practitioner must recognize

[a] Department of Diagnostic Sciences, Rutgers School of Dental Medicine, 110 Bergen Street, Room D-885A, Newark, NJ 07103, USA; [b] University of Pennsylvania School of Dental Medicine, 240 South 40th Street, Suite 214, Philadelphia, PA 19104, USA
* Corresponding author.
E-mail address: mmd@upenn.edu

Dent Clin N Am 65 (2021) 555–577
https://doi.org/10.1016/j.cden.2021.02.005
0011-8532/21/© 2021 Elsevier Inc. All rights reserved.

them so as not to identify them mistakenly as pathology. A wide range of these findings includes mostly benign entities as well as age-related calcifications and remodeling of normal anatomic structures and dystrophic calcifications. These changes often are incidental findings on dental imaging studies. On occasion, there can be bony or soft tissue changes that can alert the clinician to a more sinister disease process, such as a malignancy, but they always have other clinical findings before a radiographic appearance. This article aims to help the practitioner identify the structures found on three-dimensional imaging studies of the head and neck region so that appropriate referral can be made for intervention.

CBCT examinations often include larger sections of the head and neck region than both intraoral radiographs and panoramic imaging. Furthermore, the multiplanar reconstructions permit viewing of small structures at good contrast resolution and adequate spatial resolution for small calcified areas to be viewed. A broader range of commonly calcified structures can be viewed in CBCT examinations than in other diagnostic dental imaging studies. Contrast resolution in CT imaging is defined as "the ability of an imaging system to distinguish minor differences in tissue attenuation and to display them with different gray levels."[1] A large majority of CBCT examinations are obtained for viewing teeth and alveolar bone, are well attenuated, and are recorded as high-contrast structures relative to other head and neck structures.[2] Soft tissue calcifications tend to be incidental or serendipitous findings and not the main goal of any imaging study in dentistry.

A retrospective study by Yalcin and Ararat[3] reported the prevalence of head and neck region soft tissue calcifications found in CBCT examinations. This study found tonsilloliths to be the most prevalent soft tissue calcification in their study population and concluded that the prevalence of soft tissue calcifications was high.[3]

Khojastepour and colleagues[4] also found a high prevalence of calcifications in their study of CBCT images of the mandibular region. They found the prevalence of calcifications to be higher in males and increasing with age. It also was noted that calcifications were more common in the "posterior region."[4]

It has been stated that both physiologic and pathologic or ectopic mineralization require the coordinated actions of mineralization inhibitors and propagators.[5] Although some of the visualized calcifications are indicators of a disease process and require timely intervention, other calcified structures tend to be associated with normal aging and require merely identification and differentiation from more sinister entities. This article describes the various soft tissue calcifications, both physiologic and pathologic, and their significance.

CALCIFIED CAROTID ATHEROMAS

Calcified carotid artery atheromas (CCAAs) are noted incidentally on CBCT studies of older patients where the neck was included. These calcifications typically occur at the level of the carotid bifurcation, in the region of cervical vertebrae C3-C4 in most adults. They may be unilateral or bilateral. The shape of the calcified atheromas depends on whether the calcification is atheromatous in origin or due to medial arterial calcinosis (MAC). Calcifications that are of MAC may be circular or arc-shaped in axial reconstructions (**Fig. 1**). They also can be seen as vertical, linear, high-density structures in coronal reconstructions (**Fig. 2**). The calcified atheromas are formed by calcification of cholesterol and fat along the intima of the carotid artery. Common risk factors for CCAA include, "diabetes mellitus, hypertension, hyperlipidemia, obesity, and smoking."[6,7] They are considered risk factors and possibly markers for stroke risk.[8,9] Mupparapu and Kim[10] conducted a systematic review and concluded that CCAA is not an

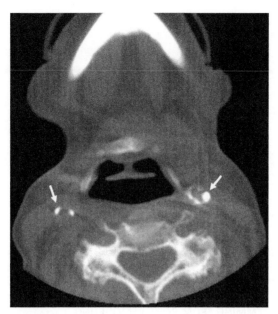

Fig. 1. Axial CBCT projection at the level of the carotid bifurcations. Arrows demonstrate bilateral calcified atheromas.

independent risk factor although associated with risk estimates related to cerebrovascular events. Recently, a meta-analysis conducted by Mupparapu and Nath[11] demonstrated that patients with Doppler ultrasound verification after a diagnosis of CCAA on panoramic radiographs showed slightly higher risk for broadened endpoints, such as stroke, cerebral vascular accident or transient ischemic attack, symptomatic plaque, stenosis greater than 70%, and endarterectomy, as demonstrated via a forest plot of random effects meta-analysis.

Calcified atheromas of the internal carotid arteries (ICAs) also are indicators of stroke risk, especially if they are atherosclerotic variety.[12] These calcifications may be seen at the foramina of the carotid canal lateral to the sella turcica and extending superiorly and posteriorly over the sphenoid sinus (**Fig. 3**). Often, the shape of the arteries is traced by the calcifications, simplifying their identification (**Fig. 4**). There are seven arterial segments for ICA as follows: C1 (cervical), C2 (petrous), C3 (lacerum),

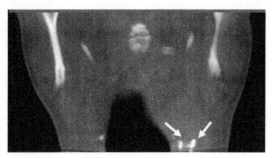

Fig. 2. CBCT coronal projection at the level of the airway. Calcifications, indicated by arrows, are seen in the left carotid bifurcation area.

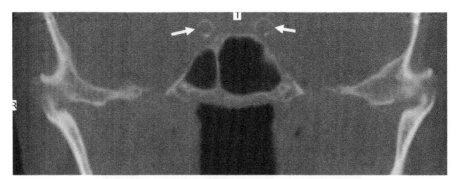

Fig. 3. Coronal CBCT projection at the level of sella turcica of calcified atheromas of the ICAs (*arrows*). The radiographic images are consistent with MAC noted at the level of C7 segment of the ICA. C7 is the communicating segment of the ICA.

C4 (cavernous), C5 (clinoid), C6 (ophthalmic), and C7 (communicating). Calcified atheromas are seen rarely in other arteries. **Fig. 5** demonstrates a calcified atheroma in the vertebral artery as it passes through the transverse foramen of C3.[13]

CALCIFICATIONS STEMMING FROM BONE REMODELING

Chronic low-grade inflammatory processes and both normal function and parafunction eventually cause remodeling of bone in the area of the joints. These conditions are referred to as degenerative joint disease or osteoarthritis. Systemic diseases, such as rheumatoid arthritis (RA), ankylosing spondylitis, psoriatic arthritis, and gout, can affect the joint.[14] The temporomandibular joint (TMJ) is a common site for this adaptive remodeling. Osteoarthritic changes to the TMJ include flattening of the anterior articulating surface of the condylar heads and posterior slopes of the articular eminences (**Fig. 6**), subchondral cyst formation on the affected cortical surfaces, thinning of the cortical bone, osteosclerosis of the medullary bone, and osteophyte

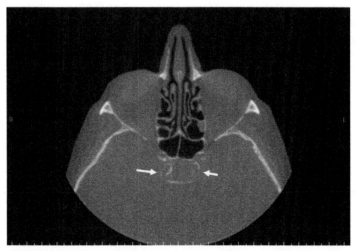

Fig. 4. CBCT axial projection at the level of the ethmoid sinuses. Bilateral MAC-related calcifications of the C7 segment of the ICAs are indicated by the arrows.

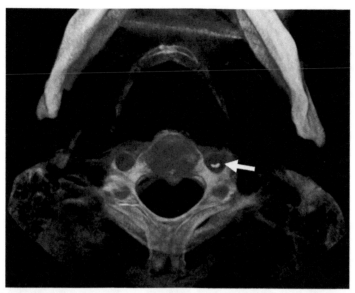

Fig. 5. Three-dimensional CBCT reconstruction of C3 with calcified atheroma of the left vertebral artery in the transverse foramina indicated by the arrow.

formation. Over time, as the articular disk (not seen in CBCT scans) is displaced or worn, the joint space diminishes. Osteophytes may break off and find their way into the joint space (**Fig. 7**). These changes take place over decades and may be accelerated with parafunctional habits, such as bruxism, as well as the loss of vertical dimension and teeth. A 2019 systematic review found high levels of association of temporomandibular disorder with both RA and osteoarthritis.[14] Tonsillar calcifications are noted on the panoramic radiographs usually in the region of the rami either unilaterally or bilaterally and should be identified as tonsilloliths (**Fig. 8**).

Osteoarthritic changes also may be seen in the cervical spine. Osteophyte formation typically is seen at the articulation between the dens and the anterior arch of

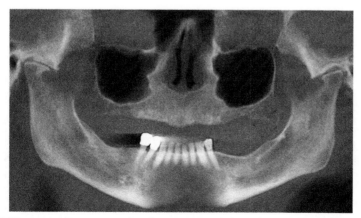

Fig. 6. CBCT panoramic reconstruction demonstrating bilateral osteoarthritic changes to the TMJs.

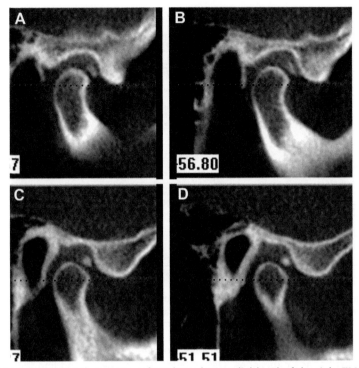

Fig. 7. Serial CBCT sagittal projections from lateral to medial (*A-D*) of the right TMJ demonstrating an osteophyte in the joint space.

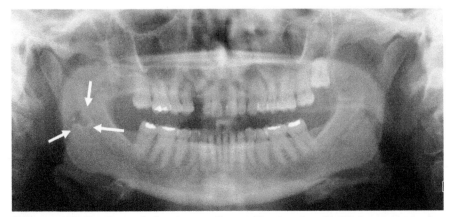

Fig. 8. Panoramic radiograph showing tonsillar calcifications (tonsilloliths) superimposed on the right ramus (*arrows*).

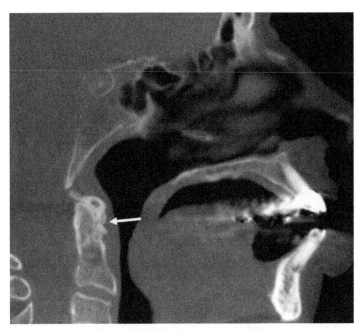

Fig. 9. CBCT sagittal projection. Arrow demonstrates osteophyte formation at the articulation be- tween the dens and anterior arch of C1.

C1 (**Fig. 9**), as well as on the anterior and posterior edges of the articulating surfaces of the vertebral bodies (**Fig. 10**). Similar to the degenerative changes to the TMJ, osteosclerosis and subchondral cyst formation also are common indicators of osteoarthritic changes to the cervical spine.

Similar destruction and remodeling of bony structures may be seen in cases of RA. In RA, the changes to the bony structures occur over a much shorter time, may be

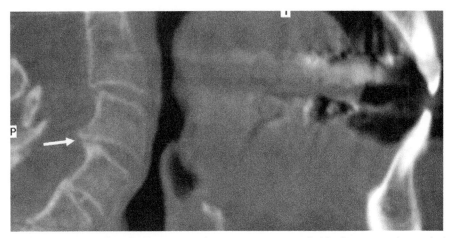

Fig. 10. CBCT sagittal projection. Arrow demonstrates osteoarthritic changes to the cervical spine include osteophyte formation, reduced joint space, and erosion of the cortical articulating surfaces of the vertebral bodies.

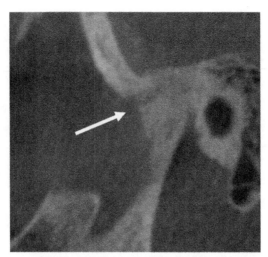

Fig. 11. CBCT sagittal projection demonstrating fibrous and bony ankylosis of the left TMJ (*arrow*).

more extreme, and may affect only one bone in the joint. Another sequela to RA (as well as trauma or other inflammatory process) in the TMJ may be fibrous union and ankylosis of the condylar head to the glenoid fossa[15,16] (**Fig. 11**).

LIMBUS VERTEBRAE

First described by Schmorl in 1927, limbus vertebra is thought to be formed due to intrabony herniation of disc material during childhood or adolescence, and, on plain radiographs, it appears as a triangular osseous fragment at the corner of the vertebral body mimicking a fracture or an infection.[17] They were found to be disc material that were calcified upon their herniation. Anterior limbus vertebra is most common compared with posterior limbus vertebra. An association was found between α1 chain

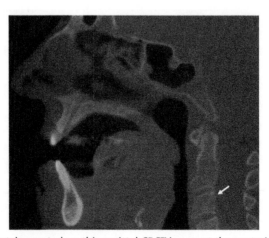

Fig. 12. Limbus vertebra noted on this sagittal CBCT image at the posterior-superior corner of the C3 vertebral body (*arrow*). Limbus vertebrae simulate fractures or infections to the untrained eye.

of type XI collagen (COL11A1) and sporting experience as risk factors for occurrence of limbus vertebrae[18] (**Fig. 12**).

DYSTROPHIC CALCIFICATION OF SOFT TISSUE ANATOMIC STRUCTURES

Deposition of calcium salts in normal anatomic structures, such as the pineal gland, choroid plexus, anterior and posterior longitudinal ligaments, petroclinoid ligament, falx cerebri, and skin, commonly is seen as high-density areas on CBCT scans exposed for such purposes as implant planning, assessment of bony lesions, and other common diagnostic and treatment planning tasks. These almost always are incidental findings. Knowledge of the general location of these structures aids in the identification of these calcifications. Typically, they are associated with normal aging and often may be visualized at an early age in a percentage of the population. For example, as many as 33% of children may demonstrate pineal calcification (**Fig. 13**) by 18 years of age.[19] Although rare, pineal gland calcification in children has been associated with conditions, including brain tumors.[20]

Calcifications and ossifications of the anterior (**Fig. 14**) and posterior longitudinal ligaments (**Fig. 15**) appear on midsagittal projections as high-density linear structures positioned anterior or posterior to the cervical spine. They may impair the normal range of motion of the cervical spine and cause pain. Clinically, the pain typically is attributed to spondylitis. Progression of the calcification of the posterior longitudinal ligament has been associated with spinal cord injury.[21] Advanced ossification of the anterior longitudinal ligament has been associated with dysphagia, sometimes requiring surgical intervention.[22] The paired choroid plexus is a site of cerebrospinal fluid production. Physiologic calcification of these structures commonly is visualized on multidetector CT (MDCT) and CBCT studies of the skull. Calcification of these structures also has been linked to schizophrenia.[23] Calcifications of the choroid plexus are often seen in pairs as irregularly shaped high-density structures in the posterior

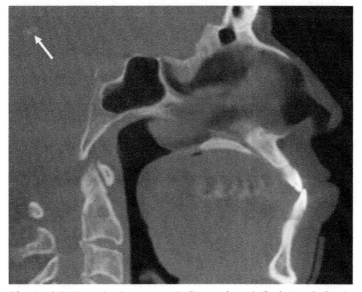

Fig. 13. Midsagittal CBCT projection. Arrow indicates the calcified pineal gland.

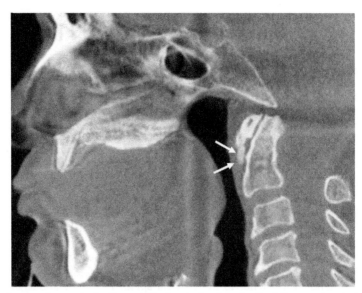

Fig. 14. Arrows demonstrate the calcified anterior longitudinal ligament anterior to the dens (of C2) on this sagittal CBCT image.

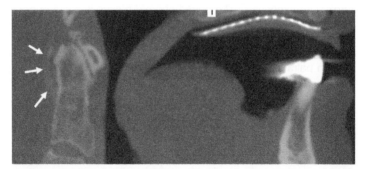

Fig. 15. Sagittal CBCT reconstruction. Arrows indicate calcification of the posterior longitudinal ligament.

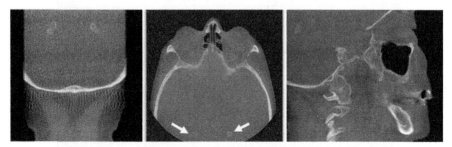

Fig. 16. Coronal (*A*), axial (*B*), and sagittal (*C*) CBCT projections. Arrows demonstrate the calcified choroid plexus.

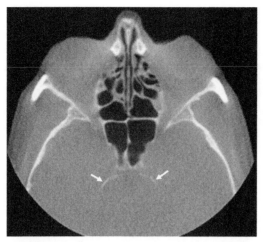

Fig. 17. Axial CBCT projection at the level of the ethmoid air cells. Arrows demonstrate the calcified petroclinoid ligaments.

cranial fossa (**Fig. 16**). They typically are found inferior to the level of the pineal gland. The rim of the calcified choroid plexus may be of higher density than the inner area.

The paired petroclinoid ligaments (**Fig. 17**) connect the apex of the petrous ridge of the temporal with the posterior clinoid process.[24] Calcification of these ligaments becomes more common with increasing age of the patient and may be unilateral or bilateral.

Osteoma cutis is a condition where small foci of calcifications or bone form in the facial skin, notably the cheek and lip areas.[25] Primary osteoma cutis is considered

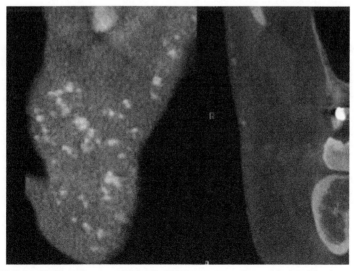

Fig. 18. Oblique (*left*) and coronal (*right*) CBCT reconstructions side by side demonstrating multiple areas of osteoma cutis in the cheek.

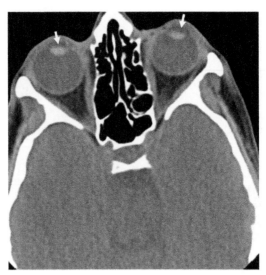

Fig. 19. Axial MDCT reconstruction in soft tissue window. Calcific plaques of the sclera (*arrows*), also known as senile calcific scleral plaques can be seen in both eyes (windows).

to be rare. Most cases can be associated with trauma, neoplasia, or inflammation[25] (**Fig. 18**).

Aging of the tissues of the eye may include dystrophic calcification, producing calcific plaques (**Fig. 19**). This is a common incidental finding on MDCT examinations of older patients when viewed in soft tissue window. The plaques typically are located anterior to the horizontal rectus muscles insertions.[26]

The falx cerebri is a soft tissue structure composed of dura mater that is located in the midline of the brain between the cerebral hemispheres (**Fig. 20**).[27] Ossification of the falx cerebri generally is an idiopathic variant of normal anatomy.

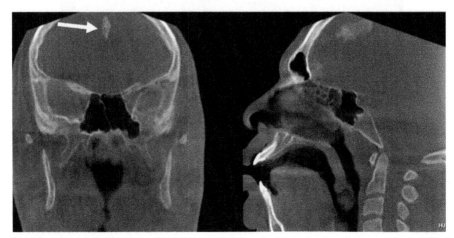

Fig. 20. Coronal (*left*) and sagittal (*right*) CBCT projections. Arrow demonstrates calcified (ossified) falx cerebri.

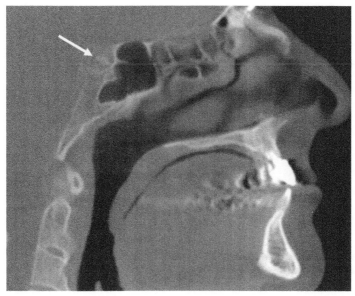

Fig. 21. Sagittal CBCT projection. Arrow shows benign pituitary calcifications within the sella.

Irregularly shaped high-density structures seen within a normal-appearing sella tur-cica can indicate benign pituitary calcifications (**Fig. 21**). These generally are idio-pathic, although they rarely may be associated with pituitary adenomas and other pituitary tumors.[28]

CALCIFIED STRUCTURES OF THE NECK

Panoramic radiographs, lateral cephalometric images, and CBCT scans may demon-strate the calcified cartilages of the neck as well as calcified atheromatous plaque in the carotid artery bifurcations. Typically, the superior cornu of the thyroid cartilage, the triticeous cartilage, and the greater cornu of the hyoid bone calcify with age (**Figs. 22 and 23**). Of these structures, the triticeous cartilage is most likely to be mistaken for calcified atheroma of the carotid bifurcation, leading to misdiagnosis.[29] The triticeous cartilage can be seen between the superior cornu of the thyroid cartilage and the

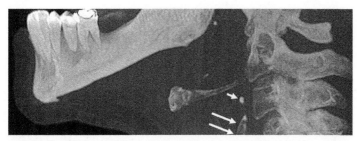

Fig. 22. CBCT maximum intensity projection (MIP) of the mandible and neck areas. The triti-ceous cartilage and superior cornu of the thyroid cartilage can be noted (*arrows*).

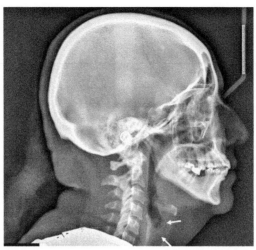

Fig. 23. Lateral cephalometric radiograph. Arrows demonstrate the calcification of the thyroid cartilage (lamina).

greater cornu of the hyoid bone. It usually is superimposed over the airway. Calcified carotid atheromas generally are located at similar height (the level of C3-C4), but further posteriorly and generally superimposed over the posterior pharyngeal wall.[29]

Also located in the neck area are the calcified or ossified stylohyoid ligaments (**Figs. 24** and **25**). Calcification of the ligaments is considered a benign and idiopathic process but may contribute to pain in the anterolateral area neck when the patient turns their head sharply.[30] If this is the case, it is diagnosed as Eagle syndrome. Extreme cases may require medical or surgical management.[31]

Calcified and enlarged lymph nodes of the submandibular chain may be an incidental finding, suggesting a history of a granulomatous disease, such as tuberculosis. These nodes can be found inferior to the angle of the mandible (**Fig. 26**). They are

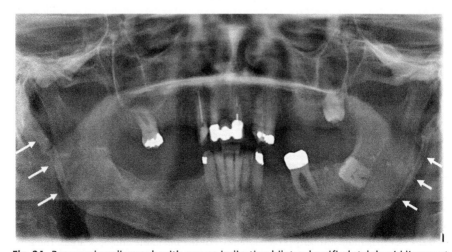

Fig. 24. Panoramic radiograph with arrows indicating bilateral ossified stylohyoid ligament.

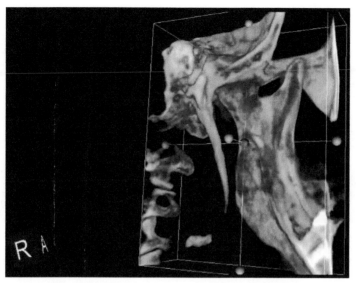

Fig. 25. Cropped CBCT of right TMJ region showing the mineralized styloid process in 3-dimensional reconstruction.

irregularly shaped and variable in size. The patients generally are asymptomatic; however, there occasionally is a complaint of pain in the neck area. In addition to tuberculosis, there are other benign and malignant conditions that may produce calcified cervical lymph nodes.[32] Calcified cervical lymph nodes (**Fig. 27**) should be differentiated from stones (sialoliths) in the salivary ducts (**Fig. 28**). Both submandibular and sublingual gland sialoliths usually are positioned at the level of the inferior border of the mandible and are found further anterior than calcified cervical nodes. They often are associated with pain at mealtimes. It has been reported that approximately 80% of sialoliths are associated with the submandibular salivary gland.[33]

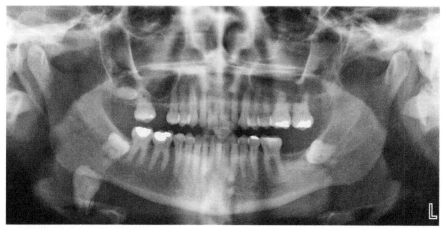

Fig. 26. Panoramic radiograph demonstrating calcified lymph node in the right submandibular area. Patient reported a history of tuberculosis.

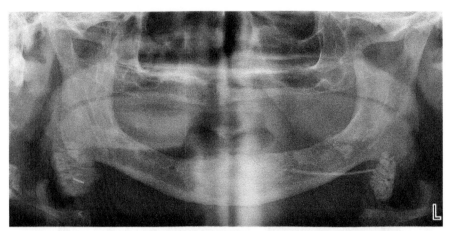

Fig. 27. Panoramic radiograph showing calcification of lymph nodes of the neck (cervical chain). Several artifacts include a ghost image on the right side, a real image of a surgical staple in the right neck and an artifact from a facial mask superimposed next to the calcified neck node on the left side.

PHLEBOLITHS

The maxillofacial region also demonstrates calcifications, known as phleboliths, due to blood flow velocity as noted in the arteriovenous malformation or a hemangioma. These are formed due to intravascular thrombus formation followed by progressive lamellar fibrosis and calcification. Radiographically, they present as layered calcifications or annular calcifications mimicking donuts (**Fig. 29**).

MALIGNANCIES DEMONSTRATING CALCIFICATIONS

Squamous cell carcinoma is by far the most common malignancy of the oral cavity and surrounding structures. Although trapped pieces of necrotic bone may be incorporated into these lesions, squamous cell carcinomas typically do not produce bone

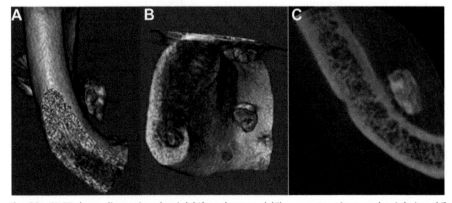

Fig. 28. CBCT three-dimensional axial (*A*) and coronal (*B*) reconstructions and axial view (*C*) of sialolith in right Wharton's duct.

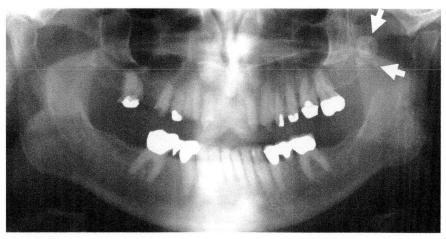

Fig. 29. Panoramic radiograph demonstrating donut-shaped phleboliths in the internal maxillary artery on the left side (*upper arrow*) just around the tip of the left coronoid process. There is a smaller phlebolith just inferior to the larger one (*lower arrow*).

and, therefore, remain radiolucent. Sarcomas represent only 1% of malignancies of the head and neck region.[34]

Osteosarcomas are the most common type of sarcoma. Although most malignancies of the oral cavity and surrounding structures are radiolucent or seen as low-density on CT scans, osteosarcomas and chondrosarcomas produce bone and cartilage, respectively, in characteristic sunray patterns, once they have expanded beyond the periosteum. Other malignant lesions that are known to produce bone include metastatic lesions of prostate and breast cancers. Although mixed-density benign lesions, such as ossifying fibroma, cemento-osseous dysplasias, and fibrous dysplasia, may demonstrate similar fully or partially calcified internal structures, the destructive effects on the structures adjacent to sarcomas aid in the radiographic differential diagnosis of sarcomas. In the examples (**Figs. 30** and **31**), destruction of the cortical borders of the

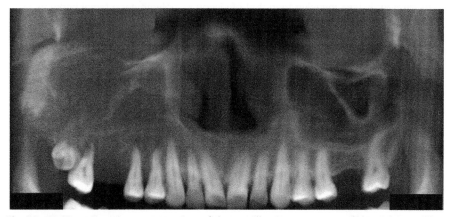

Fig. 30. CBCT panoramic reconstruction of the maxilla. Osteosarcoma of the right maxillary sinus showing the bone destruction.

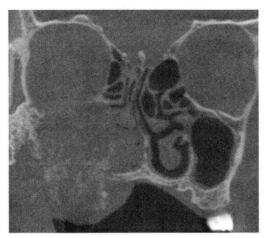

Fig. 31. CBCT coronal image of osteosarcoma. Destruction of the right hard palate, sinus walls, and the floor of the orbit are noted.

maxillary sinus, significant expansion, and effacement of the lamina dura of the maxillary teeth demonstrate that this is an extremely aggressive lesion. The radiographic diagnosis always is confirmed by histopathologic examination.

IMPLANTED HIGH-DENSITY STRUCTURES

High-density structures may be implanted in the skin for cosmetic purposes. Their purpose may be as fillers to provide a more youthful appearance to the skin, or to compensate for a more significant defect, such as a retrognathic appearance of the chin, or deficiencies of the malar processes or the mandible. Biocompatible materials, such as hydroxyapatite and silicon or polyethylene, may be used. It is optimal that the material used is of a greater degree of radiopacity than the surrounding skin and muscles. Calcium hydroxyapatite fillers typically disperse and/or resorb after approximately 2 years. They still may be radiographically visualized after their desired effects have diminished. They have become popular recently, because the procedure for placement is less invasive than that of silicon or polyethylene facial implants.[35]

Calcium hydroxyapatite fillers often are used in the malar area (**Fig. 32**). They can be visualized most readily on axial CBCT projections. They are seen as multiple linear high-density strands located in the skin by the anterior walls of the maxillary sinuses and the malar process of the maxilla. Silicon or polyethylene implants often are initially near isodense with the surrounding soft tissues. Over time, the surface facing bone acquires a layer of calcification, making their presence more radiographically apparent (**Fig. 33**). Complications with these implants include displacement of the implant and infection.

SUSUK

Susuk are implanted needles, usually gold, that are implanted in the skin to act as talismans.[36] They often are planted in the subcutaneous tissues of the face as well as other areas of the body. This practice apparently is common among women in the countries of Southeast Asian. Men have susuk needles implanted less frequently. Benefits ascribed to susuk include good fortune, beauty, and relief of pain. Susuk is an incidental

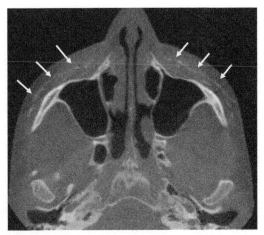

Fig. 32. Axial CBCT projection at the level of the malar processes. Calcium hydroxyapatite midface injectable filler (*arrows*) is seen underneath the skin near the maxilla and the zygomatic (malar) processes of the maxilla.

radiographic finding. It apparently is taboo in some modern cultures, and, therefore, patients may be reluctant to discuss their susuk. In panoramic, periapical, and bitewing radiographs, the needles may be seen as 1-mm to 3-mm long, straight or curved linear opacities positioned over the cheek areas and appear superimposed over the posterior teeth and mandible (**Fig. 34**). Panoramic radiographs may not show the full complement of susuk needles, because some of the needles may be out of the panoramic focal trough.

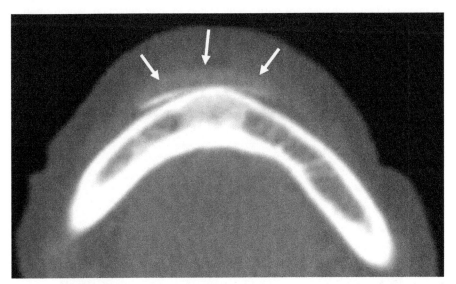

Fig. 33. Axial CBCT image at the level of the mandible. Chin graft can be seen in the soft tissues of the skin (*arrows*). The graft surface closer to the buccal cortical surface is calcified.

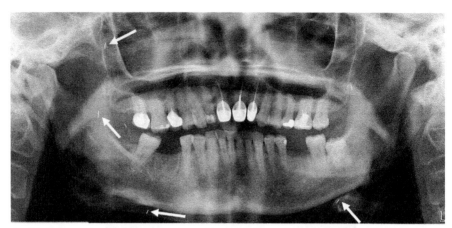

Fig. 34. Panoramic projection. Susuk needles can be noted scattered across the facial region (*arrows*).

ANTROLITHS

Antroliths are calcifications that occur in the maxillary sinuses (antra). They usually form by ongoing deposition of calcium salts around a nidus.[37] They may be associated with chronic sinus inflammatory processes, such as sinusitis and fungal sinus infections.[37] Typically, mucosal thickening can be seen radiographically along the sinus floor, often surrounding the antrolith. The size and shape of maxillary antrolith can vary from small stones to larger structures of several centimeters in largest dimension. The internal appearance ranges from uniformly high-density to targetoid, with a high-density outer layer. They may be seen singly or with multiple structures and may be present in one or both maxillary sinuses.[37] Although antroliths may be seen on plain film imaging, CBCT studies are particularly suited to their detection, which often is an incidental finding (**Fig. 35**). They also can be seen on panoramic radiographs.[38]

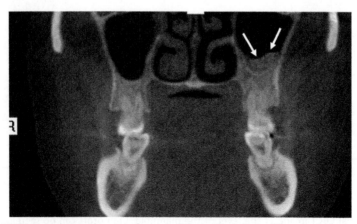

Fig. 35. CBCT coronal view showing the antroliths in the left maxillary sinus on the floor (*arrows*) as an incidental finding.

SUMMARY

With broader use of CBCT for dental diagnosis and treatment planning, knowledge of the calcified structures visualized in the volumes becomes imperative. CBCT is designed primarily as a relatively low-dose imaging modality and is limited in its usefulness in discriminating soft tissue densities. Deposition of calcium salts in the soft tissue structures makes them highly visible in CBCT imaging studies. Although most soft tissue calcifications are benign, most likely of little consequence to the well-being of the patient, and minimally impactful to the treatment of dental disease, some of these calcified structures may be more sinister and require further attention.

Many of the calcified soft tissue structures represent physiologic calcifications that generally are associated with normal aging. These include most calcifications of the pineal gland, petroclinoid ligament, and cartilages of the neck. These often may be simply documented in the radiology report and not considered further. Other findings, such as calcifications of the artery walls and intima, require correlation with a patient's medical history and may demand referral to the patient's physician for further testing. Occasionally, serious issues, such as primary or metastatic malignant disease, may present as soft tissue calcifications and require immediate intervention. It should be emphasized that CBCT seldom is the primary method for detecting diseases affecting the soft tissues of the head and neck.

CLINICS CARE POINTS

- In CBCT, a larger range of commonly calcified structures can be viewed compared with other diagnostic dental imaging studies
- Subtle alterations of normal bony anatomy should not be mistaken as pathology.
- Many of the calcified soft tissue structures represent physiologic calcifications that generally are associated with normal aging. These include calcifications of the pineal gland, petroclinoid ligament, and cartilages of the neck.
- Other findings, such as calcifications of the artery walls and intima, require correlation with a patient's medical history and may demand referral to the patient's physician for further testing.
- Occasionally, bony or soft tissue changes may indicate a malignancy. Such changes always have other clinical findings before changes appear on radiographs.
- CBCT is seldom the primary method for detecting diseases affecting the soft tissues of the head and neck.

DISCLOSURE

The authors have nothing to disclose.

REFERENCES

1. Angelopoulos C, Scarfe WC, Farman AG. A comparison of maxillofacial CBCT and medical CT. Atlas Oral Maxillofac Surg Clin North Am 2012;20(1):1–17.
2. Pauwels R, Beinsberger J, Stamatakis H, et al. Comparison of spatial and contrast resolution for cone-beam computed tomography scanners. Oral Surg Oral Med Oral Pathol Oral Radiol 2012;114(1):127–35.
3. Yalcin ED, Ararat E. Prevalence of soft tissue calcifications in the head and neck region: A cone-beam computed tomography study. Niger J Clin Pract 2020;23(6): 759–63.

4. Khojastepour L, Haghnegahdar A, Sayar H. Prevalence of Soft Tissue Calcifications in CBCT Images of Mandibular Region. J Dent (Shiraz) 2017;18(2):88–94.
5. Kirsch T. Determinants of pathological mineralization. Curr Opin Rheumatol 2006; 18(2):174–80.
6. Levy C, Mandel L. Calcified carotid artery imaged by computed tomography. J Oral Maxillofac Surg 2010;68(1):218–20.
7. Atalay Y, Asutay F, Agacayak KS, et al. Evaluation of calcified carotid atheroma on panoramic radiographs and Doppler ultrasonography in an older population. Clin Interv Aging 2015;10:1121–9.
8. Wakhloo AK, Lieber BB, Seong J, et al. Hemodynamics of carotid artery atherosclerotic occlusive disease. J Vasc Interv Radiol 2004;15(1 Pt 2):S111–21.
9. Cohen SN, Friedlander AH, Jolly DA, et al. Carotid calcification on panoramic radiographs: an important marker for vascular risk. Oral Surg Oral Med Oral Pathol Oral Radiol Endod 2002;94(4):510–4.
10. Mupparapu M, Kim IH. Calcified carotid artery atheroma and stroke: a systematic review. J Am Dent Assoc 2007;138(4):483–92.
11. Mupparapu M, Nath S. Calcified Carotid Artery Atheroma and Stroke risk assessment. Use of doppler ultrasonography as a secondary marker: A meta- analysis. Quintessence Int 2020. https://doi.org/10.3290/j.qi.a45604.
12. Lee JI, Jander S, Oberhuber A, et al. Stroke in patients with occlusion of the internal carotid artery: options for treatment. Expert Rev Neurother 2014;14(10): 1153–67.
13. Singer SR, Mupparapu M. Cone beam computed tomography detection of extracranial vertebral artery (EVA) calcification and ectasia. J Orofac Sci 2019;11: 65–70.
14. Pantoja LLQ, de Toledo IP, Pupo YM, et al. Prevalence of degenerative joint disease of the temporomandibular joint: a systematic review. Clin Oral Investig 2019; 23(5):2475–88.
15. Cunha CO, Pinto LM, de Mendonça LM, et al. Bilateral asymptomatic fibrousankylosis of the temporomandibular joint associated with rheumatoid arthritis: a case report. Braz Dent J 2012;23(6):779–82.
16. Bénateau H, Chatellier A, Caillot A, et al. 'ankylose temporo-mandibulaire [Temporo-mandibular ankylosis]. Rev Stomatol Chir Maxillofac Chir Orale 2016; 117(4):245–55.
17. Mupparapu M, Vuppalapati A, Mozaffari E. Radiographic diagnosis of Limbus vertebra on a lateral cephalometric film: report of a case. Dentomaxillofac Radiol 2002;31(5):328–30.
18. Koyama K, Nakazato K, Min S, et al. COL11A1 gene is associated with limbus vertebra in gymnasts. Int J Sports Med 2012;33(7):586–90.
19. Helmke K, Winkler P. Die Häufigkeit von Pinealisverkalkungen in den ersten 18 Lebensjahren [Incidence of pineal calcification in the first 18 years of life]. Rofo 1986;144(2):221–6.
20. Tuntapakul S, Kitkhuandee A, Kanpittaya J, et al. Pineal calcification is associated with pediatric primary brain tumor. Asia Pac J Clin Oncol 2016;12(4):e405–10.
21. Shin J, Choi JY, Kim YW, et al. Quantification of risk factors for cervical ossification of the posterior longitudinal ligament in korean populations: a nationwide population-based Case-control Study. Spine (Phila Pa 1976) 2019;44(16): E957–64.
22. Ohara Y. Ossification of the ligaments in the cervical spine, including ossification of the anterior longitudinal ligament, ossification of the posterior longitudinal

ligament, and ossification of the ligamentum flavum. Neurosurg Clin N Am 2018; 29(1):63–8.

23. Bersani G, Garavini A, Taddei I, et al. Choroid plexus calcification as a possible clue of serotonin implication in schizophrenia. Neurosci Lett 1999;259(3):169–72.

24. Cederberg RA, Benson BW, Nunn M, et al. Calcification of the interclinoid and petroclinoid ligaments of sella turcica: a radiographic study of the prevalence. Orthod Craniofac Res 2003;6(4):227–32.

25. Syed AZ, Torres M, Rathore S, et al. Radiographic diagnosis of osteoma cutis of the face: a case series. J Mich Dent Assoc 2016;100(11):56–8.

26. Alorainy I. Senile scleral plaques: CT. Neuroradiology 2000;42(2):145–8.

27. Tsitouridis I, Natsis K, Goutsaridou F, et al. Falx Cerebri Ossification: CT and MRI Evaluation. Neuroradiol J 2006;19(5):621–8.

28. Ogiwara T, Nagm A, Yamamoto Y, et al. Clinical characteristics of pituitary adenomas with radiological calcification. Acta Neurochir (Wien) 2017;159(11): 2187–92.

29. Carter LC. Discrimination between calcified triticeous cartilage and calcified carotid atheroma on panoramic radiography. Oral Surg Oral Med Oral Pathol Oral Radiol Endod 2000;90(1):108–10.

30. Badhey A, Jategaonkar A, Anglin Kovacs AJ, et al. Eagle syndrome: A comprehensive review. Clin Neurol Neurosurg 2017;159:34–8.

31. Khan HM, Fraser AD, Daws S, et al. Fractured styloid process masquerading as neck pain: Cone-beam computed tomography investigation and review of the literature. Imaging Sci Dent 2018;48(1):67–72.

32. Paquette M, Terezhalmy GT, Moore WS. Calcified lymph nodes. Quintessence Int 2003;34(7):562–3.

33. Stelmach R, Pawłowski M, Klimek L, et al. Biochemical structure, symptoms, location and treatment of sialoliths. J Dent Sci 2016;11(3):299–303.

34. de Carvalho WRS, de Souza LL, Pontes FSC, et al. A multicenter study of oral sarcomas in Brazil. Oral Dis 2020;26(1):43–52.

35. Rojas YA, Sinnott C, Colasante C, et al. Facial Implants: Controversies and Criticism. A Comprehensive Review of the Current Literature. Plast Reconstr Surg 2018;142(4):991–9.

36. Arishiya Thapasum F, Mohammed F. Susuk - black magic exposed "white" by dental radiographs. J Clin Diagn Res 2014;8(7):ZD03–4.

37. Cho BH, Jung YH, Hwang JJ. Maxillary antroliths detected by cone-beam computed tomography in an adult dental population. Imaging Sci Dent 2019; 49(1):59–63.

38. Aoun G, Nasseh I. Maxillary antroliths: a digital panoramic-based study. Cureus 2020;12(1):e6686.

Radiographic Diagnosis of Systemic Diseases Manifested in Jaws

Eugene Ko, DDS, Temitope Omolehinwa, BDS, DScD,
Sunday O. Akintoye, BDS, DDS, MS,
Mel Mupparapu, DMD, MDS, DABOMR*

KEYWORDS

- Dental anomalies • Syndromes • Hematologic diseases • Metabolic
- Medication-related

KEY POINTS

- Systemic diseases can have oral and maxillofacial radiographic changes.
- General dentists are likely to encounter one of many systemic diseases that present with oral and maxillofacial radiologic changes.
- The scope of differential diagnoses of radiographic changes should involve systemic as well as traditional dental etiologies.

Systemic disease can be manifested in the jaws in multiple ways (**Table 1**). The manifestations can be limited to the teeth or may extend to involve the soft and hard tissues that form the oral cavity. Mandibular and maxillary bone often is the target. In this article, individual disease entities that have both systemic and dental manifestations and a summary of the most common jaw affected, radiographic and pathognomonic findings, and management aspects is listed in a table format within this article. Images for many conditions are provided to illustrate the jaw involvement.

AMELOGENESIS IMPERFECTA

Amelogenesis imperfecta is a group of hereditary enamel defects that occur in the absence of a generalized syndrome.

Clinical and Radiographic Presentation

In general, enamel malformations fall into 3 categories: hypoplastic, hypomature, and hypocalcified. Hypoplastic enamel presents as pathologically thin and rough, and there is lack of contact between teeth that are yellowish. The most severe form of

Department of Oral Medicine, University of Pennsylvania, School of Dental Medicine, 240 South 40th Street, Philadelphia, PA 19104, USA
* Corresponding author.
E-mail address: mmd@upenn.edu

Dent Clin N Am 65 (2021) 579–604
https://doi.org/10.1016/j.cden.2021.02.006
0011-8532/21/© 2021 Elsevier Inc. All rights reserved.

Table 1
Summary of clinicopathologic features of systemic diseases

Disorder	Commonly Affected Part (Jaws)	Radiographic Category	Radiopathognomic Sign	Treatment Strategy
Gorlin syndrome	Mandible >> maxilla	Decreased bone density	Multiple radiolucent lesions	Surgical intervention
Cherubism	Mandible and maxilla	Decrease bone density	Symmetric radiolucent lesions	Spontaneous regression
Brown tumor of primary hyperparathyroidism	Mandible >> maxilla	Radiolucent bone cavities	Radiolucent lesion	Surgical removal of affected parathyroid gland. Resection of affected bone may be necessary.
MRONJ	Mandible >> maxilla	Radiolucency (plain images); osteolytic lesions (CT)	Osteomyelitic-like lesions surrounded by dense sclerotic bone	Stage specific treatment-débridement and antibiotics
Sickle cell anemia	Mandible >> maxilla	Altered trabeculation	Extreme enlargement of bone marrow spaces	Prevention; blood transfusions
Thalassemia	Maxilla	Altered trabeculation	Extreme enlargement of bone marrow spaces	Prevention; blood transfusions
Osteoporosis	Mandible >> maxilla	Decreased bone density (lucent)	Absence or reduction of trabeculae with thinning of inferior cortex	Medication to increase bone density
Gardner syndrome	Both mandible and maxilla are affected	Increased bone density	Osteomas, supernumerary teeth	Surgical and symptomatic intervention
FD	Both maxilla and mandible	Mixed radiolucent/ radiopaque density	Jaw expansion, dental malocclusion	Surgery and medications to control bone pain

Renal osteodystrophy	Both maxilla and mandible	Osteolytic (lucent) lesions	Subperiosteal bone resorption, decreased bone trabeculation, reduced cortical bone thickness; ground-glass opacities; jaw enlargement, increased interdental spaces	Medical correction of hyperphosphatemia and lowering of PHT levels
Osteopetrosis	Both maxilla and mandible	Generalized increased bone density	Prognathic mandible, increased skull size, intracranial calcifications	Calcitriol, aesthetic, and functional treatment
Paget disease of bone	Both maxilla and mandible	Radiolucent	Cotton wool–like irregular opaque lesions, loss of lamina dura, hypercementosis	Surgery for early lesions, drug therapy
Acromegaly	Mandible	Increased BMD	Mandibular prognathism, dental malocclusion, dense skull bones, enlarged pituitary fossa	Both surgical (transsphenoidal resection) and medical
CCD	Mandible and maxilla	Mixed densities	Hypoplastic or absent clavicles, supernumerary teeth and missing teeth	Symptomatic, aesthetic, and functional
Papillon-Lefèvre syndrome	Maxilla and mandible	Periapical radiolucency, alveolar resorption	Free floating teeth, premature loss of primary and permanent dentition	Periodontal therapy, medications
AI	Maxilla and mandible	Alterations to enamel thickness and density	Thinning of enamel and/or decreased radiodensity of enamel	Multidisciplinary approach for preventative measures, malocclusion, and aesthetics

(continued on next page)

Table 1
(continued)

Disorder	Commonly Affected Part (Jaws)	Radiographic Category	Radiopathognomic Sign	Treatment Strategy
Dentinogenesis imperfecta types II and III	Maxilla and mandible	Alterations in tooth morphology and density	Type II: bulbous crowns and obliteration of pulp and root canals Type III: hypoplastic dentin, described as shell teeth	Treatment of infections and restoring aesthetics
Dentin dysplasia type II	Maxilla and mandible	Alterations in tooth morphology and density	Primary teeth resemble features seen in dentinogenesis types II and III. Permanent teeth: may appear normal, but with pulpal chamber abnormalities, described as thistle/flame-shaped	Treatment of infections and restoring aesthetics
Regional odontodysplasia	All or part of maxillary quadrant	Decreased density of enamel and dentin with enlarged pulp chamber	Ghostlike teeth	Early extraction or conservative management of teeth

>> more commonly affected.

hypoplastic amelogenesis imperfecta (AI) is enamel agenesis.[1] Hypomature forms of AI present with dental crowns that are normal in size and contact adjacent teeth, but the mottled, brownish-yellow enamel is soft and has a radiodensity similar to dentin.[1] Lastly, in hypocalcified teeth, the enamel layer may be of normal thickness but is rough and soft and wears away quickly following tooth eruption.[1] Radiographically, mineral deficient enamel is marked by the lack of contrast between enamel and dentin[2] (**Fig. 1**).

Diagnostic Approach

Environmental factors and systemic diseases, such as fever, can be associated with enamel disorders that do not represent isolated AI.[3] Thus, diagnosis requires family history, pedigree plotting, and clinical observations for a diagnosis of AI.[4]

Management

Treatment of teeth usually depends on the state of enamel and likely requires a multi-disciplinary approach. Crowns may be used to improve the appearance of teeth and protect from damage.[5] Malocclusions occur in AI, so a treatment plan includes orthodontic consultation.[4]

DENTINOGENESIS IMPERFECTA TYPES II AND III

Dentinogenesis imperfecta describes a group of nonsyndromic, hereditary defects in dentin formation and pulp morphology.

Clinical and Radiographic Presentation

In general, both types II and III can involve primary and permanent teeth, and teeth are marked by a bluish to opalescent amber/brown discoloration.[6] Radiographically, teeth are bulbous with cervical constriction, with complete pulpal obliteration, including the root canals[6,7] (**Fig. 2**). Specifically, for type III, there may be multiple pulp exposures and periapical radiolucencies in noncarious teeth. Moreover, type III teeth present with hypotrophy of the dentin, and this appearance has been described as "shell" teeth.[6]

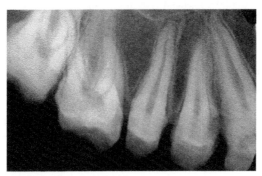

Fig. 1. Periapical radiograph showing features of AI (hypoplastic type). (*From* Al Zamel G, Odell S, Mupparapu M. Developmental disorders affecting jaws. Dental Clinics of North America 2016;60:39-90. (Figure 12 in original); with permission.)

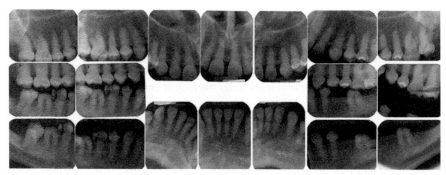

Fig. 2. Intraoral full mouth radiographic series demonstrating dentinogenesis imperfecta. (*From* Al Zamel G, Odell S, Mupparapu M. Developmental disorders affecting jaws. Dental Clinics of North America 2016;60:39-90. (Figure 13 in original); with permission.)

Diagnostic Approach

Historically, the Shields classification has divided inherited dentin defects in 5 types.[8,9] Despite overlap in clinical features, however, genetic studies have revealed distinctions within these groupings. Specifically, mutations in dentin sialophosphoproprotein (*DSPP*) have been mapped in dentinogenesis imperfecta types II and III and also in dentin dysplasia type II,[6,8] whereas dentinogenesis type I (osteogenesis imperfecta) demonstrates mutations in COL1A1 and presents with skeletal abnormalities not seen in types II and III. Notwithstanding the classification systems, diagnosis is based on history, clinical examination, and radiographic features.

Management

Aims of treatment are to remove sources of infection or pain, restore aesthetics, and protect posterior teeth from wear.[6]

DENTIN DYSPLASIA TYPE II

Dentin dysplasia type II is a nonsyndromic, hereditary defect that affects dentin formation and pulp morphology.

Clinical and Radiographic Presentation

Clinical features for dentin dysplasia type II overlap features seen in dentinogenesis imperfecta types II and III. In the permanent teeth, however, the teeth are normal in color, and on radiographs, the pulp chamber has a thistle/flame-shaped morphology and contains pulp stones.[6,8]

Diagnostic Approach

Based on a shared *DSPP* mutation between dentin dysplasia type II and dentinogenesis imperfecta types II and III, the clinical features seen may represent a spectrum along the same disease. Thus, dentin dysplasia type II may represent a milder clinical phenotype compared with dentinogenesis imperfecta type III.[3] Nevertheless, diagnosis is based on history, clinical examination, and radiographic features.

Management

Aims of treatment are to remove sources of infection or pain, restore aesthetics, and protect posterior teeth from wear.[6]

REGIONAL ODONTODYSPLASIA

Regional odontodysplasia is a nonhereditary disorder of root development that is associated with enamel and dentin dysplasia.

Clinical and Radiographic Presentation

Clinically, teeth are rough with a discolored crown surface, and all or part of a quadrant is affected, more often the maxilla than the mandible.[7,10] Both deciduous and/or permanent teeth can be affected.[11] Often, the most common clinical presentation is failure or delay of dental eruption.[10,12] Radiographically, affected teeth are hypoplastic with reduced radiodensity and enlarged pulp chamber, which have been described as "ghostlike"[10,12] (**Fig. 3**).

Diagnostic Approach

Although clinical and radiographic features, described previously, are diagnostic, histologic examination of affected teeth can be further supportive for diagnosis.

Management

Treatment of regional odontodysplasia involves early extraction of teeth, the rationale being that affected teeth are nonrestorable and susceptible to dental abscess formation after eruption.[10,13] Conversely, conservative management entails retaining noninfected teeth to help maintain alveolar bone.[13]

CLEIDOCRANIAL DYSPLASIA

Cleidocranial dysplasia (CCD) is a rare genetic disorder, reported in 1 in every 100,0000 cases, and is inherited as an autosomal dominant genetic trait. CCD represents several skeletal abnormalities.[14]

Clinical and Radiographic Presentation

Also known as cleidocranial dysostosis, this is a rare skeletal disorder with defective or absent clavicles causing sloping shoulders, moderately short stature, delayed eruption of teeth, incomplete development or absence of teeth, hypoplastic enamel, and supernumerary teeth (**Figs. 4** and **5**) apart from other features like delayed closure of fontanels, deformations of chest, and abnormal pelvic and pubic bones, which are common among other skeletal deformities. Individuals with CCD have increased

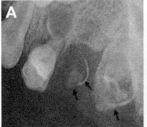
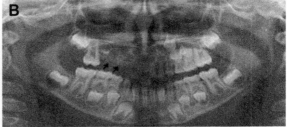

Fig. 3. Regional odontodysplasia. (*A*) Periapical radiograph showing ghostlike teeth (*arrows*). (*B*) Panoramic image shows thin shell of hypoplastic enamel and dentin (*arrows*). (*From* Masood F, Benavides E. Alterations in tooth structure and associated systemic conditions. Radiologic Clinics of North America 2018;56:125-140. (Figure 13 in original); with permission.)

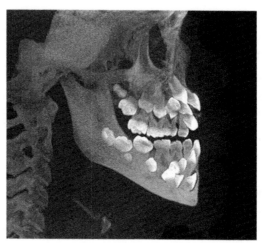

Fig. 4. Maximum intensity projection–rendered lateral skull reconstruction of the right side in a patient with CCD showing multiple unerupted supernumerary teeth in maxilla and mandible.

risk for recurrent ear and sinus infections and upper respiratory tract problems as well as hearing loss.

Diagnostic Approach and Management

Failure of resorption of overlying alveolar bone as well as mechanical interference from impacted supernumerary teeth leads to noneruption of many teeth.[15] Serial

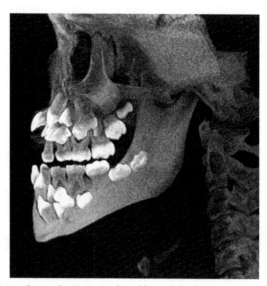

Fig. 5. Maximum intensity projection–rendered lateral skull reconstruction of the left side in a patient with CCD showing multiple unerupted supernumerary teeth in maxilla and mandible.

uncovering of teeth is suggested that would accelerate the eruption of these teeth. Interceptive and traditional orthodontics and selective osteotomies, all are part of the management of these patients.

- Genetic disorder inherited as an autosomal dominant trait
- Absent or defective clavicles, delayed eruption of teeth, supernumerary teeth
- Chest deformation, abnormal pelvis, short stature
- Recurrent ear and sinus infections
- Serial uncovering of teeth inducing eruption, selective osteotomies, orthodontics when possible are the treatments of choice,

OSTEOPOROSIS

Osteoporosis is a degenerative or metabolic bone disease associated with increased fracture risk, if left untreated or undiagnosed for long periods of time. Patients with this condition present with low bone mineral density (BMD) as well as changes in bony tissue structure. Osteoporosis is more prevalent in populations with deficiency in sex hormone, estrogen depletion (usually in postmenopausal women), and advanced age.

Clinical and Radiographic Findings

Patients who have low trauma fractures in bones not easily susceptible to fracture raise a suspicion for osteoporosis. The exception, however, is those with other previously diagnosed bone diseases like multiple myeloma. Postmenopausal women over the age 50 years also are more likely to have osteoporosis as are men and women over the age of 65 years. Other clinical risk factor, include alcoholism, smoking, and low body weight (<57.6 kg). Panoramic radiographic findings include an alteration in trabecular pattern of the bone and thinning of the mandibular cortex (**Fig. 6**).

Diagnosis

Diagnosis of osteoporosis is attained by assessing BMD. The most accurate assessment of BMD is with the use of dual-energy x-ray absorptiometry (DXA) scan. A T-score of less than −2.5, which compares the BMD of the patient to that of healthy

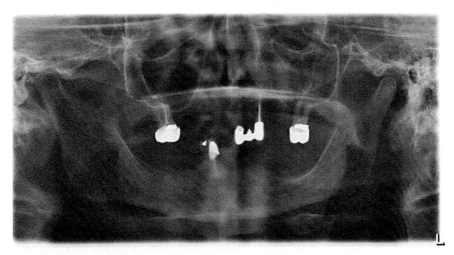

Fig. 6. Panoramic radiograph shows trabecular bone pattern consistent with decreased BMD within the body of the mandible bilaterally.

adults, is diagnostic for osteoporosis. When BMD is evaluated via computed tomography (CT), a procedure called quantitative CT is performed for BMD in lumbar spine, hip, and limbs. This is considered more specific compared with DXA.[16]

Management

Management of osteoporosis is dependent on disease severity.[17] The goal of treatment is to reduce fracture risk as well as maintain quality of life for patients with osteoporosis. Pharmacologic management includes the consecutive use of bone-building agents, such as teriparatide with bisphosphonates (oral or intravenous) or denosumab. Supplements like calcium and vitamin D as well as exercises, including those that focus on weight bearing and improving balance, can be used as preventive measures.

MEDICATION-RELATED OSTEONECROSIS OF THE JAW

Medication-related osteonecrosis of the jaw (MRONJ) can be described as persistent nonspecific odontogenic symptoms without exposed bone or exposed bone in the jaws of at least 8 weeks' duration in a patient treated with antiresorptives or antiangiogenic agents. Exclusion criteria for an MRONJ diagnosis include previous radiation treatment and primary or metastatic cancer to the head and neck.[18]

Clinical and Radiographic Findings

Clinical findings can vary from nonspecific presentation, such as periodontitis and mobile teeth, to more specific findings of fistulas, exposed bone, infection with purulent discharge, and pathologic fractures in severe cases. Radiologic findings also vary depending on stage of disease (**Table 2**), with CT being able to accurately identify

Table 2
Table showing clinical and radiographic findings in various stages of medication-related osteonecrosis of the jaw

Stage of Disease	Clinical Findings	Radiographic Findings
0	No exposed bone. Nonspecific pain symptoms, loose teeth in absence of diagnosed periodontitis, unexplained loss of alveolar bone	Sclerosis of the bone, thickening of lamina dura
1	Exposed bone or fistula. Absence of infection	Medullary/trabeculae sclerosis, interruption of the bony trabeculae (see **Fig. 7**), thickened lamina dura, widening of PDL, and osteolysis
2	Exposed bone with pain and evidence of infection	Periosteal reaction, widening of PDL. Cortical bone perforation, bone sequestrum, mucosal thickening in maxillary sinus
3	Exposed bone with pain and evidence of infection with 1 or more of the following: • Presence of pathologic fracture • Oroantral communication • Extraoral fistula	Fractures, bone sequestrum, cortical bone perforation, periosteal reaction, thickened lamina dura, distinct appearance of inferior alveolar nerve canal, mucosal thickening in maxillary sinus

Adapted from Omolehinwa TT, Akintoye SO. Chemical and radiation-associated jaw lesions. *Dent Clin North Am* 2016;60:265-277; and Ruggiero SL. Diagnosis and staging of medication-related osteonecrosis of the jaw. *Oral Maxillofac Surg Clin North Am* 2015;27:479-487 with permission.

disease extent at an early stage compared with panoramic radiographs (**Fig. 7**). Although MRONJ can affect either the maxilla or mandible, it is reported more commonly in the mandible.[19]

Diagnosis

A diagnosis is arrived at based on careful medical history as well as a patient meeting the inclusion and exclusion criteria for diagnosis based on definition of MRONJ.

Management

Treatment of MRONJ depends on stage/grade of the disease. This ranges from conservative treatment of stages 0 and 1 to surgical removal of the involved bone (stage 3).

OSTEITIS FIBROSA CYSTICA (BROWN TUMOR OF PRIMARY HYPERPARATHYROIDISM)

Primary hyperthyroidism (PHPT) is a condition that occurs from a primary problem in the parathyroid gland, usually a parathyroid adenoma, hyperplasia of the parathyroid

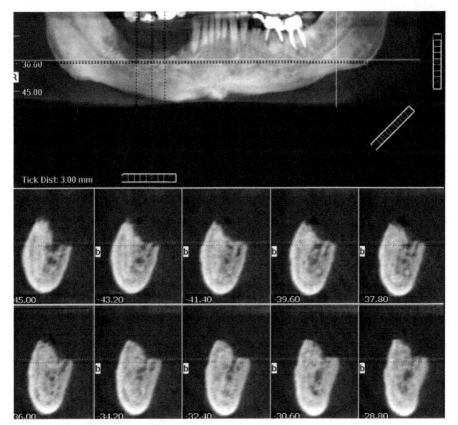

Fig. 7. CBCT scan depicting MRONJ in the right body of the mandible. The orthogonal sections of the mandibular right premolar and molar regions show the alveolar bone destruction and potential involvement of the inferior alveolar nerve canal in the region (sections 30.60 and 28.80).

gland, or, less commonly, a metastatic lesion affecting 1 or more of the parathyroid glands. PHPT results in excess secretion of parathyroid hormone (PTH) as well as increased calcium in the blood, that is, hypercalcemia, as a result of calcium resorption from the bones, kidneys, and small intestine. Brown tumor is a late complication of PHPT, which occurs in different body site as a result of calcium breakdown from the bone, resulting in bone resorption. In the head and neck, it occurs more commonly in the mandible.

Clinical and Radiographic Findings

Brown tumor of the jaw closely resembles giant cell tumor. Short teeth crowns and roots as well as enamel discoloration also frequently are noted radiographically. Patients with this condition also could present with burning mouth as a result of the anemia.[20]

Diagnosis

Blood work showing high levels of PTH and hypercalcemia and low phosphate levels helps with diagnosing this condition.

Management

Surgical resection of the involved parathyroid gland as well as the affected bone. Bone resection depends on the level of bone destruction.

CHERUBISM

Cherubism is a rare familial bone disease characterized by resorption limited to the jaws.

Clinical and Radiographic Presentation

Cherubism is defined by the appearance of symmetric, multilocular radiolucent lesions of the mandible and/or maxilla (**Fig. 8**) that typically appear at the age of 2 years to 7 years.[21] Clinically, this can manifest as a cherubic appearance—full round cheeks with the upward casting of eyes[21]—and enlargement of cervical lymph nodes, a high arched palate, and early loss of primary teeth. Moreover, supernumerary and missing teeth are common findings in patients with cherubism.[21]

Diagnostic Approach

Radiographic findings should raise suspicion for the disease. Common findings include bilateral multiloculated areas of the jaws that can clinically cause expansion. Additionally, radiographic findings can include multiple unerupted, impacted teeth in varying stages of development (see **Fig. 8**). Genetic testing may determine the presence of mutation in the cherubism gene SH3BP2.[22,23]

Management

Most cases regress spontaneously after puberty.[24] Surgical interventions are performed in individuals who have jaw expansion associated with complications, such as difficulty swallowing, tongue displacement, and upper respiratory dysfunction.[25]

THALASSEMIA

Thalassemia is a genetic hemoglobin disorder. It affects the alpha or beta chains of the globin component of hemoglobin, resulting in ineffective erythropoiesis as well as hemolysis. This results in malfunctioning hemoglobin and varying degrees of hemolytic anemia, depending on disease severity.

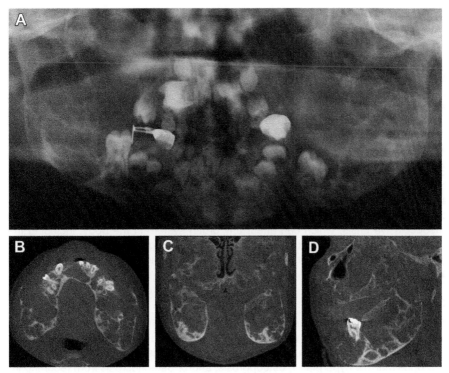

Fig. 8. (*A*) Panoramic radiograph of a child with cherubism shows bilateral, multilocular, expansile lesions in the posterior mandible and maxilla are evident and characteristic of the condition. Multiple teeth have been displaced largely in an anterior direction. (*B*) Axial, (*C*) coronal, and (*D*) sagittal CBCT sections demonstrate significant bony expansion bilaterally in both jaws. Note the multilocular appearance of the lesions. (*From* Ahmad M, Gaalaas L. Fibro-osseous and other lesions of bone in the jaws. Radiologic Clinics of North America 2018; 56:91-104. (Figure 7 in original); with permission.)

Clinical and Radiographic Presentation

Patients with this condition typically present with maxillary protrusion, teeth spacing, and class II malocclusion due to enlargement of bone marrow cavity from bone marrow hyperplasia to compensate for anemia.[26] On radiographs, the mandibular cortical bone is notably thin. Patients also have a higher caries rate from reduced amounts of immunoglobulin A and phosphorous in saliva and may present with gingivitis if their spleen has been removed. Short teeth crowns and roots also frequently are noted radiographically. Patients with this condition also could present with burning mouth as a result of the anemia. Systemically, they present with splenomegaly, hepatomegaly, jaundice, and osteoporosis.

Diagnostic Approach

Suspicion of thalassemia is higher in those of certain endemic areas and ancestry, including Africans, Middle Easterners, Asians, Italians, and those of Greek ancestry. Diagnosis of this condition is by blood/genetic testing, especially in patients with persistent anemia. This includes mean corpuscular volume (<80 fL), and mean corpuscular hemoglobin (<27 pg).[27,28] In most cases, diagnosis is achieved before the age of

2 years. Prenatal screening also should be considered in pregnant patients who have a diagnosis of thalassemia.

Management

Management of thalassemia involves blood transfusion and chelation therapy, particularly when there is iron overload from transfusion. In severe cases, hematopoietic stem cell transplantation is considered.

SICKLE CELL DISEASE

Sickle cell disease (SCD) is an inherited autosomal recessive disorder of the red blood cells, in which the disc shape of red blood cells is replaced by less flexible sickle-shaped cells. These abnormally shaped cells are fragile and sequester together, obstructing blood flow through the vessel wall. This results in hemolytic anemia and vasoocclusive crisis, which can affect any organ system in the body, including the bones of the head and neck, with a consequence of organ failure. This condition is most common in sub-Saharan Africa. Other areas include the Middle East, India, and Mediterranean area.

Clinical and Radiographic Presentation

The mandible is the second most common site of bone involvement in the head and neck region, with the orbital wall the most common head and neck site. Bone infarction/ischemia from vasoocclusion as well as osteomyelitis can occur in acute phases and bone marrow hyperplasia, osteoporosis, and/or osteonecrosis from recurring infarctions; transfusion-induced iron deposition in the bone is noted in chronic phases. Neuropathies also have been reported after a vasoocclusive crisis as a result of involvement of the inferior alveolar nerve. Radiographically, abnormal bony trabeculae pattern is noted as wide spacing and decreased radiodensity, commonly referred to as stepladder changes (**Fig. 9**). Osteosclerosis is seen in 15% of cases, and osteolysis may be noted in areas of bony infarcts (see **Fig. 9**). Osteoporosis/osteopenia is the finding reported most frequently in patients with SCD.[29] Avascular necrosis, noted most commonly in the femoral head, is the most debilitating bone complication of SCD. Osteomyelitis, although reported in less than 5% of patients with SCD, has been reported. When it does occur, it tends to affect the mandible. On magnetic resonance imaging (MRI), areas of bony infarcts may present with high signal intensity, whereas areas of iron deposits in bone may present with low to intermediate signal intensity.

Diagnosis

Based on blood group tests with detection of large amounts of hemoglobin S relative to fetal hemoglobin and hemoglobin A, neonatal screening usually is carried out at birth. For patients who are carriers of the hemoglobin S trait who also are married to carriers, fetal screening of the amniotic food also can be carried out.

Management

Blood transfusions and pharmacologic management with hydroxyurea are used in managing patients with SCD. Hematopoietic stem cell transplant currently is the only curative option. Gene therapy is being explored and results so far seem promising.

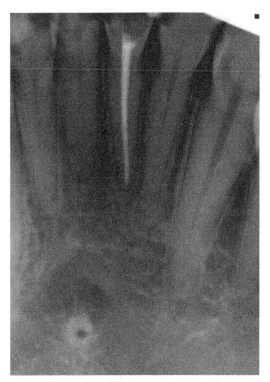

Fig. 9. SCD showing abnormal bony trabecular pattern in this mandibular central incisor posteroanterior radiograph. Note the prominent lingual foramen in this radiograph surrounded by large expanded bone marrow spaces suggestive of the underlying pathology. It is not common to find such a clear representation of the sickle cell–related findings in intraoral radiographs.

FIBROUS DYSPLASIA

Fibrous dysplasia (FD) is a genetically mosaic skeletal disorder caused by somatic missense mutations of the alpha-subunit of the stimulatory G protein encoded at the GNAS locus on chromosome 20q13.3.[30] The result is a gain-of-function mutation that impairs intrinsic activity of GTPase, leading to excessive production of intracellular cAMP. FD is an uncommon skeletal disorder with a broad spectrum of clinical presentation that ranges from incidental radiographic discovery in adulthood to a severely handicapping disease that presents early in life. FD is classified as monostotic FD when it involves 1 bone, polyostotic FD when it involves multiple bones, or panostotic FD when the entire skeleton is affected. FD often is associated with a wide range of extraskeletal manifestations that include café au lait skin hyperpigmentation and hyperfunctioning endocrinopathies, such as growth hormone excess, precocious puberty, hyperthyroidism, and Cushing syndrome. McCune-Albright syndrome (MAS) is a combination of FD with café au lait skin pigmentation and 1 or more endocrinopathies.[31] Although less common than MAS, polyostotic FD in the absence of endocrinopathies is referred to as Jaffe-Lichtenstein syndrome and association of FD with intramuscular myxomas is called Mazabraud syndrome.[31] Production of excessive fibroblast growth factor 23 (FGF-23) by dysplastic FD bone cells can lead to renal phosphate wasting,[32] and FD within the context of MAS has been associated with disorders of the pancreas, heart, liver, and other organs.[33]

Clinical Presentation and Radiographic Presentations

Clinical presentation of FD is variable depending on the severity of the FD lesions and skeletal sites affected, which could be a combination of craniofacial, appendicular, and axial skeletons. FD lesions can cause severe bone pain. Craniofacial bones commonly are affected with extensive expansion of the skull, maxilla, and mandible, resulting in severe facial disfigurement. Additionally, dental features associated with jaw FD may include enamel hypoplasia and hypomineralization, dentin dysplasia, odontoma, taurodontic pulp, and high caries index.[34–37] Panoramic radiograph and CT display homogeneous jaw FD lesion as ground-glass appearance whereas a heterogeneous lesion appears sclerotic with a mixed radiolucent/radiopaque regions (**Fig. 10**).[34,35,38] Although rare, sarcomatous change of FD should be suspected in a rapidly expanding FD lesion.

Management

A combination of clinical, radiographic, and histologic features is needed to diagnose, establish disease burden, and treat FD. Surgery is the main approach to severe FD. Bisphosphonates to control pain may be beneficial but should be used with caution due to the risk of osteonecrosis of the jaw.[31]

OSTEOPETROSIS (ALBERS-SCHÖNBERG DISEASE)

Albers-Schönberg disease is a rare inherited disorder, clinical manifestations of which include abnormally expansile jaw bones and skull due to abnormal bone growth and increased density. Three types are noted: osteopetrosis congenita and osteoporosis tarda, which are infantile, and adult-type marble bone disease (Albers-Schönberg disease). The 2 infantile forms are autosomal recessive and the adult type is autosomal dominant.[39]

Clinical and Radiographic Presentation

This disease is characterized by increasing bone density and abnormal bone growth. Patients present with delayed growth, hearing impairment, increased skull size,

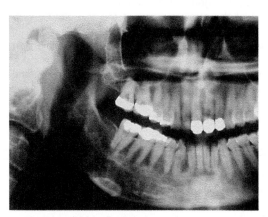

Fig. 10. Cropped panoramic radiograph showing a heterogeneous sclerotic lesion with mixed radiolucent/radiopaque areas on this right mandible.

intracranial calcifications, bone infection, increased incidence of caries, and mandibular prognathism. Symptoms vary from person to person.

Diagnostic Approach

In a dental setting, a panoramic radiograph reveals any gross abnormalities of the jaws, and skull views like posteroanterior skull, lateral skull, and Waters view add to the dental radiograph images. Cone beam CT (CBCT) is the choice of radiographic investigation because it is easier to localize dental disease and appropriate symptomatic treatment can be instituted.[39]

Management

Symptom-specific treatment can be given. Infantile osteoporosis can be treated with calcitriol, interferon gamma, erythropoietin, and bone marrow transplantation. Adult forms of osteopetrosis require treatment only for aesthetic or functional reasons.

- Rare inherited disorder manifested by expansile jaws and skull
- Due to increased thickness of jaws and skull, patients may present with prognathism, hearing impairment, bone infections.
- Panoramic radiographs and CBCT or CT are required for a diagnosis.
- Treated with calcitriol, interferon gamma, erythropoietin, and bone marrow transplants in severe cases

PAGET DISEASE OF BONE

Paget disease is a disorder of bone remodeling initiated by increased osteoclast-mediated bone resorption with compensatory increased formation of new bone and abnormal bone turnover.

Skeletal sites affected by Paget disease display an expansion of disorganized mosaic of woven and lamellar bone that is less compact, more vascular, and more susceptible to deformity and fracture. Paget disease may affect 1 bone (monostotic) or multiple bones (polyostotic).

Clinical Manifestations and Radiographic Presentations

Clinical presentations of Paget disease vary from patient to patient and from one skeletal site to the other. Although some patients may be asymptomatic, others may experience bone pain, deformity, fracture, compression of adjacent nerves, and excessive warmth due to bone hypervascularity. The skull bones commonly are affected and the disease could extend to the maxillofacial bones, causing facial disfigurement and dental malocclusions (**Fig. 11**). Most Paget disease patients are asymptomatic, so the disease may be discovered due to incidental radiographic findings and abnormal markers of bone turnover. Radiographically, the early-stage Paget disease is radiolucent as bone resorption occurs. This can transition to granular radiographic pattern that eventually may become irregular distributed radiopaque appearance. The maxilla and mandible often are enlarged while the teeth also could display loss of the lamina dura. These radiographic changes in the jaw present as a spotty cotton wool–like appearance in the trabecular and periapical regions. Some posterior teeth could display hyperplasia of the cementum and hypercementosis.[40,41]

Management

Treatment goals are to reduce symptoms and complications, but mild forms of Paget disease do not require treatment. High-potency bisphosphonates are the treatment of choice.[42] Occurrence of Paget disease at an early age often requires surgery and

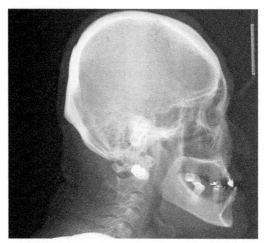

Fig. 11. Lateral cephalometric view of a patient whose chief complaint was anterior malocclusion and mandibular prognathism that recently was noticed.

bisphosphonate therapy. Dosing regimen of bisphosphonates should be monitored cautiously to prevent the complication of osteonecrosis of the jaw.[43]

ACROMEGALY

Acromegaly is a rare, progressive, acquired disorder affecting adults due to excessive secretion of growth hormone from the pituitary gland. Excess growth hormone production prior to puberty leads to gigantism in children.[44]

Clinical and Radiographic Skull Presentation

Prominent facial bones, enlarged skull due to increased calvarial thickening, frontal bossing (see **Fig. 13**), mandibular prognathism, and dental malocclusion are common features, with unusually thick and full lips. The sinuses are enlarged. The patients develop a deep husky voice due to thickening of vocal cords. Patients are prone to osteoarthritis, arthralgia, and myalgia. Patients also may have kyphoscoliosis and be prone to carpal tunnel syndrome, among many other symptoms. Some of the metabolic abnormalities include hypertension, type 2 diabetes mellitus, and obstructive sleep apnea.[45] In addition, the terminal phalangeal tufts become hypertrophied, giving the appearance of a spade, leading to a radiographic sign, known as the spade phalanx sign (**see Fig. 14**).

Diagnostic Approach

Patients are tested for elevated levels of insulinlike growth factor 1 that is associated with acromegaly. MDCT or MRI can reveal the presence of pituitary tumor. Because patients with acromegaly also are at increased risk for bone fractures, a DXA can be done for assessment of BMD.[45] In a dental setting, CBCT can be obtained to identify some of the skeletal changes, discussed previously.

Management

Both medical and dental therapeutic approaches are present but generally acromegaly is treated by transsphenoidal resection of all or part of the pituitary gland.

- Prominent facial bones, mandibular prognathism, and dental malocclusion can be found.
- Thickened vocal cords may lead to husky voice.
- DXA bone scan is recommended for assessment of bone density.
- CBCT may be useful in dental settings.
- Acromegaly is treated with transsphenoidal resection of all or part of pituitary gland.

RENAL OSTEODYSTROPHY

Renal osteodystrophy refers to the pathologic alterations of bone morphology associated with chronic kidney diseases. Because the kidneys play important roles in the regulation of calcium, phosphate, PTH, calcitriol (1,25-dihydroxyvitamin D), and FGF-23; chronic kidney disease causes dysregulation of mineral metabolism that in turn results in pathologic alterations of bone growth, modeling, and remodeling. The phosphate retention (hyperphosphatemia) in chronic kidney disease results in hypocalcemia and hyperparathyroidism. The damaged kidneys are unable to convert inactive vitamin D to the active form; this further stimulates PTH secretion in an effort to maintain serum calcium level. The response of the parathyroid gland causes a cascade of events that results in bone disease, extraskeletal calcifications, and cardiovascular outcomes.

Clinical Presentation and Radiographic Presentations

Renal osteodystrophy may present with normal, reduced, or elevated bone turnover, whereas bone mineralization may be either normal or impaired. Bone pain and joint pains are common and may be severe. Early radiographic features of renal osteodystrophy are subperiosteal bone resorption of the phalanges. There are generalized decrease in bone trabeculation and reduced cortical bone thickness at multiple skeletal sites.[46] Craniofacial radiological features include the salt and pepper skull displaying blurred demarcation between the inner and outer tables and granular cranial vault caused by trabecular bone resorption and osteosclerosis within the diploe.[47] Due to the initial subperiosteal bone resorption, there is thinning of the jaw cortical bones and loss of the lamina dura.[48] The secondary hyperparathyroidism with progression of bone turnover leads to osteolytic lesions, known as brown tumors of hyperparathyroidism. Some patients also can display diffuse generalized ground-glass opacities due to loss of bone trabeculation, whereas others may display extreme enlargement of the jaw caused by expansion of the malar processes, widening of the nares, and increased interdental spaces.[49,50]

Management

The therapeutic approach is to correct the hyperphosphatemia and lower PTH levels with the goal of limiting the cascade of events resulting from kidney damage.

GARDNER SYNDROME

Gardner syndrome is a clinical subgroup of familial adenomatous polyposis with autosomal dominant genetic transmission.[51]

Clinical and Radiographic Presentation

This condition is characterized by gastrointestinal polyps and extraintestinal manifestations like multiple osteomas in the mandible, skull, and long bones; desmoid tumors;

epidermal cysts on face, scalp, and extremities; and tissue tumors like lipomas, fibromas, and leiomyomas. Hypercementosis and odontomas also are noted. Dental abnormalities (**Fig. 12**) are noted in approximately 22% to 30% of familial adenomatous patients on the panoramic radiographs.[52] Increased alveolar bone density, presence of supernumerary teeth, and widened periodontal ligament (PDL) space are well depicted on CBCT imaging (**Fig. 13**).

Diagnostic Approach

Multiple impacted teeth can be identified through panoramic radiography and advanced imaging (CT). Radiographic evidence of osteomas and multiple unerupted and supernumerary teeth and colonoscopy showing multiple dysplastic polyps are diagnostic tests for Gardner syndrome.[52]

Management

Management of Gardner syndrome primarily involves surgical intervention for function and aesthetics. Because the polyps have a high malignant potential, they should be followed-up via their primary care physician.

- Multiple unerupted and supernumerary teeth, multiple dysplastic polyps are noted.
- Multiple osteomas of mandible, skull, and long bones are noted.
- Dermoid cysts and soft tissue tumors may be present.
- CT and colonoscopy are diagnostic tests.

PAPILLON-LEFÈVRE SYNDROME

Papillon-Lefèvre syndrome is an autosomal recessive disorder characterized by destructive periodontal disease of primary and permanent dentitions and hyperkeratosis of the palms of the hands and soles of the feet. It is attributed to a point mutation of the cathepsin C gene and alterations of the host defense due to defective functions of lymphocytes, leukocytes, and monocytes responsible for the body's defense against infections.[53]

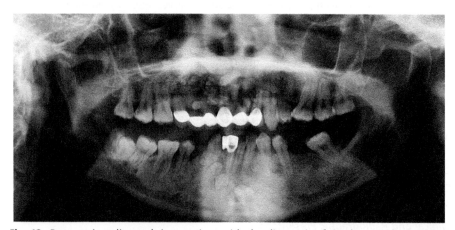

Fig. 12. Panoramic radiograph in a patient with the diagnosis of Gardner syndrome. Note the presence of multiple osteomas as well as unerupted permanent and supernumerary teeth. (Image courtesy of Dr. Steven Singer, DDS, Newark, NJ.)

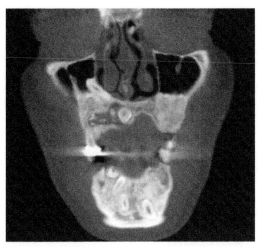

Fig. 13. Coronal CBCT at the level of maxillary sinuses showing several impacted permanent and supernumerary teeth, osteomas in both mandible and maxilla (homogenous densities noted on the left) as well as hypoplastic maxillary sinuses. (Image courtesy of Dr. Steven Singer, DDS, Newark, NJ.)

Clinical Management and Radiographic Presentations

Onset of the disease is associated with eruption of the primary dentition after which gingiva becomes inflamed and combined with rapid destruction of the periodontal tissues and exfoliation of primary teeth. After eruption of the permanent dentitions, the aggressive periodontal destruction is repeated, leading to rapid loss of the permanent dentition during the teenage years. Radiographically, maxillary and mandibular teeth display periapical radiolucency, alveolar bone resorption, and free-floating teeth.[54]

Management

Palmoplantar hyperkeratosis is treated with anti-inflammatory emollients and keratolytic agents like topical steroids and salicylic acid. Conventional periodontal therapy combined with use of adjunctive use of antibiotics and antimicrobial oral rinses are used mainly to stabilize the aggressive periodontitis of Papillon-Lefèvre syndrome. Placement of dental implants after loss of the permanent dentition has been found successful.[55,56]

NEVOID BASAL CELL CARCINOMA SYNDROME (GORLIN SYNDROME)

Nevoid basal cell carcinoma syndrome is an autosomal dominant inherited syndrome characterized by tumor formation and skeletal abnormalities.

Clinical and Radiographic Presentation

Nevoid basal cell carcinoma syndrome (NBCCS) has a wide range of clinical manifestations. There have been no studies to define the sensitivity and specificity of which phenotypic combination is most accurate for diagnosis.[57] Diagnosis can be reasonably made, however, based on major and minor criteria (discussed later). Most patients develop multiple odontogenic keratocysts (OKCs) within the first and second decades of life. There is continuous development of new and recurring cysts, which can number up to 30 cysts.[58] The mandible is affected more commonly than the maxilla.[58] Radiographically, OKCs can present as unilocular or multilocular radiolucencies with a smooth or scalloped border (**Fig. 14**).[58]

Diagnostic Approach

The genetic basis of the syndrome involves mutations in several genes in the sonic hedgehog signaling pathway, including PTCH1 and SUFU.[57,59] Diagnosis of NBCS involves (1) 1 major criterion and molecular confirmation; (2) 2 major criteria; or (3) 1 major and 2 minor criteria[57–59]:

Major criteria
1. Multiple basal cell carcinomas (BCCs) prior to age 20 years old or excessive BCCs out of proportion to prior sun exposure and skin type
2. OKCs of the jaws prior to age 20 years old
3. Palmar or plantar pitting
4. Lamellar calcification of the falx cerebri
5. First degree relatives with NBCCS
6. Medulloblastoma (desmoplastic)

Minor criteria
1. Rib anomalies
2. Other specific skeletal malformations and radiologic changes: vertebral anomalies, kyphoscoliosis, short fourth metacarpals, postaxial polydactyly
3. Macrocephaly
4. Cleft/lip palate
5. Ovarian/cardiac fibroma
6. Lymphomesenteric cysts
7. Ocular abnormalities: strabismus, hypertelorism, congenital cataracts, glaucoma, coloboma

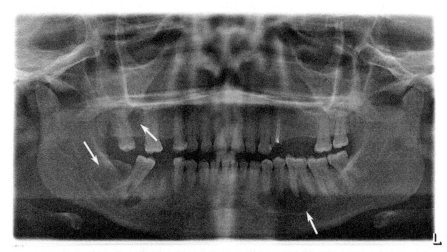

Fig. 14. OKCs in a 42-year-old woman. Panoramic radiograph shows OKC in the right maxillary molar region (*middle arrow*), another OKC in the mandibular right posterior region (*left arrow*), and another OKC in the left mandibular body (*right arrow*). Multiple OKCs are seen in a patient with basal cell nevus syndrome. (*From* Gohel A, Villa A, Sakai O. Benign jaw lesions. Dental Clinics of North America 2016;60:125-141. (Figure 6 in original); with permission.)

Management

A multidisciplinary approach is needed to address the diversity of issues in patients with NBCCS.

CLINICS CARE POINTS

- Systemic diseases can present with radiographic changes in jaws and teeth that do not correspond to common entities of an everyday dental practice.

- In general, radiographic changes range from alterations in enamel, dentin, and bone trabeculation.

- Based on the amount of bone involvement, the radiographic changes can vary from radiolucencies to complete opacifications and mixed density appearances.

- Radiographic appearances or changes in a systemic disease can be due to environmental factors or metabolic dysfunction or be syndromic.

DISCLOSURES

The authors have nothing to disclose.

REFERENCES

1. Hu JCC, Chun YHP, Al Hazzazzi T, et al. Enamel formation and amelogenesis imperfecta. Cells Tissues Organs 2007;186:78–85.
2. Collins MA, Mauriello SM, Tyndall DA, et al. Dental anomalies associated with amelogenesis imperfect: a radiographic assessment. Oral Surg Oral Med Oral Pathol Oral Radiol Endod 1999;88:358–64.
3. Neville BW, Damm, DD, Allen CM, et al. Oral and maxillofacial pathology. Fourth edition. St Louis, (MO): Elsevier; 2016.
4. Crawford PJM, Aldred M, Bloch-Zupan A, et al. Amelogenesis imperfecta. Orphanet J Rare Dis 2007;2:17.
5. Dashash M, Yeung CA, Jamous I, et al. Interventions for the restorative care of amelogenesis imperfect in children and adolescents. Cochrane Database Syst Rev 2013;6:CD007517.
6. Barron MJ, McDonnell ST, MacKie I, et al. Hereditary dentine disorders: dentinogenesis imperfect and dentine dysplasia. Orphanet J Rare Dis 2008;3:31.
7. Luder HU. Malformations of the tooth root in humans. Front Physiol 2015;6:307.
8. Bailleul-Forestier I, Molla M, Verloes A, et al. Genetic basis of inherited anomalies of the teeth: part 1: clinical and molecular aspects of non-syndromic dental disorders. Eur J Med Genet 2008;51:273–91.
9. Kim JW, Simmer JP. Hereditary dentin defects. J Dent Res 2007;86:392–9.
10. Spini TH, Sargenti-Neto S, Cardoso SV, et al. Progressive dental development in regional odontodysplasia. Oral Surg Oral Med Oral Pathol Oral Radiol Endod 2007;104:e40–5.
11. Cunha JLS, Santana AVB, da Mota Santana LA, et al. Regional odontodysplasia affecting the maxilla. Head Neck Pathol 2020;14:224–9.
12. Tervonen SA, Stratmann U, Mokrys K, et al. Regional odontodysplasia: a review of the literature and report of four cases. Clin Oral Investig 2004;8:45–51.
13. Cho SY. Conservative management of regional odontodysplasia: case report. J Can Dent Assoc 2006;72:735–8.

14. Mundlos S. Cleidocranial dysplasia: clinical and molecular genetics. J Med Genet 1999;36:177–82.
15. Farrar EL, Van Sickels JE. Early surgical management of cleidocranial dysplasia: a preliminary report. J Oral Maxillofac Surg 1983;41:527–9.
16. Pauwels R, Jacobs R, Singer SR, et al. CBCT-based bone quality assessment: are Hounsfield units applicable? Dentomaxillofac Radiol 2015;44:20140238.
17. Camacho PM, Petak SM, Binkley N, et al. American association of clinical endocrinologists/american college of endocrinology clinical practice guidelines for the diagnosis and treatment of postmenopausal osteoporosis-2020 update. Endocr Pract 2020;26(Suppl 1):1–46.
18. Omolehinwa TT, Akintoye SO. Chemical and radiation-associated jaw lesions. Dent Clin North Am 2016;60:265–77.
19. Rosella D, Papi P, Giardino R, et al. Medication-related osteonecrosis of the jaw: Clinical and practical guidelines. J Int Soc Prev Community Dent 2016;6:97–104.
20. Dos Santos B, Koth VS, Figueiredo MA, et al. Brown tumor of the jaws as a manifestation of tertiary hyperparathyroidism: A literature review and case report. Spec Care Dentist 2018;38:163–71.
21. Papadaki ME, Lietman SA, Levine MA, et al. Cherubism: best clinical practice. Orphanet J Rare Dis 2012;7(Suppl 1):S6.
22. Ueki Y, Tiziani V, Santanna C, et al. Mutations in the gene encoding c-Abl-binding protein SH3BP2 cause cherubism. Nat Genet 2001;28:125–6.
23. Rechenberger EJ, Levine MA, Olsen BR, et al. The role of SH3BP2 in the pathophysiology of cherubism. Orphanet J Rare Dis 2012;7(Suppl 1):S5.
24. Kozakiewicz M, Perczynska-Partyka W, Kobos J. Cherubism – clinical picture and treatment. Oral Dis 2001;7:122–30.
25. Tekin AF, Unal OF, Goksel S, et al. Clinical and radiological evaluation of cherubism: a rare case report. Radiol Case Rep 2020;15:416–9.
26. Helmi N, Bashir M, Shireen A, et al. Thalassemia review: features, dental considerations and management. Electron Physician 2017;9:4003–8.
27. Lee YK, Kim HJ, Lee K, et al. Recent progress in laboratory diagnosis of thalassemia and hemoglobinopathy: a study by the Korean red blood cell disorder working party of the Korean society of hematology. Blood Res 2019;54:17–22.
28. Saito N, Nadgir RN, Flower EN, et al. Clinical and radiologic manifestations of sickle cell disease in the head and neck. Radiographics 2010;30:1021–35.
29. De Luna G, Ranque B, Courbebaisse M, et al. High bone mineral density in sickle cell disease: prevalence and characteristics. Bone 2018;110:199–203.
30. Bianco P, Riminucci M, Majolagbe A, et al. Mutations of the GNAS1 gene, stromal cell dysfunction, and osteomalacic changes in non-McCune-Albright fibrous dysplasia of bone. J Bone Miner Res 2000;15:120–8.
31. Foster BL, Ramnitz MS, Gafni R, et al. Rare bone diseases and their dental, oral, and craniofacial manifestations. J Dent Res 2014;93(7 Suppl):7S–19S.
32. Collins MT, Chebli C, Jones J, et al. Renal phosphate wasting in fibrous dysplasia of bone is part of a generalized renal tubular dysfunction similar to that seen in tumor-induced osteomalacia. J Bone Miner Res 2001;16:806–13.
33. Shenker A, Weinstein LS, Moran A, et al. Severe endocrine and nonendocrine manifestations of the McCune-Albright syndrome associated with activating mutations of stimulatory G protein GS. J Pediatr 1993;123:509–18.
34. Akintoye SO, Boyce AM, Collins MT. Dental perspectives in fibrous dysplasia and McCune-Albright syndrome. Oral Surg Oral Med Oral Pathol Oral Radiol 2013; 116:e149–55.

35. Akintoye SO, Lee JS, Feimster T, et al. Dental characteristics of fibrous dysplasia and McCune-Albright syndrome. Oral Surg Oral Med Oral Pathol Oral Radiol Endod 2003;96:275–82.
36. Burke AB, Collings MT, Boyce AM. Fibrous dysplasia of bone: craniofacial and dental implications. Oral Dis 2017;23:697–708.
37. Akintoye SO, Chebli C, Booher S, et al. Characterization of gsp-mediated growth hormone excess in the context of McCune-Albright syndrome. J Clin Endocrinol Metab 2002;87:5104–12.
38. Akintoye SO, Otis LL, Atkinson JC, et al. Analyses of variable panoramic radiographic characteristics of maxilla-mandibular fibrous dysplasia in McCune-Albright syndrome. Oral Dis 2004;10:36–43.
39. Carolino J, Perez JA, Popa A. Osteopetrosis. Am Fam Physician 1988;57:1293–6.
40. Ahmad M, Gaalaas. Fibro-osseous and other lesions of bone in the jaws. Radiol Clin North Am 2018;56:91–104.
41. Bender IB. Paget's disease. J Endod 2003;29:720–3.
42. Reid IR, Miller P, Lyles K, et al. Comparison of a single infusion of zoledronic acid with risedronate for Paget's disease. N Engl J Med 2005;353:898–908.
43. Khosla S, Burr D, Cauley J, et al. Bisphosphonate-associated osteonecrosis of the jaw: report of a task force of the American Society for Bone and Mineral Research. J Bone Miner Res 2007;22:1479–91.
44. Melmed S. Medical progress: acromegaly. N Engl J Med 2006;355:2558–73.
45. Melmed S. Acromegaly pathogenesis and treatment. J Clin Invest 2009;119:3189–202.
46. You M, Tang B, Wang ZJ, et al. Radiological manifestations of renal osteodystrophy in the orofacial region: a case report and literature review. Oral Radiol 2018;34:262–6.
47. Kanjevac T, Bijelic B, Brajkovic D, et al. Impact of chronic kidney disease mineral and bone disorder on jaw and alveolar bone metabolism: a narrative review. Oral Health Prev Dent 2018;16:79–85.
48. Chang JI, Som PM, Lawson W. Unique imaging findings in the facial bones of renal osteodystrophy. AJNR Am J Neuroradiol 2007;28:608–9.
49. Collum J, Jones RH, Lynham A, et al. Leontiasis ossea: a presentation of hyperparathyroidism in an indigenous Australian man secondary to chronic renal failure. J Oral Maxillofac Surg 2013;71:56–61.
50. Raubenheimer EJ, Noffke CE, Mohamed A. Expansive jaw lesions in chronic kidney disease: review of the literature and a report of two cases. Oral Surg Oral Med Oral Pathol Oral Radiol 2015;119:340–5.
51. Gardner EJ. Follow-up study of a family group exhibiting dominant inheritance for a syndrome including intestinal polyps, osteomas, fibromas and epidermoid cysts. Am J Hum Genet 1962;4:376–90.
52. Wolf J, Jarvinen HJ, Hietanen J. Gardner's dento-maxillary stigmas in patients with familial adenomatosis coli. Br J Oral Maxillofac Surg 1986;24:410–6.
53. Dhanrajani PJ. Papillon-Lefevre syndrome: clinical presentation and a brief review. Oral Surg Oral Med Oral Pathol Oral Radiol Endod 2009;108:e1–7.
54. Jose J, Bartlett K, Salgado C, et al. Papillon-Lefèvre syndrome: review of imaging findings and current literature. Foot Ankle Spec 2015;8:139–42.
55. Ullbro C, Crossner CG, Lundgren T, et al. Osseointegrated implants in a patient with Papillon-Lefevre syndrome: a 4-1/2–year follow-up. J Clin Periodontol 2000;27:951–4.
56. Senel FC, Altintas NY, Bagis B, et al. A 3-year follow-up of the rehabilitation of Papillon-Lefèvre syndrome by dental implants. J Oral Maxillofac Surg 2012;70:163–7.

57. Bree AF, Shah MR. Consensus statement from the first international colloquium on basal cell nevus syndrome (BCNS). Am J Med Genet A 2011;155A:2091–7.
58. Lo Muzio. Nevoid basal cell carcinoma (Gorlin syndrome). Orphanet J Rare Dis 2008;3:32.
59. Fujii K, Miyashita. Gorlin syndrome (nevoid basal cell carcinoma syndrome): update and literature review. Pediatr Int 2014;56:667–74.

Radiographic Evaluation of Prosthodontic Patients

Eva Anadioti, DDS, MS, FACP[a],*, Heidi Kohltfarber, DDS, MS, PhD, FADI, FICD[b]

KEYWORDS

- CBCT • Prosthodontics • Implant planning • Virtual planning • Guided surgery
- Radiographic guide • 3D imaging

KEY POINTS

- Prosthetically driven implant planning enables and ensures esthetic, functional, and long-lasting restorative outcomes.
- Cone-beam computed tomography is the preferred imaging method for pretreatment dental implant treatment planning.
- The prosthodontically driven implant planning includes evaluation of adjacent anatomy, three-dimensional measurements of the edentulous sites, anterior-posterior spread considerations, and restorative space assessment.
- Restorative space assessment is necessary to ensure adequate space for optimum physical and mechanical properties of all components/materials required in the prosthesis.

Implant imaging for the rehabilitation of the partially and completely edentulous patient.

INTRODUCTION

Prosthodontics is the dental specialty pertaining to the diagnosis, treatment planning, rehabilitation, and maintenance of the oral function and esthetics of patients with missing or deficient teeth by using prosthetic substitutes.[1] Prosthodontic patients may be completely dentate and interested in improving the esthetics and/or function of their existing dentition. They could also be missing 1 or more teeth (partially edentulous) or all of their teeth (completely edentulous) and seeking to replace their missing dentition. The prosthetic substitutes that prosthodontists use to restore and/or replace the deficient tissues may be divided into 4 categories depending on the type of support that is used:

---

[a] Department of Preventive and Restorative Sciences, University of Pennsylvania School of Dental Medicine, 240 South 40th Street, Philadelphia, PA 19104, USA; [b] Division of Diagnostic Sciences, University of North Carolina School of Dentistry, 385 S Columbia St, Chapel Hill, NC 27599, USA
* Corresponding author.
E-mail address: evanad@upenn.edu

Dent Clin N Am 65 (2021) 605–621
https://doi.org/10.1016/j.cden.2021.02.007
0011-8532/21/© 2021 Elsevier Inc. All rights reserved.

1. Fixed prostheses supported on remaining teeth, which cannot be removed by the patient, such as veneers, onlays, inlays, full-coverage crowns, and fixed dental prostheses (FDPs).
2. Removable prostheses supported mainly on soft tissues, which can be removed by the patient, such as complete or partial dental prostheses (dentures) and overdentures.
3. Fixed or removable prostheses that are supported mainly by dental implants.
4. Maxillofacial prostheses, intraoral or extraoral, and are supported on hard and/or soft tissues and/or dental implants.

The evolution of implant dentistry has expanded the prosthetic rehabilitation options for completely and partially edentulous patients and those dentate patients with indications for tooth extraction.[2] The patient selection criteria along with thorough clinical and radiographic evaluation of areas indicated for implant therapy play a major role in the planning process that greatly affects the prosthetic result. Therefore, it is of paramount importance to begin the planning process with the end in mind. Prosthetically driven implant planning enables and ensures esthetic, functional, and long-lasting prosthodontic outcomes.[3] This article focuses on the radiographic evaluation with regard to planning, treating, and maintaining partially and completely edentulous prosthodontic patients with dental implants.

BACKGROUND
Cone-Beam Computed Tomography

Sir Godfrey Hounsfield introduced a technology that used image reconstruction developed by Alan Cormack in the 1960s. This discovery became known as computed tomography (CT) and its three-dimensional (3D) capabilities revolutionized medicine; it is now the standard of care for diagnostic imaging in medicine. Similarly, the advent of implant dentistry fueled a desire for a 3D imaging system that had lower radiation dose than medical CT as well as lower cost to the patient. Cone-beam CT (CBCT) was introduced in 1998 by Mozzo and colleagues[4] when they described the NewTom-9000 as a low-dose alternative to medical CT for implant planning purposes. CBCT units can be dedicated machines for only 1 field of view (FOV) or may be able to image a variety of FOVs within the same unit. Example of the various FOVs associated with corresponding diagnostic tasks are as follows:

1. FOV 4 to 10 cm (2"–4"): adequate for imaging the dentoalveolar region for a more local or endodontic purpose.
2. FOV 10 to 15 cm (4"–6"): adequate for imaging the maxillary and mandibular region for implants and dentoalveolar concerns.
3. FOV 15 to 23 cm (6"–9"): desirable for the maxillofacial and craniofacial regions for orthodontic and oral surgery, and evaluation of the temporomandibular joints.

One of the well-known advantages of CBCT is its ability to provide isotropic voxels (a cuboidal volume element that is geometrically equal in the x, y, and z planes). Therefore, it provides geometric accuracy, minimal distortion, as well as a 1:1 measurement ratio of objects within the volumetric images.[4–6] However, it is not able to differentiate between soft tissue densities such as fluid and soft tissue disorders because of its lack of gray-scale sensitivity,[7] but it is able to clearly and accurately visualize high-contrast osseous structures in the maxillofacial region.[4,8–10] The advantages and disadvantages of various imaging modalities used in the evaluation and treatment planning for potential implant sites, such as panoramic radiography and CBCT, are compared in **Table 1**.[7,11–13]

Table 1
Advantages and disadvantages of panoramic images and cone-beam computed tomography

Imaging Modalities	Advantages	Disadvantages
Panoramic radiography	• Most common dental radiograph available • Low cost • Low radiation dose • Broad coverage of facial hard tissues • High patient tolerance	• Image distortions • Panoramic parallax • Superimposition of structures • Low efficacy when evaluating the maxillary sinuses • Poor soft tissue detail • Low resolution
CBCT	• Evaluation of anatomy in 3 planes (axial, coronal, sagittal) • Excellent hard tissue detail • Isotropic voxels • High spatial resolution • No superimpositions of structures	• Poor soft tissue contrast • Imaging artifacts such as beam hardening and streak artifacts from high-contrast objects such as cortical bone and dental metallic restorations • Image noise caused by cone-beam geometry • Higher cost and dose compared with panoramic imaging

Table 2
Dosimetry of multiple cone-beam computed tomography units and a multidetector computed tomography

CBCT/CT	Effective Dose (μSv)[c]	Digital Panoramic Equivalent[d]	Annual Per Capita Background Radiation (d)[e]
CBCT examination (average dose for small-FOV protocols)[b]	84	6	10
CBCT examination (average dose for medium-FOV protocols)[b]	177	13	21
CBCT examination (average dose for large-FOV protocols)[b]	212	15	25
Medical CT maxillomandibular: skull[a]	2100	150	247
Comparison with Somatom Sensation32 row/64 slice MultiDetector CT[a]	860	61	101
Comparison with Somatom 32-row/64-slice multidetector CT with CARE dose 4 D[a]	534	38	63

Effective Doses from CBCT and Medical CT Compared with Digital Panoramic Equivalent and Days of Per Capita Background Radiation

Small-FOV CBCT scan doses range from 5 to 652 μSv for all protocols. Medium-FOV CBCT scan doses range from 9 to 560 μSv for all protocols. Large-FOV CBCT scans doses range from 46 to 1073 μSv for all protocols. The CARE dose is the pediatric dose.
[a] Ludlow and colleagues,[15,16] Ludlow and Ivanovic.[17]
[b] Ludlow and colleagues.[18]
[c] Effective dose calculated with International Commission on Radiological Protection 2007 tissue weights.
[d] Median of published effective dose for digital dental panoramic radiography = 14 μSv.
[e] Annual per capita = 3.1 mSv (3100 μSv) per annum or approximately 8.5 μSv/d in the United States.

Cone-Beam Computed Tomography Dosimetry

Low-level ionizing radiation is used with CBCT. Dental practitioners are taught to observe the principle of as low as reasonably achievable as well as selection criteria in the use of ionizing radiation.[14] However, a discussion of dosimetry is important when deciding whether an image is justified for a particular diagnostic purpose. The effective dose is used to calculate radiation dose and represented in microsieverts (μSv). This method can give a broad indication of the level of detriment to health from radiation exposure by expressing the risk to the whole body. The effective dose takes into consideration both the volume as well as the sensitivity of the tissues involved.[15–18] It is estimated that the population in the United States receives approximately 3100 μSv of ubiquitous background radiation a year, which equates to approximately 8.5 μSv/d. An additional average annual dose from medical sources of approximately 3100 μSV to the population has been cited, bringing the total average yearly dose from both background radiation and medical sources to 6200 μSv/y.[19] **Table 2** shows the various FOVs and effective doses of CBCT units with a comparison with digital panoramic units as well as days of per capita background radiation in the United States. Medical CT radiation dose is also observed for comparison purposes.[14–18]

DISCUSSION

The American Academy of Oral and Maxillofacial Radiology (AAOMR) recommends cross-sectional imaging for dental implant treatment planning and that CBCT is the preferred imaging method for obtaining the pretreatment images.[20] In addition, it is advised that a panoramic radiograph with supplemented intraoral images should be taken for the initial pretreatment evaluation to determine whether the patient is a candidate for implants before taking a CBCT scan (**Fig. 1**).

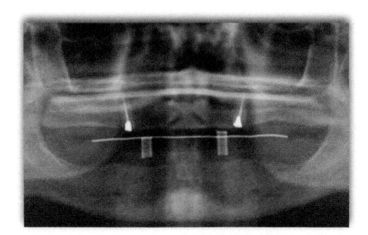

Fig. 1. Panoramic radiograph with guide to determine implant location and need for pre-prosthetic surgery. A metal wire was used on the occlusal/incisal surface of the mandibular interim prosthesis, which is at the correct occlusal vertical dimension, to illustrate radiographically the occlusal plane and therefore measure the restorative space. Alveoloplasty is needed to create 10 to 12 mm of restorative space for unsplinted implant overdenture.

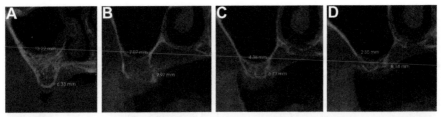

Fig. 2. Residual bone height using the classification by Jensen and colleagues.[21] (A) Class A (≥10 mm), no sinus augmentation needed; (B) class B (7–9 mm), small crestal osteotomy with immediate implant placement; (C) class C (4–6 mm), sinus elevation with a lateral approach and immediate or delayed implant; (D) class D (1–3 mm), sinus elevation with a lateral approach and a second procedure for implant placement.

Diagnosis and Treatment Planning for Prosthodontic Patients

Anatomy

The anatomy surrounding the potential implant site should be thoroughly evaluated. Before focusing on the height and width of the residual alveolar bone to measure the dimensions for implant placement, the entire volume should be reviewed to rule out pathologic entities. Sinus augmentation procedure recommendations using the residual alveolar bone height classification is used as a reference for predictable implant treatment planning (**Fig. 2**).[21,22] The following localized anatomy should be evaluated in the pretreatment assessment of the CBCT based on the position of the desired implant[23–26]:

Maxilla (**Figs. 3–5**)
1. Maxillary tuberosity
2. Maxillary sinuses
   a. Thickness and angle of the lateral cortical borders
   b. Topography of the sinus floor and bony septations
   c. The height and width of the maxillary sinus
   d. Location of the maxillary sinus ostium to ensure that sinus augmentation will not result in blockage of the sinus drainage pathway
   e. Vascularization along the floor of the maxillary sinus: posterior superior alveolar artery, infraorbital artery, and the anastomosis between the 2 arteries known as the alveolar antral artery

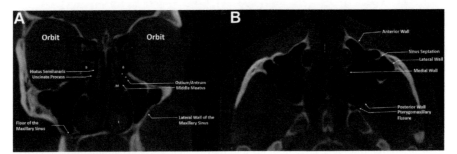

Fig. 3. Maxillary sinus anatomy. (A) Coronal image showing the M (middle turbinate), I (inferior turbinate), B (ethmoidal bulla), and asterisk (infundibulum). (B) Axial image of the maxillary sinus anatomy.

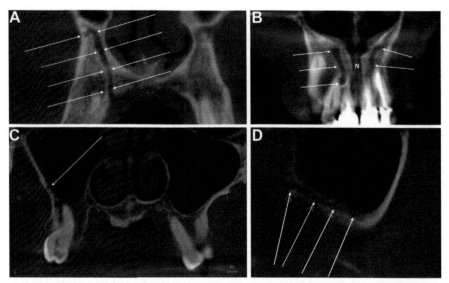

Fig. 4. Maxillary neurovascular bundles. (*A*) Anterior superior alveolar nerve canal descending in the canine region, and (*B*) within the lateral incisor regions along with the location of the nasopalatine canal (N). (*C* and *D*) The location of the posterior superior alveolar artery and nerve canal as it extends anteriorly along the lateral cortical border of the maxillary sinus to anastomose with the infraorbital neurovascular canal.

> f. Posterior superior alveolar nerve canal
> g. Common incidental findings that may complicate sinus augmentation, such as mucosal thickenings/sinus disease, mucus retention pseudocysts, and antroliths
> 3. Nasopalatine canal

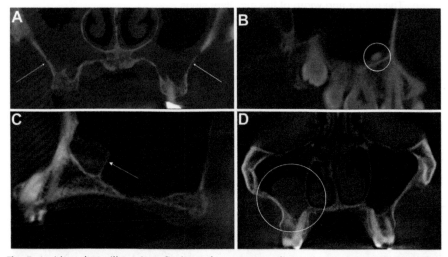

Fig. 5. Incidental maxillary sinus findings that may complicate sinus augmentation, such as (*A*) bilateral mucosal thickenings (*arrows*) indicating acute rhinosinusitis, (*B*) antrolith (*circled*), (*C*) sinus septation(*arrow*), and (*D*) mucus retention pseudocyst (*circle*). Note that the ostium is patent (*red arrow*) in the volume at this time.

4. Anterior superior alveolar nerve canal
5. Pathologic findings such as tumor or cysts

Mandible (**Fig. 6**)

1. Submandibular fossa and mylohyoid ridge
2. Mandibular foramen and lingula
3. Mandibular canal location as well as potential bifurcation and anterior loop
4. Mental foramen location as well as potential accessory foramina
5. Lingual canal location and anatomic variants
6. Genial tubercles
7. Pathologic findings such as tumors or cysts

In general, a minimum of 1 mm of circumferential bone is required to allow sufficient volume to stabilize an implant.[27] A 2-mm margin of safety is recommended next to all pertinent anatomic structures.[28] The presurgical radiographic evaluation also determines the need for additional surgical procedures before or at the time of implant placement to ensure appropriate distance from adjacent anatomy and adequate surrounding bone volume for implant stability, such as indirect or direct sinus augmentation, inferior alveolar nerve repositioning, and bone graft (**Fig. 7**).

Radiographic measurements of the partially edentulous site

1. Mesial-distal (MD) dimension: between an implant and a tooth at least 1.5 mm and between 2 implants at least 3 mm are required to preserve adequate blood supply and maintain healthy hard and soft tissues.[29,30]
2. Buccal-palatal/lingual (BP/L) dimension: at least 1.5 mm from the buccal bone is recommended to maintain tissue architecture after tooth extraction and implant placement.[31] To facilitate that, the implant should be placed 2 mm palatal/lingual to the planned gingival zenith.[32]
3. Incisal-apical (IA) dimension: the bone crest to the interproximal contact point should be less than 6 mm to support papilla formation.[33] The implant-abutment

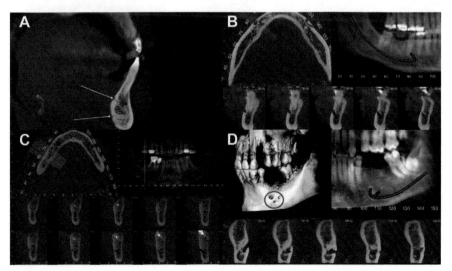

Fig. 6. Mandibular anatomy normal variants that may complicate implant placement, such as (*A*) multiple lingual canals (*arrows*), (*B*) anterior loop of the mandibular canal, (*C*) mandibular canal bifurcations and accessory canals, and (*D*) multiple mental foramina.

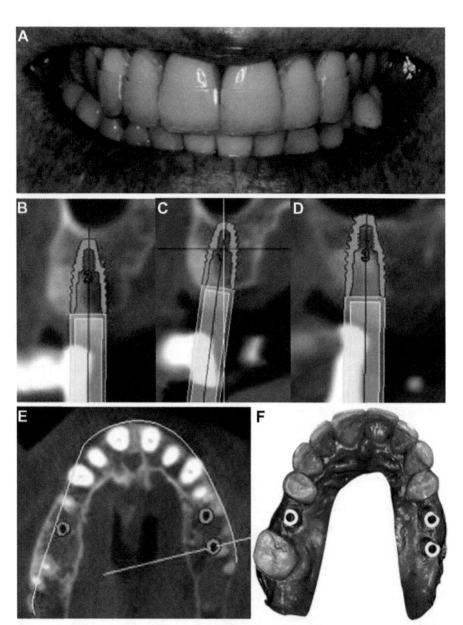

Fig. 7. (*A*) Radiographic guide try-in for posterior maxillary implants. Denture teeth were inserted in a thermoplastic guide made on a stone cast. Gutta-percha was used as a radiopaque marker at the middle of each denture tooth, shown on CBCT cross sections (*B*). Implant planning site #3, (*C*) site #13, and (*D*) site #14. Need for indirect sinus augmentation at the time of placement was also determined from this 3D plan. (*E*) Horizontal cross section of the proposed implant positions to measure the distance from adjacent teeth and between the implants. The radiographic stent was then converted into a pilot surgical guide with the removal of the gutta-percha. (*F*) Intraoral scan using scan bodies to record implant position for single crown fabrication. The standard triangulation language (.stl) file was shared with the dental laboratory to mill the screw-retained single implant crowns. Note the final implant positions are the same as the 3D planned ones.

interface should be approximately 3 mm apical to the adjacent tooth cement-enamel junction (**Fig. 8**).[32]

Radiographic measurements of the completely edentulous arch

For a complete arch rehabilitation, the number of implants required to support the desired prosthesis should be taken into consideration during the radiographic evaluation of the residual alveolar bone (**Fig. 9**). Adequate anterior-posterior (A-P) spread for fixed and removable prostheses may sometimes be offset by the abovementioned anatomic structures. Therefore, in order to avoid extensive grafting procedures, nowadays, fewer implants are recommended to restore a full-arch. At least 4 implants are recommended for maxillary and mandibular full-arch fixed or maxillary removable prosthesis.[34–37] For mandibular complete removable prosthesis, at least 2 implants are advocated (**Fig. 10**).[38]

Radiographic measurement of restorative space

Restorative space is calculated from the implant platform to the occlusal surface of the planned restoration, and it depends on the type of prosthesis planned. This measurement is necessary to ensure adequate space for optimum physical and mechanical properties of all components/materials required in the prosthesis. Each prosthesis requires different restorative space, which is why the selection of the final prosthesis should be determined before implant surgery. Adjunctive treatments may be required before or during implant placement, such as alveoloplasty or alveolectomy, to ensure that the prosthetic components/materials will have adequate space/thickness for long-lasting results (**Fig. 11**). If residual alveolar bone volume is limited and alveoloplasty cannot be performed, increase in occlusal vertical dimension may be considered in order to achieve the recommended vertical restorative space or alternative restoration/materials should be planned. Therefore, a template of the final prosthesis at the correct restorative dimensions is required during CBCT imaging.

Based on the available literature and contemporary biomaterials, the minimum vertical restorative space for different implant-supported prostheses is[39]:

- Fixed screw-retained prosthesis (crown or FDP) (implant level): 4 to 5 mm
- Fixed screw-retained prosthesis (crown or FDP) (abutment level): 7.5 mm
- Fixed cement-retained prosthesis (crown or FDP): 7 to 8 mm
- Unsplinted implant overdenture: 7 to 17 mm
- Splinted (bar-supported) implant overdenture: 13 to 14 mm
- Screw-retained fixed complete denture (abutment level): greater than 15 mm

Importance of Radiographic Guides for Planning of all Prosthodontic Patients

As mentioned earlier, for prosthodontically driven implant imaging, the definitive prosthesis position is represented by an appropriately designed and fabricated radiographic guide. Radiographic templates containing radiopaque materials and/or fiducial markers transfer both the proposed prosthesis design and desired implant location for appropriate CBCT scan.[40] There are several approaches available to conventionally or digitally fabricate radiographic stents, which include the use of:

1. An existing prosthesis with ideal teeth position with added radiopaque fiduciary markers.
2. A thermoplastic stent with incorporated radiopaque markers and/or made out of radiopaque acrylic material such as barium sulfate. This stent is made using a duplicate cast of the diagnostic wax-up.

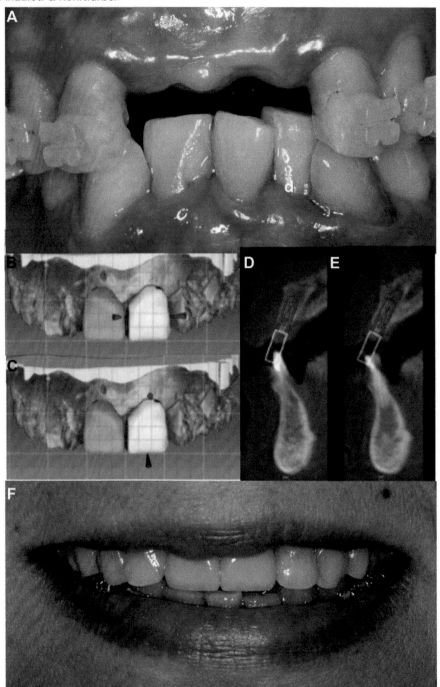

Fig. 8. (*A*) Missing maxillary central incisors. 3D clinical and radiographic analysis of the edentulous space was performed to determine MD, BP, IA dimensions as well as distance from incisive canal and restorative space. (*B*, *C*) Digital design software was used for a virtual wax-up to determine ideal tooth dimensions to prosthetically coordinate the orthodontic treatment. (*D*, *E*) CBCT scan and implant planning software were used to plan the implants' positions to prosthetically drive the surgical phase of the treatment. (*F*) Definitive cement-retained single crowns on #8 and 9 implants with optimal esthetic and functional result.

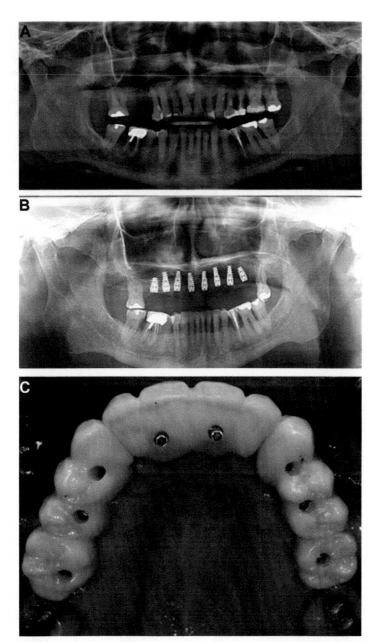

Fig. 9. (*A*) Terminal maxillary dentition caused by severe periodontal disease. The patient elected to proceed with maxillary implant–supported prostheses. (*B*) Postoperative panoramic to evaluate the 8 implants placed to support 3 FDPs. (*C*) Maxillary arch rehabilitation with 3 FDPs.

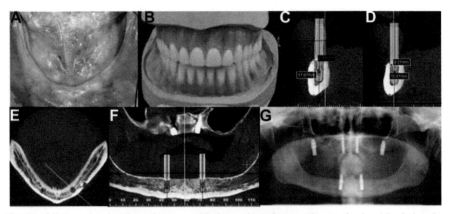

Fig. 10. (*A*) Completely edentulous mandibular arch with severely resorbed residual alveolar bone. (*B*) Definitive prostheses tooth setup at correct occlusal vertical dimension was used as a radiographic guide to plan the implant position. (*C, D*) Sagittal cross sections of the implant sites with measurements of the height and width of the residual bone to determine ideal implant dimensions. (*E, F*) Horizontal and frontal cross sections of planned implant positions. (*G*) Postoperative panoramic radiograph for evaluation of implant placement.

3. Radiopaque teeth at the position of the planned restoration in a mucosa-supported or tooth-supported stent.
4. Digital design software is used to determine ideal prosthesis/teeth position via virtual wax-up. Based on that design, a diagnostic model, a radiographic template or even a surgical guide may be fabricated.[41]

After planning, the radiographic guide may be converted to a pilot surgical stent by modification.[42,43] It has been shown that the combined use of a prosthodontic stent and 3D imaging is an effective technique in achieving an ideal position of dental implants.[44]

CONTEMPORARY PROSTHODONTICS

CBCT is an excellent modality that has resulted in an increase in diagnostic accuracy and has become a foundation for implant prosthodontics and digital dentistry. Contemporary prosthodontics includes integration of digital technology with implant

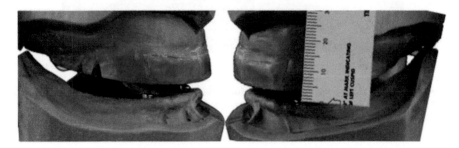

Fig. 11. Lack of prosthetic planning before implant placement led to inadequate restorative space for mandibular implant-retained overdenture.

imaging, planning software, and guided surgical implant placement along with virtual design and digital fabrication of prostheses. For partially edentulous patients, planning is accomplished by merging the Digital Imaging and Communications in Medicine (DICOM) file from the CBCT and the standard tessellation language or standard triangulation language (.stl) file from the digital wax-up. Subsequently, the surgical guide can be fabricated, either by milling or printing for pilot or fully guided surgery (**Fig. 12**). For completely edentulous patients, the dual-scan technique is used, where the first scan is made of the patient with the radiographic guide in place and the second scan is made of the radiographic guide separately. Both scans are merged in the planning software using the fiducial markers in order to plan and fabricate a surgical guide (**Fig. 13**). When comparing the placed implant position to the planned one, fully guided surgery has demonstrated higher accuracy and reliability than conventional protocol.[45,46]

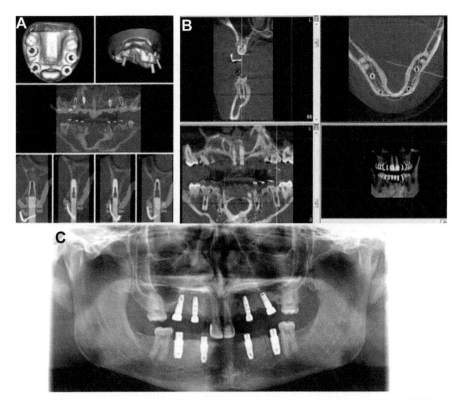

Fig. 12. (*A*) Contemporary prosthodontics includes integration of DICOM file from CBCT and .stl file from digitalization of the stone cast. 3D virtual implant planning for 4 maxillary implants to support 2 FDPs. Guided surgery performed because of limited available residual bone. Tooth-supported surgical guide was designed using design software. (*B*) Same software was used for virtual implant planning of the 4 mandibular implants to support 1 fixed dental prosthesis. Note that the removable interim prosthesis was converted into radiographic guide with the use of lead foil strip applied over sticky wax on each denture tooth. (*C*) Maxillary and mandibular postoperative panoramic radiograph to verify implant placement. Note the inclination of the maxillary posterior implants to avoid the maxillary sinuses.

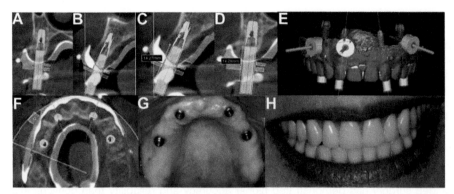

Fig. 13. (A–D) 3D virtual implant planning for 4 implants with radiographic guide. Sagittal views of each implant with measurement of the restorative space (implant platform to occlusal plane/surface). The patient's immediate interim denture was used as a radiographic guide with fiduciary markers. Dual-scan technique was performed to superimpose the DI-COM file of the denture with the DICOM file of the patient while wearing the prosthesis. The round fiduciary markers were used to superimpose the 2 scans together. Note that the implants are placed subcrestally to allow enough restorative space for the removable prosthesis and remaining components. Also, alveoloplasty was performed to reduce the buccal undercuts and facilitate insertion of removable prosthesis. (E) Virtual design of the surgical guide. (F) Horizontal cross section of planned implant positions. (G) Intraoral view of the maxillary attachments (implant locations same as virtually planned). (H) Inserted definitive prostheses with adequate esthetics and function because of prosthetically driven implant planning.

Maintenance

The success of all prosthodontic treatment depends on regular maintenance and patient compliance.[47,48] Periodic postoperative evaluation with intraoral or panoramic imaging is suggested to help determine bone levels around implants over time in asymptomatic patients. However, any postoperative complications, such as implant mobility or neurosensory deficits, should be evaluated with CBCT to better assess possible impingement on the surrounding anatomic structures.[49,50]

CLINICS CARE POINTS

> • Preprosthetic implant imaging and planning lead to predictable prosthetic, esthetic, and functional results.

ACKNOWLEDGMENTS

The authors gratefully acknowledge Dr Nupur Patel, Dr Lucie Yin, Dr Abdulrahman Almalki, and Dr Bill Scruggs for their contributions and photographs.

DISCLOSURE

The authors have nothing to disclose.

REFERENCES

1. The Glossary of Prosthodontic Terms: Ninth Edition. J Prosthet Dent 2017; 117(5S):e1–105.

2. Morton D, Gallucci G, Lin W, et al. Group 2 ITI Consensus Report: Prosthodontics and implant dentistry. Clin Oral Implants Res 2018;29(S16):215–23.

3. Scherer MD. Presurgical Implant-Site Assessment and Restoratively Driven Digital Planning. Dent Clin North Am 2014;58(3):561–95.

4. Mozzo P, Procacci C, Tacconi A, et al. A new volumetric CT machine for dental imaging based on the cone-beam technique: preliminary results. Eur Radiol 1998;8(9):1558–64.

5. Pinsky H, Dyda S, Pinsky R, et al. Accuracy of three-dimensional measurements using cone-beam CT. Dentomaxillofac Radiol 2006;35(6):410–6.

6. Mischkowski RA, Zinser MJ, Ritter L, et al. Intraoperative navigation in the maxillofacial area based on 3D imaging obtained by a cone-beam device. Int J Oral Maxillofac Surg 2007;36(8):687–94.

7. Scarfe W, Li Z, Aboelmaaty W, et al. Maxillofacial cone beam computed tomography: essence, elements and steps to interpretation: Maxillofacial cone beam computed tomography. Aust Dent J 2012;57:46–60.

8. Stratemann SA, Huang JC, Maki K, et al. Comparison of cone beam computed tomography imaging with physical measures. Dentomaxillofac Radiol 2008; 37(2):80–93.

9. Yu L, Vrieze TJ, Bruesewitz MR, et al. Dose and image quality evaluation of a dedicated cone-beam ct system for high-contrast neurologic applications. AJR Am J Roentgenol 2010;194(2):W193–201.

10. Bamba J, Araki K, Endo A, et al. Image quality assessment of three cone beam CT machines using the SEDENTEXCT CT phantom. Dentomaxillofac Radiol 2013; 42(8):20120445.

11. Perschbacher S. Interpretation of panoramic radiographs. Aust Dent J 2012; 57(Suppl 1):40–5.

12. Mahesh M. The essential physics of medical imaging, third edition. Med Phys 2013;40(7):077301.

13. Constantine S, Clark B, Kiermeier A, et al. Panoramic radiography is of limited value in the evaluation of maxillary sinus disease. Oral Surg Oral Med Oral Pathol Oral Radiol 2019;127(3):237–46.

14. Ludlow JB, Davies-Ludlow LE, White SC. Patient risk related to common dental radiographic examinations: the impact of 2007 International Commission on Radiological Protection recommendations regarding dose calculation. J Am Dent Assoc 2008;139(9):1237–43.

15. Ludlow J, Davies-Ludlow L, Brooks S. Dosimetry of two extraoral direct digital imaging devices: NewTom cone beam CT and Orthophos Plus DS panoramic unit. Dentomaxillofac Radiol 2003;32(4):229–34.

16. Ludlow J, Davies-Ludlow L, Brooks S, et al. Dosimetry of 3 CBCT devices for oral and maxillofacial radiology: CB Mercuray, NewTom 3G and i-CAT. Dentomaxillofac Radiol 2006;35(4):219–26.

17. Ludlow JB, Ivanovic M. Comparative dosimetry of dental CBCT devices and 64-slice CT for oral and maxillofacial radiology. Oral Surg Oral Med Oral Pathol Oral Radiol Endod 2008;106(1):106–14.

18. Ludlow JB, Timothy R, Walker C, et al. Effective dose of dental CBCT-a meta analysis of published data and additional data for nine CBCT units. Dentomaxillofac Radiol 2015;44(1):20140197.

19. National Council on Radiation Protection and Measurements, editor. Ionizing radiation exposure of the population of the United States: recommendations of the National Council on radiation Protection and measurements. National Council on Radiation Protection and Measurements; 2009.

20. Tyndall DA, Price JB, Tetradis S, et al. Position statement of the American Academy of Oral and Maxillofacial Radiology on selection criteria for the use of radiology in dental implantology with emphasis on cone beam computed tomography. Oral Surg Oral Med Oral Pathol Oral Radiol 2012;113(6):817–26.

21. Jensen OT, Shulman LB, Block MS, et al. Report of the Sinus Consensus Conference of 1996. Int J Oral Maxillofac Implants 1998;13(Suppl):11–45.

22. Krasowski J. Essentials of maxillary sinus augmentation. CRANIO 2018; 36(4):273.

23. Ilgüy D, Ilgüy M, Dolekoglu S, et al. Evaluation of the posterior superior alveolar artery and the maxillary sinus with CBCT. Braz Oral Res 2013;27(5):431–7.

24. Sonneveld KA, Mai PT, Hogge M, et al. Bifid Mandibular Canal: A Case Review and Retrospective Review of CBCTs. Implant Dent 2018;27(6):682–6.

25. Vieira CL, Veloso S do AR, Lopes FF. Location of the course of the mandibular canal, anterior loop and accessory mental foramen through cone-beam computed tomography. Surg Radiol Anat 2018;40(12):1411–7.

26. Nithya J, Aswath N. Assessing the Prevalence and Morphological Characteristics of Bifid Mandibular Canal Using Cone-Beam Computed Tomography – A Retrospective Cross-Sectional Study. J Clin Imaging Sci 2020;10:30.

27. Bryington M, De Kok IJ, Thalji G, et al. Patient Selection and Treatment Planning for Implant Restorations. Dent Clin North Am 2014;58(1):193–206.

28. Fokas G, Vaughn VM, Scarfe WC, et al. Accuracy of linear measurements on CBCT images related to presurgical implant treatment planning: A systematic review. Clin Oral Implants Res 2018;29(S16):393–415.

29. Grunder U, Gracis S, Capelli M. Influence of the 3-D bone-to-implant relationship on esthetics. Int J Periodontics Restorative Dent 2005;25(2):113–9.

30. Wang T, De Kok I, Zhong S, et al. The Role of Implant-Tooth Distance on Marginal Bone Levels and Esthetics. Int J Oral Maxillofac Implants 2019;34(2):499–505.

31. Vera C, De Kok IJ, Reinhold D, et al. Evaluation of buccal alveolar bone dimension of maxillary anterior and premolar teeth: a cone beam computed tomography investigation. Int J Oral Maxillofac Implants 2012;27(6):1514–9.

32. Cooper LF, Pin-Harry OC. "Rules of Six"-diagnostic and therapeutic guidelines for single-tooth implant success. Compend Contin Educ Dent 2013;34(2):94–8, 100-101.

33. Tarnow DP, Magner AW, Fletcher P. The effect of the distance from the contact point to the crest of bone on the presence or absence of the interproximal dental papilla. J Periodontol 1992;63(12):995–6.

34. Heydecke G, Zwahlen M, Nicol A, et al. What is the optimal number of implants for fixed reconstructions: a systematic review. Clin Oral Implants Res 2012; 23(Suppl 6):217–28.

35. Daudt Polido W, Aghaloo T, Emmett TW, et al. Number of implants placed for complete-arch fixed prostheses: A systematic review and meta-analysis. Clin Oral Implants Res 2018;29(Suppl 16):154–83.

36. de Luna Gomes JM, Lemos CAA, Santiago Junior JF, et al. Optimal number of implants for complete-arch implant-supported prostheses with a follow-up of at least 5 years: A systematic review and meta-analysis. J Prosthet Dent 2019; 121(5):766–74.

37. Di Francesco F, De Marco G, Gironi Carnevale UA, et al. The number of implants required to support a maxillary overdenture: a systematic review and meta-analysis. J Prosthodont Res 2019;63(1):15–24.

38. Feine JS, Carlsson GE, Awad MA, et al. The McGill consensus statement on over-dentures. Mandibular two-implant overdentures as first choice standard of care for edentulous patients. Gerodontology 2002;19(1):3–4.
39. Carpentieri J, Greenstein G, Cavallaro J. Hierarchy of restorative space required for different types of dental implant prostheses. J Am Dent Assoc 2019;150(8): 695–706.
40. De Kok IJ, Thalji G, Bryington M, et al. Radiographic Stents. Dent Clin North Am 2014;58(1):181–92.
41. Morton D, Phasuk K, Polido WD, et al. Consideration for Contemporary Implant Surgery. Dent Clin North Am 2019;63(2):309–29.
42. Schneider D, Sancho-Puchades M, Benic GI, et al. A Randomized Controlled Clinical Trial Comparing Conventional and Computer-Assisted Implant Planning and Placement in Partially Edentulous Patients. Part 1: Clinician-Related Outcome Measures. Int J Periodontics Restorative Dent 2018;38(Suppl):s49–57.
43. Sancho-Puchades M, Alfaro F, Naenni N, et al. A Randomized Controlled Clinical Trial Comparing Conventional And Computer-Assisted Implant Planning and Placement in Partially Edentulous Patients. Part 2: Patient Related Outcome Measures. Int J Periodontics Restorative Dent 2019;39(4):e99–110.
44. Talwar N, Chand P, Singh BP, et al. Evaluation of the Efficacy of a Prosthodontic Stent in Determining the Position of Dental Implants: Efficacy of Stents. J Prosthodont 2012;21(1):42–7.
45. Schneider D, Sancho-Puchades M, Schober F, et al. A randomized controlled clinical trial comparing conventional and computer-assisted implant planning and placement in partially edentulous patients. part 3: time and cost analyses. Int J Periodontics Restorative Dent 2019;39(3):e71–82.
46. Schneider D, Sancho-Puchades M, Mir-Marí J, et al. A randomized controlled clinical trial comparing conventional and computer-assisted implant planning and placement in partially edentulous patients. part 4: accuracy of implant placement. Int J Periodontics Restorative Dent 2019;39(4):e111–22.
47. Bidra AS, Daubert DM, Garcia LT, et al. Clinical practice guidelines for recall and maintenance of patients with tooth-borne and implant-borne dental restorations: clinical practice guidelines. J Prosthodont 2016;25(S1):S32–40.
48. Bidra AS, Daubert DM, Garcia LT, et al. A systematic review of recall regimen and maintenance regimen of patients with dental restorations. part 2: implant-borne restorations: recall and maintenance of implant-borne restorations. J Prosthodont 2016;25(S1):S16–31.
49. European Commission. Cone Beam CT for dental and maxillofacial radiology. Radiat Prot 2012;172:1–156.
50. Renvert S, Hirooka H, Polyzois I, et al. Working Group 3. Diagnosis and non-surgical treatment of peri-implant diseases and maintenance care of patients with dental implants - Consensus report of working group 3. Int Dent J 2019; 69(Suppl 2):12–7.

Imaging in Orthodontics

Nipul K. Tanna, DMD, MS[a],*,
Anwar A.A.Y. AlMuzaini, DDS, MS, BDM, MSOB[b], Mel Mupparapu, DMD, MDS, DABOMR[c]

KEYWORDS

- Intraoral scans • Orthodontic imaging • 2D and 3D cephalometric analysis
- Skeletal maturation • TMJ evaluation • Airway analysis • Obstructive sleep apnea

KEY POINTS

- Historically, 2D imaging first provided a method for evaluating the relationship between the cranium and the dentition.
- Standardized methods allowed for research in growth and development.
- 3D intraoral scanning and imaging techniques are a game changer and have paved the path for:
  - 3D analysis, diagnosis, and virtual treatment planning.
  - Determination of the biologic boundaries of orthodontic treatment.
  - 3D evaluation of the TMJ.
  - Airway analysis methodology.

INTRODUCTION

According to the current practice guidelines published by the American Association of Orthodontists[1] the following diagnostic imaging in orthodontics are considered as part of the diagnostic records:

1. Intraoral and/or panoramic radiographs to assess the condition and developmental status of the teeth and hard tissue supporting structures, and to identify any dental anomalies or pathology.
2. Radiographic imaging to permit relative evaluation of the size, shape, and positions of the relevant hard and soft tissue craniofacial structures including the dentition, and to aid in the identification of skeletal anomalies and/or pathology.
3. Posterior-anterior (PA) cephalometric and lateral cephalometric radiographs may be considered as part of the diagnostic imaging. Three-dimensional (3D) cone-beam computed tomography (CBCT) may be used as an imaging source to obtain this information.

[a] Postdoctoral Periodontics/Orthodontics Program, University of Pennsylvania School of Dental Medicine, 240 South 40th Street, Philadelphia, PA 19104, USA; [b] Ministry of Health, Government Office, Jasim Boodai Street, Kuwait City, Kuwait; [c] University of Pennsylvania School of Dental Medicine, 240 South 40th Street, Suite 214, Philadelphia, PA 19104, USA
* Corresponding author.
E-mail address: nipul77@upenn.edu

Dent Clin N Am 65 (2021) 623–641
https://doi.org/10.1016/j.cden.2021.02.008
0011-8532/21/© 2021 Elsevier Inc. All rights reserved.

dental.theclinics.com

Additionally, for patients still in the growth and development stage, a hand-wrist film for evaluating the level of skeletal maturation can also be considered.

In the age of the digital workflow era, intraoral scanners have permitted clinicians to replace impressions and plaster casts with accurate virtual casts (e-models) that become part of the diagnostic record. These can also be used to print 3D models for appliance fabrication and so forth. 3D radiographic imaging merged with intraoral scanned stereolithography files have become a powerful technological tool for 3D virtual planning of orthodontic and orthognathic surgery cases.

In recent years, the introduction of CBCT imaging has provided clinicians with the option to extract two-dimensional (2D) images from a full-volume CBCT. Although 3D analysis is gaining popularity, it does have a learning curve in that accurate positioning and proper landmark identification is challenging. With further studies, standardized methodology with new norms may be required. With the introduction of more sophisticated software, the incorporation of artificial intelligence methods, and the value-added information gained from 3D analysis, using this powerful tool for 3D diagnosis will continue to gain acceptance as a routine part of orthodontic diagnosis and treatment planning.

As Ricketts[2] stated in 1960, you cannot know how to treat a case until you know what you are treating. The purpose of a through clinical examination combined with appropriate diagnostic records is to provide the clinician with enough information to "know what you are treating."

DIGITAL INTRAORAL SCANS

As part of the diagnostic record, intraoral scans are replacing impressions and plaster models with "digital impressions," "e-models," and 3D printed casts. There are many advantages to this diagnostic record modality. Scans are electronically stored with patient records, thus eliminating model storage and allowing authorized users to view patient records when not physically present in the office. Files are sent electronically to authorized dental laboratories, eliminating concerns of proper disinfection and saving delivery time. Virtual diagnostic setups can be digitally completed, and treatment plans are viewed by multiple clinicians simultaneously without being physically present when treatment planning multidisciplinary cases. In the current age of COVID, this provides the additional advantage of minimizing in person contact (**Figs. 1–3**).

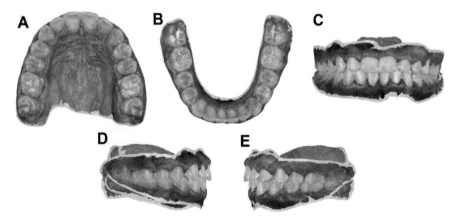

Fig. 1. Images captured from an intraoral scanner. (*A*) Maxilla. (*B*) Mandible. (*C*) Frontal view of occlusion. (*D*) Right lateral view of occlusion. (*E*) Left lateral view of occlusion. (*Courtesy of* Dr. Justin Orr, DDS, University of Pennsylvania School of Dental Medicine.)

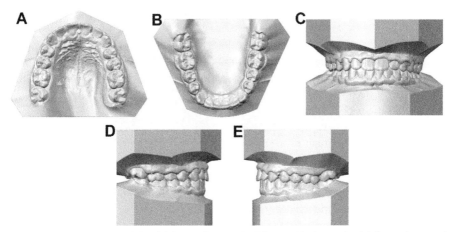

Fig. 2. Virtual casts/e-models of (*A*) maxillary arch, (*B*) mandibular arch, (*C*) frontal view of occlusion both arches, (*D*) right lateral occlusion, and (*E*) left lateral occlusion. (*Courtesy of* Dr. Justin Orr, DDS, University of Pennsylvania School of Dental Medicine.)

PANORAMIC RADIOGRAPH

Although magnification and distortion factors must be taken into consideration, a properly exposed panoramic radiograph provides the clinician with valuable 2D information to view normal structures and to identify the presence of any abnormalities or pathologic conditions. It provides an overview of the cervical vertebrae and areas adjacent to the hyoid bone, areas of calcifications may be visible, condylar shape, ramus heights, the inferior alveolar canal and mental foramen, the maxillary sinuses, the nasal cavity and septum, the orbit, dental development, pattern of eruption, the dentition and a broad overview of the supporting structures associated with it. Asymmetrical growth may also be detected first on a panoramic radiograph when there are large differences in ramus heights between the right and left sides. Any area that does not appear normal or there is suspicion of an underlying pathologic condition requires further investigation. **Fig. 4** shows the panoramic image of a 13-year-old patient in the permanent dentition stage with condylar resorption and asymmetric ramus heights. Roots of the premolars are shorter and the developing third molars will require further evaluation later. Rotation

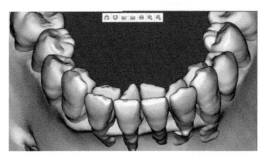

Fig. 3. 3D orthodontic planning based on intraoral scans merged with CBCT images. This virtual diagnostic setup allows clinicians to determine if the orthodontic movement is even biologically possible. (*Courtesy of* Dr. Eric Howard, DMD, Private Practice, Levittown, Pennsylvania.)

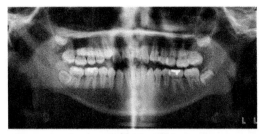

Fig. 4. Panoramic radiograph of a 13-year-old patient in the permanent dentition stage with condylar resorption and asymmetric ramus heights.

of the mandibular canines, lower incisor crowding, prominent marginal ridges, and prominent cingulum of the maxillary incisors is also observed.

SKELETAL MATURATION INDICATORS
Hand-Wrist Radiograph

It has been recognized and well established that chronologic and skeletal maturation ages do not necessarily correlate. As Fishman[3] noted in 1979, all too often, the timing of orthodontic treatment was determined by chronologic age and the stage of dental development, neither of which are reliable to establish a child's skeletal age.

In 1959, Pyle and coworkers[4] established a radiographic atlas of skeletal development using hand-wrist films. Practitioners have used this as a reference to estimate the age of their patients. Bjork and Helm[5] reported a close association between the age at maximal growth and the age when ossification of the ulnar metacarpophalangeal sesamoid of the thumb occurred. In 1981 Fishman established a clinically oriented method based on hand-wrist films to determine skeletal maturation. Fishman's SMI method uses four stages of bone maturation using six anatomic sites on the thumb, third finger, fifth finger, and the radius. From these anatomic sites, 11 discrete stages of skeletal maturation (SMI 1–11) have been established. The 11 stages of skeletal maturation are described in **Box 1**. This method continues to be

---

Box 1
Fishman's 11 stages of skeletal maturation

Width of epiphysis as wide as the diaphysis:
  SMI 1: Third finger-proximal phalanx
  SMI 2: Third finger-middle phalanx
  SMI 3: Fifth finger-middle phalanx

Ossification:
  SMI 4: Adductor sesamoid of thumb

Capping of epiphysis:
  SMI 5: Third finger-distal phalanx
  SMI 6: Third finger-middle phalanx
  SMI 7: Fifth finger-middle phalanx

Fusion of epiphysis and diaphysis:
  SMI 8: Third finger-distal phalanx
  SMI 9: Third finger-proximal phalanx
  SMI 10: Third finger-middle phalanx
  SMI 11: Radius

used by many clinicians today and the reader is referred to Steven Wang and Brian Ford' article, "Imaging in Oral and Maxillofacial Surgery," in this issue. Fishman's[6] work for a more detailed understanding of this methodology.

The hand-wrist radiograph in **Fig. 5** is that of an adolescent patient. When this radiograph is obtained, it is preferable to have a clear image of the hand-wrist complex, including the radius and the ulna. In the image for this patient, the capping stage on the middle phalanx of the fifth digit is not as clearly visible, most probably caused by the fifth finger positioning during the exposure. The abductor sesamoid is visible, capping is seen on the middle phalanx of the third finger, and there is no fusion on the distal phalanx of the third finger. Most probably, this patient would be categorized as an SMI 7 based on Fishman's work.

Other methods for determining the level of skeletal maturity have been reported. McNamara and Franchi[7] reported using the cervical vertebral maturation method as a guide to determine the skeletal maturation stage. With this method, data from the second, third, and fourth cervical vertebrae are used based on the morphology. In summary, the vertebral bodies generally have a flat inferior border in the prepubertal stage and transform to a more concave inferior border with C3 and C4 remaining vertically shorter in the circumpubertal stage and elongation of C3 and C4 is evident in the postpubertal stage. The reader is referred to the work of McNamara and Franchi[7] for a more detailed understanding of this methodology.

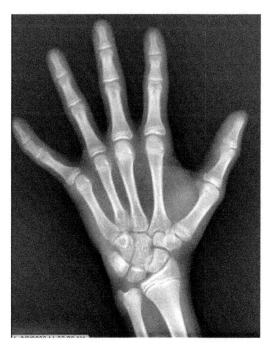

Fig. 5. Hand-wrist radiograph. In the image, the capping stage on the middle phalanx of the fifth digit is not as clearly visible, most probably caused by the fifth finger positioning during the exposure. The abductor sesamoid is visible, capping is seen on the middle phalanx of the third finger, and there is no fusion on the distal phalanx of the third finger. Most probably, this patient would be categorized as an SMI 7 based on Fishman's work.

Two-Dimensional Lateral Cephalometric Analysis

The application of anthropometric measurements was introduced to orthodontic clinicians in the early part of the twentieth century. Most orthodontists at the time were evaluating dental discrepancies primarily by the interrelation of the teeth within the jaws. In 1931, the advent of the cephalostat by Broadbent[8] enabled clinicians to accurately use established craniometric landmarks to evaluate skeletal and dental relationships and also introduce soft tissue findings as it relates to the position of the jaws and the dentition.

The Miriam-Webster dictionary defines cephalometric as the science of measuring the head in living individuals. This definition is further elaborated as the measurement and study of craniofacial proportions, the dentition, and the soft tissues as they relate to one another. In the skeletally immature patient, this also includes growth and development. The concept of using angles and linear measurements for evaluating facial proportions dates back to the fifteenth century when Leonardo da Vinci used it to study facial form. The first truly scientific attempt of a cranial measurement was reported by Spigel in the sixteenth century and was coined the term "lineae cephalometricae." The measurement consisted of four lines: (1) facial, (2) occipital, (3) frontal, and (4) the sincipital. In a well-proportioned skull, it was believed that these lines should be equal to one another.[9]

From the sixteenth to the twentieth century, numerous craniologists developed various types of analysis (eg, Camper, DeSchamps, Daubeuton, Broca, Bell, Gibson, Soemmerring, Blumenbach, Retzius, Barclay, Huxley, and Topinard). At the meeting of the thirteenth general congress of the German Anthropological Society, contributions were made that led to the development of what is referred to today as the Frankfort horizontal plane.

Roentgen's development of X-rays in 1895 paved the path for development of the cephalostat by Hofrath in Dusseldorf and Broadbent in Cleveland. This development was a significant breakthrough because most orthodontists at the time were evaluating dental discrepancies primarily by the interrelation of the teeth using plaster models. Dental casts have limitations in that the articulation of casts may provide a reasonably good evaluation of how the teeth interrelate with each other but do not provide an accurate assessment of their relationship with the cranium. Additionally, this can provide a misrepresentation of the dental position relative to the jaw position. It is possible for teeth to be projected differently depending on how the dentition is oriented on a plaster model. Another limitation is that the growth and development cannot be assessed by dental casts. A standardized method using a cephalostat provided a great opportunity for researchers to study growth and development. Therefore, the advent of the cephalostat allowed clinicians to use radiographs for the purpose of evaluating growth and for the evaluation of interrelationships between the dentition, the jaws, the cranium, and the face and thus provide a method for determining skeletal diagnosis, treatment planning, monitoring of treatment, evaluation of the post-treatment outcome, and the detection of asymmetric growth patterns.

The dynamic pattern of growth and development also has a differential component. Based on the postnatal growth and development reported by Scammon[10,11] the brain case follows the neural growth curve gradient, whereas the face and the dentition more closely follow the general growth pattern. With this information it is possible to identify which landmarks may remain stable and can be used for comparison purposes to study growth, diagnose and treat, monitor treatment, and evaluate the post-treatment results based on superimposition of determined stable structures.

Cephalometric analysis first requires a thorough understanding of internal and external skull anatomy and the overlying soft tissue before anatomic landmarks consisting of hard and soft tissue structures are identified. The reader is referred to any major textbook of anatomy or an anatomic atlas to review this information. Although the introduction of numerous analyses has resulted in identifying additional landmarks, many of the important anthropometric points still used today were defined by the first cephalometric workshop held in 1957 at Western Reserve University.[12] The purpose of the workshop was primarily to define cephalometric points and planes, to standardize the technique, to clarify interpretation, and to evaluate clinical applications. Contributions by Krogman and Sassouni[13] were also studied during this workshop, the proceedings of which went on to define and validate the skeletal cephalometric landmarks (**Table 1**).

Supplementing the workshop-identified skeletal landmarks, currently there are additional cephalometric landmarks that are used by clinicians as noted in **Table 2**.

Robert Ricketts expanded this further with the addition of skeletal landmarks, such as the cranium center, DC point, suprapogonion, and point Xi (**Table 3**). Several soft tissue landmarks are often used for cephalometric analysis as shown in **Table 4**.

Since the original workshop, the total number of identified landmarks has significantly increased, and numerous analyses have been introduced. It is beyond the scope of this article to list all landmarks and review all available analyses. The landmarks that are commonly used along with their respective angles, planes (actually lines in 2D), and measurements are described further and identified in **Fig. 6**.

For the experienced clinician, identifying all landmarks and reviewing all reported analyses for each patient is not practical. The objectives of a lateral cephalometric analysis are primarily to evaluate:

1. The relationship of the maxilla to the cranium
2. The relationship of the mandible to the cranium
3. The interrelationship of the maxillomandibular complex
4. The relationship of the dentition to the maxilla
5. The relationship of the dentition to the mandible
6. The relationship between the entire complex and the soft tissue that drapes it

On a calibrated cephalometric radiograph, the described points are used for measuring lengths, defining planes (a line in 2D), and calculating the angles associated with them to evaluate the craniofacial complex.[14,15] Several of the cephalometric analyses used are shown in **Fig. 6A–F** and the corresponding tracings in **Fig. 6A1–F1**. However, most clinicians use a combination of measurements from various analyses. In summary, the lateral cephalometric in this case would be interpreted as a retrognathic maxilla and mandible with a high angle, clockwise growth pattern, deficient posterior facial height, open bite pattern, and proclined upper incisors.

Two-Dimensional Posterior-Anterior Cephalometric Analysis

In the transverse dimension, there are limitations with 2D cephalometry. Although the PA frontal radiograph has been used traditionally in orthodontics for capturing the transverse measurements, these measurements do have errors created by magnification, patient positioning, and landmarks are sometimes difficult to see because of superimposition of structures of interest. When gross asymmetries are present, PA frontal radiographs worked well for skeletal diagnosis. Most practitioners do not routinely use PA cephalometric radiographs; however, this modality is useful for evaluation of transverse discrepancies and facial asymmetries. In identifying skeletal transverse discrepancies of the jaws, width measurements are calculated between

Table 1
Krogman and Sassouni modification to skeletal cephalometric landmarks

A point	Subspinale	The deepest, most posterior midline point on the premaxilla between the anterior nasal spine and prosthion (alveolar point) [Downs].
ANS	Anterior nasal spine	The tip of the anterior nasal spine seen on the radiograph film from norma lateralis. Also referred to as the sharp bony process of the anterior maxilla at the lower margin of the anterior nasal opening.
Ar	Articulare	The point of intersection of the dorsal contours of process articularis mandibulae and the occipital bone (os temporale) [Björk]. A junction point between the posterior border of the ramus and the inferior border of the posterior cranial base.
B	Supramentale	The most posterior point in the concavity between infradentale and pogonion [Downs].
Ba	Basion	The lowermost point on the anterior margin of the foramen magnum in the midsagittal plane.
Bo	Bolton point	The highest point in the upward curvature of the retrocondylar fossa [Broadbent] located at the intersection of the outline of the occipital condyle and foramen magnum.
Gn	Gnathion	The most inferior point in the contour of the chin usually between pogonion and menton.
Go	Gonion	The point that on the jaw angle is the most inferiorly, posteriorly, and outwardly directed. Located on the outer curvature of the angle of the mandible. Constructed gonion is located at the intersection formed by the lines tangent to the posterior ramus and the inferior border of the mandible.
Me	Menton	The lowermost point on the symphyseal shadow in norma lateralis.
Na	Nasion	The intersection of the internasal suture with the nasofrontal suture in the midsagittal plane.
Or	Orbitale	The lowest point on the lower margin/inferior border of the bony orbit.
PNS	Posterior nasal spine	The tip of the posterior spine of the palatine bone in the hard palate.
Po	Porion	The midpoint on the upper edge of the porus acusticus externus located by means of the metal rods on the cephalometer [Björk]. It is the most superiorly positioned point of the external auditory meatus. This is a very important landmark still used routinely; however, the metal rods may not allow for accurate location of anatomic porion and it may be significantly further away.[12,14]

(*continued on next page*)

Table 1
(continued)

Pog	Pogonion	Most anterior point in the contour of the chin.
Ptm	Pterygomaxillary fissure	The lowest point on the teardrop shape of the projected contour of the fissure; the anterior wall represents closely the retromolar tuberosity of the maxilla, and the posterior wall represents the anterior curve of the pterygoid process of the sphenoid bone.
"R"	Broadbent registration point	The midpoint of the perpendicular from the center of sella turcica to the Bolton plane.
S	Sella turcica	The midpoint of sella turcica, as determined by inspection. Identified as the geometric center of the pituitary fossa.
SO	Sphenooccipital synchondrosis	The upper most point of the suture.

the upper and lower jaws and maxillomandibular differences in conjunction with molar angulation may serve as a guide to determine the amount of required orthopedic correction. It is important, however, to note that ethnic norms in this dimension have not been well established. PA frontal radiographs have also been used for evaluation of the frontal sinuses, the nasal cavity, and the orbital area. Currently, this imaging modality is being used less frequently. With the advent of 3D imaging, any diagnostic information gained from a PA cephalometric image is viewed in much greater detail on a CBCT image. **Fig. 7** shows a PA cephalometric image and the cephalometric tracing associated with it. **Table 5** shows the cephalometric landmarks associated with the PA cephalometry.

Three-Dimensional Analysis

Anthropometric measurements based on dry skulls were introduced to orthodontic clinicians in the early part of the twentieth century. Broadbent's cephalostat enabled clinicians to use established craniometric landmarks that were identified on dry skulls and transfer many of the landmarks onto a standardized radiograph. This allowed for the evaluation of skeletal and dental relationships and also introduced soft tissue findings as it related to the position of the jaws and the dentition. There were, however, limitations in that some landmarks were difficult to identify on a 2D image, some landmarks between the right and left side were superimposed, and magnification errors were introduced and had to be accounted for.[16] Nonetheless, once established, cephalometric radiographs provided valuable information for many research endeavors and perhaps the most well-known of these are the growth and development studies

Table 2
Additional cephalometric landmarks currently used by clinicians

LMT	Mesial cusp of the lower first molar
UMT	Mesial cusp of the upper first molar
Ag	Antegonion (also referred to as the antegonial notch)
LIA	Lower incisor root apex
UIA	Upper incisor root apex
LIE	Incisal tip of the lower incisor
UIE	Incisal tip of the upper incisor

Table 3	
Robert Ricketts's modification of skeletal landmarks	
CC	Cranium center: A point formed at the intersection of 2 lines, basion-nasion and pterygoid-gnathion
DC	DC point: A point identified at the center of the condylar neck along the basion-nasion line
PM	Suprapogonion: Point at which shape of symphysis changes from convex to concave
Xi	Xi constructed point located at the center of the ramus; the intersection of 2 diagonals as described next:
	R1: Line drawn at the deepest point on the anterior border of the ramus and parallel point vertical
	R2: located on posterior border of the ramus parallel to R1
	R3: deepest point of the coronoid notch, perpendicular to R1 and R2
	R4: located opposite and parallel to R3 on the inferior border of the mandible at the antegonial notch
	In the resulting rectangle draw 2 diagonals, the intersection of which is the constructed Xi point

at numerous well-known institutions. With time and wider acceptance, the lateral cephalometric radiographic became a standard in orthodontic treatment.

With technological advances occurring at such a rapid pace, CBCT imaging has allowed for more accurate extraction of cephalometric images from a full-volume CBCT. However, there are many practices that are still in the early stages of incorporating true 3D cephalometry on a routine basis.

Table 4		
Soft tissue landmarks used for cephalometric analysis		
Tri	Trichion	Intersection of the normal hairline and the midline of the forehead
G	Glabella	The anterior most prominent point on the soft tissue forehead
N	Soft tissue nasion	Soft tissue profile's most concave point between the forehead and bridge of the nose
Bn	Bridge of nose	Midpoint from soft tissue nasion to tip of nose
Pn	Pronasale	Most prominent point on the anterior curve of the nose
Sn	Subnasale	Point along the midsagittal plane where the nose connects to the center of the upper lip
A'	Soft tissue A point	Most concave point between subnasale and the anterior part of the upper lip
St	Stomion	Superius is the most inferior part on the curve of the upper lip and inferius is the most superior part on the curve of the lower lip
Ls	Labrale superius or upper lip	Most anterior part on the curve of the upper lip
Li	Labrale inferius or lower lip	Most anterior part on the curve of the lower lip
B'	Soft tissue B point	Most concave point on the anterior curve of the upper lip
Gn'	Soft tissue gnathion	The midpoint between the most anterior and inferior points of the soft tissue chin in the midsagittal plane
Me'	Soft tissue menton	Most inferior point of the soft tissue chin

A Steiner analysis	
SNA	72°
SNB	70°
ANB	2°
1/ TO NA	30°
1/ TO NA	7 mm
/1 TO NB	3 mm
/1 TO NB	21°
1/1 ANGLE	128°
OP to SN	26°
GoGn to SN	42°
Pog to NB	3 mm

B Tweed/Wits appraisal	
FMA	31°
FMIA	64°
IMPA	86°
Wits appraisal	
A'O B'O	-2

C Ricketts analysis	
Max. Depth. (FH-Na)	86°
Max. Height (N-Cf-A)	58°
SN to PP	12°
Facial Angle (FH-NPg)	86°
Facial Axis (BaN-PtGn)	84°
Facial Taper (N-Gn-Go)	64°
MPA (FH-GoGn)	30°
Corpus Length (Xi-Pm)	65°
Mand Arc (Dc-Xi-Pm)	24°
Convexity (A-NPg)	0
LFH (ANS-Xi-Pg)	51°
1/ to APO	8
6/ to PTV	15
to APO	1 mm
Hinge Axis (DC-/1)	90°
1/1 Angle	128°
OJ	7
OB	0
Upper Lip E-line	-3 mm
Lower Lip E-line	-2 mm

D Bjork-Jarabak analysis	
Saddle Angle	124°
Articular Angle	148°
Gonial Angle	133°
Sum of Angles	405°
Upper Go	52°
Lower Go	81°
A Cranial Base	63 mm
P Cranial Base	32 mm
Ramus Height	34 mm
Mand Body	66 mm
PFH	63 mm
AFH	111 mm
PFH/AFH	58%
ACB: Mand Body	63:66
1/ to SN	102
1/ to FH	116
UFH	43%
LFH	57%

E McNamara analysis	
Max Skeletal	-4 mm
Max Dental	7 mm
Mand Skeletal	-8 mm
Mand Dental	1 mm
Mand Length	101 mm
Midface Length	73 mm
Mx-Md Diff	28 mm
LFH-ok	64 mm
Mand Plane	28°
Facial Axis	-7°

F Down's analysis	
Facial Angle (FH-Npog)	86°
Convexity (N-A-Pog)	0
AB Plane (AB-Npog)	-4°
Md Plane	30°
Y Axis (SGn-FH)	62°
Occl Plane to FH	12°
Interincisal	**128°**
L1-Occl Pl	76°
L1-Md Plane	-6°
U1-Apog	7 mm

Fig. 6. Identification of common hard and soft tissue landmarks on a cephalometric tracing. (*A–F*) Several of the cephalometric analyses commonly used are shown as a composite image. Corresponding tracings in *A1–F1*. Cephalometric tracings that correspond to cephalometric analysis: *6A1*, Steiner tracing; *6B1*, Tweed tracing; *6C1*, Ricketts tracing; *6D1*, Bjork-Jarabak tracing; *6E1*, McNamara tracing; and *6F1*, Downs tracing.

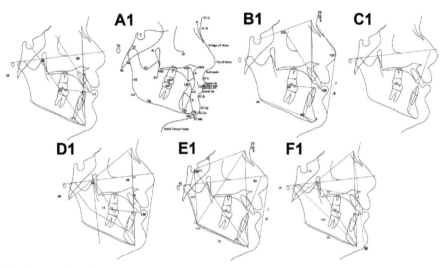

Fig. 6. (continued)

Until recently, most clinicians who used CBCT technology extracted 2D images for lateral cephalometric analysis purposes and for evaluation of transverse discrepancies. Today, advanced technology with the advent of the CBCT merged with intraoral scanning technology and sophisticated software have opened a whole new era in 3D cephalometric analysis, 3D diagnosis of the craniofacial structures, and 3D planning of orthodontic treatment. Virtual planning of orthognathic surgical treatment and the subsequent 3D printed splint fabrication is becoming routine. This methodology is covered in more detail elsewhere in this issue. 3D diagnosis and treatment

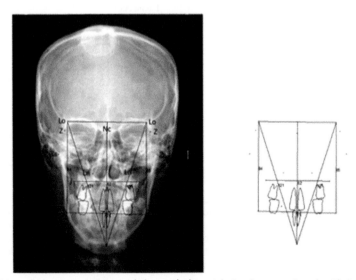

Fig. 7. PA cephalometric image and the cephalometric tracing associated with it.

Table 5 Cephalometric landmarks associated with the PA cephalometry		
Nc	Christa galli	The constricted upper part of the perpendicular plate of the ethmoid bone
Ln	Lateral nasal	The lateral wall of the nasal cavity at its widest point
Lo	Latero-orbitale	Lateral wall of the orbit
Z	Z point	Frontozygomatic suture
Za	Zygomatic arch	The right and left zygomatic arches
J	Jugal process	Midpoint on the curve of the jugal process
Me	Menton	Point on the inferior border of the symphysis
A	A point	Point on the premaxilla between the anterior nasal spine and prosthion

planning have truly been a game changer not just in orthodontics but also in all aspects of dentistry.

Although the adaptation of 3D analysis does require a learning curve, it continues to be accepted more and more by clinicians. Many 2D landmarks do not equate the same when transferred to a 3D image. For example, a line on a 2D film may become a 3D space on a 3D image. Further studies are required, which will allow for the introduction of new landmarks, new measurements, and the establishment of new planes. As more data are collected, new norms will also be established.

Fig. 8 shows a 3D cephalometric analysis constructed from a full-volume CBCT image. One can appreciate the high-quality image and the clear identification of most structures. Once appropriate landmarks have been properly identified, accurate measurements without magnification are made. It is important to note that although the images in this document cannot be rotated, within the image analysis software, these images can be rotated in all three dimensions.

ORTHODONTIC DIAGNOSIS, TREATMENT, AND THE TEMPOROMANDIBULAR JOINT

Temporomandibular joint (TMJ) morphology and symmetry plays a vital role in the development of occlusion. Changes within the TMJ can define the orthodontic diagnosis and management. The positioning of the condyle within the glenoid fossa is critical in the initial orthodontic evaluation and subsequent work-up. The condyles are generally located centrally within the glenoid fossa in healthy joints. Disk discrepancies and occlusal disturbances may affect the condylar position. In growing children, a history of trauma is elicited in many cases. If condyles are malformed or hypoplastic because of developmental disturbances, they will affect the way occlusion is presented in an orthodontic patient. When occlusion is normal initially and the patient develops an open bite progressively, the condyles must be evaluated. **Figs. 9** and **10** show the condylar anatomy in a patient who developed anterior open bite several years after she initially underwent orthodontic treatment.

If the condyles show evidence of hypoplasia, destruction, and/or morphologic changes that are significant to orthodontic diagnosis, it is imperative that the practitioner takes measures to overcome this issue without which the orthodontic treatment might fail.

AIRWAY ANALYSIS IN ORTHODONTICS

The respiratory system in humans allows for the conduction and exchange of inhaled gases. The airway (or respiratory tract) is anatomically classified into the upper and

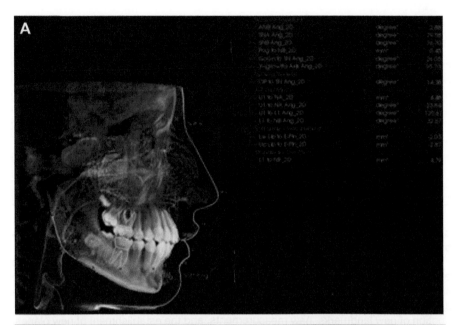

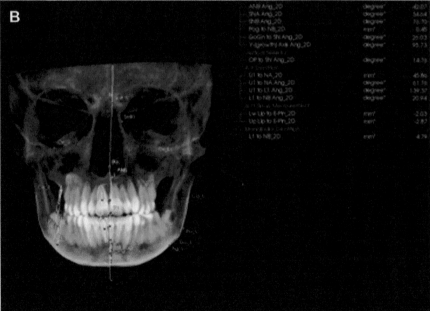

Fig. 8. (A, B) A 3D cephalometric analysis constructed from a full-volume CBCT image. (*Courtesy of* Dr. Grace Simco, DMD, MSD, Private Practice, Levittown, Pennsylvania.)

lower airway. Organs comprising the upper airway include the nose, pharynx, and larynx, whereas the lower airway includes the trachea and lungs.[17] The flow of air through the nasal cavity during sleep increases ventilation and thus stimulates breathing.[18]

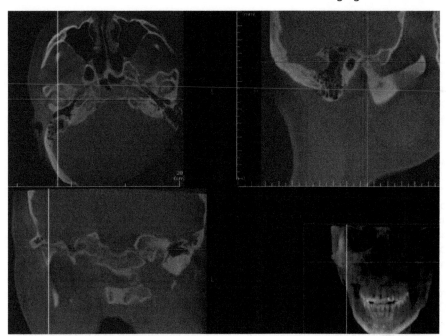

Fig. 9. CBCT in multiplanar reformatting showing the right TMJ and the condylar anatomy in a patient who developed anterior open bite several years after the patient initially underwent orthodontic treatment.

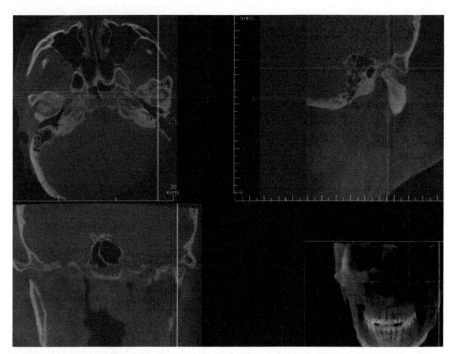

Fig. 10. CBCT in multiplanar reformatting showing the left TMJ and the condylar anatomy in a patient who developed anterior open bite several years after the patient initially underwent orthodontic treatment.

Obstructive Sleep Apnea

Obstructive sleep apnea (OSA) is a sleep breathing disorder that occurs as a result of upper airway obstruction. This obstruction can be caused by insufficient airway dilator muscle or tongue motor tone. Because of the person's inability to breath while sleeping, OSA frequently results in disturbed sleep.[19] This, in turn, leads to sleepiness and fatigue during the day.[20] OSA is highly prevalent among adults and has been related to obesity and age.[21]

According to The International Classification of Sleep Disorders–Third edition, polysomnography revealing more than five events per hour of obstructive respiratory disturbance index along with the previously mentioned symptoms, or a respiratory disturbance index of more than 15 events per hour without symptoms, is diagnostic of OSA.[22] In addition, the most recent American Academy of Sleep Medicine guidelines recommend diagnosis of OSA with an adequate home sleep apnea test or polysomnography for adults at risk of moderate-severe OSA.[20] This is important because complications of OSA can include coronary artery disease, stroke, heart failure, and arrythmias.[23]

Craniofacial structures can also be affected with resultant crossbite, mandibular retrognathia, and a narrow maxillary arch reported in mouth breathers and patients with OSA.[24] A recent systematic review and meta-analysis found a strong correlation between morphologic changes of the craniofacial structures and OSA in adults.[25] In attempts to facilitate OSA diagnosis, CBCT has been investigated as a potential reliable imaging modality in assessing the upper airway. A study found that the airway morphology and anatomy is more accurately depicted on CBCT when compared with sagittal and transverse measurements (which are typically used on lateral cephalograms).[26] A systematic review assessing 3D segmentation of the upper airway and its reliability found it difficult to conclude whether a CBCT study is accurate or reliable in modeling the airways because the evidence was lacking.[24]

Diagnosis of Obstructive Sleep Apnea and the Role of Orthodontists in the Diagnosis and Management of Obstructive Sleep Apnea

The Board of Trustees of the American Association of Orthodontists tasked a panel of medical and dental experts to create a document for guidance regarding the diagnosis and management of OSA for practicing orthodontists. A white paper was published in 2019 that summarizes the task force's findings and its recommendations.[27]

As the child grows into adolescence and adulthood, there are changes happening to the skeletal tissues, such as growth and expansion and shrinkage of the oropharyngeal lymphoid tissues, contributing to the expansion of the oropharyngeal airway. Based on current available literature, orthodontic movement of teeth does not in any way affect the nasopharyngeal airway volume.

The gist of the recommendations is outlined here:

1. The diagnosis of OSA is performed by a physician specializing in sleep medicine by performing an overnight sleep study (polysomnography).
2. The American Academy of Sleep Disorders developed several sets of criteria, primary and secondary to diagnose OSA.[22]
3. Conventional orthodontic therapy has never been proven to be an etiologic factor for the development of OSA.
4. If nasal tissues are potentially the causative factors contributing to OSA, then nasal surgery including correction of deviated nasal septum and turbinate reduction are considered. This goes to prove that nasal airway plays a vital role in the overall diagnosis and management of OSA. Because OSA analysis includes volumetric

assessment of the airway to identify the changes in the airway volume, perhaps quantifying nasal airway via segmentation might be able to give a better understanding of the overall volume of the nasal and nasopharyngeal airway. A recent study by Mupparapu and colleagues[28] demonstrated the quantification of nasal airway via segmentation.

SUMMARY

The advent of the cephalostat in 1931 and the identification of anthropometric landmarks on radiographic images initiated the process through which diagnostic methods in orthodontics changed with inclusion of the craniofacial complex and its relationship to the dentition. For many decades, skeletal diagnosis by means of cephalometric analysis became a standard in orthodontic diagnosis. Growth and development research in conjunction with methods of identifying skeletal maturation levels determined the timing of treatment. In the past two decades, technological developments have propelled orthodontic imaging methods into the digital era with improved and accurate methods of computerized 3D diagnosis while at the same time providing the added benefit of less exposure to ionizing radiation.

3D diagnosis and virtual planning of cases with consideration given to periodontal limitations, the TMJ, and the airway are becoming the new standard. This methodology is truly a game changer and has added an entirely new dimension to dentistry. Although the introduction of advanced technology and newer diagnostic capabilities has provided a wealth of information, it does come with caveats. The information output is only as reliable as the user input, meaning that there is a learning curve in the process as clinicians familiarize themselves with the use of advanced diagnostic methods. Accurate skeletal landmark identification, for example, still has concerns and limitations. One must be cognizant that a skeletal landmark identified on a 2D image may differ from that identified on a 3D image. With further research, there may be a need to establish new norms that would be more applicable to a 3D analysis. It is also important to mention and emphasize that with the added information comes the additional responsibility and obligation to identify abnormalities and pathologic conditions that are within the field of view but may be outside of the practitioner's realm and therefore collaboration with colleagues may be advisable. With time, as this methodology continues to evolve, more clinicians will continue to embrace it and with continued research, further insight will be gained to assist in accurate diagnosis to provide guidance toward a well-designed and executed treatment plan.

CLINICS CARE POINTS

- Orthodontic imaging in conjunction with the clinical evaluation allows the clinician to diagnose skeletal, facial and dental relationships. In addition to this, it allows for monitorin of growth and development, evaluation of the TMJ and analysis of the airway.

- Digital stereolithography files generated via an intraoral scanner can be combined with CBCT data to generate 3D images which can be used for 3D diagnosis and treatment simulation.

REFERENCES

1. American Association of Orthodontists: Clinical practice guidelines for orthodontics and dentofacial orthopedics 1996; amended 2017. Available at: https://www. aaoinfo.org/d/apps/get-file?fid=12939. Accessed October 8, 2020.

2. Ricketts RM. A foundation for cephalometric communication. Am J Orthod 1960; 41:330–57.

3. Fishman LS. Chronological versus skeletal age, an evaluation of craniofacial growth. Angle Orthod 1979;49:181–9.

4. Pyle SI, Waterhouse AM, Greulich WW. Radiographic standard of reference for the growing hand and wrist. 2nd edition. Cleveland (OH): The Press of the Case Western Reserve Univ Orthop; 1971. p. 1–91.

5. Bjork A, Helm S. Prediction of the age of maximum pubertal growth in body height. Angle Orthod 1967;37:134–43.

6. Fishman L. Radiographic evaluation of skeletal maturation a clinically oriented method based on hand-wrist films. Angle Orthod 1981;52:88–112.

7. McNamara J Jr, Franchi L. The cervical vertebral maturation method: a user's guide. Angle Orthod 2018;88:133–43.

8. Broadbent H. A new x-ray technique and its application to orthodontia. Angle Orthod 1931;2:45–66.

9. Finlay L. Craniometry and cephalometry: a history prior to the advent of radiography. Angle Orthod 1980;50:312–21.

10. Scammon RE. The first seriatim study of human growth. Am J Phys Anthropol 1927;10:329–33.

11. Harris JA, Jackson CM, Patterson DG, et al. The measurement of man. Minneapolis (MN): University of Minnesota Press; 1930. p. 1–215.

12. Graber TM. Implementation of the roentgenographic cephalometric technique. Am J Orthod 1958;44:906–32.

13. Krogman WM, Sassouni V. A syllabus in roentgenographic cephalometry. Philadelphia, PA: Philadelphia Center for Research in Child Growth; 1957. p. 1–366.

14. Ricketts RM. Perspectives in the clinical application of cephalometrics. Angle Orthod 1981;51:115–50.

15. Jacobson A, Jacobson R. Radiographic cephalometry from basics to 3-D imaging. 2nd edition. Chicago: Quintessence; 2006. p. 1–320.

16. Kula K, Ghoneima A. Cephalometry in orthodontics: 2D and 3D. Chicago: Quintessence; 2018. p. 17–73, 89–99.

17. Patwa A, Shah A. Anatomy and physiology of respiratory system relevant to anaesthesia. Indian J Anaesth 2015;59:533–41.

18. Sahin-Yilmaz A, Naclerio RM. 2011. Anatomy and physiology of the upper airway. Proc Am Thorac Soc 2011;8:31–9.

19. Park JG, Ramar K, Olson EJ. Updates on definition, consequences, and management of obstructive sleep apnea. Mayo Clin Proc 2011;86:549–54.

20. Kapur VK, Auckley DH, Chowdhuri S, et al. Clinical practice guideline for diagnostic testing for adult obstructive sleep apnea: an American Academy of Sleep Medicine clinical practice guideline. J Clin Sleep Med 2017;13:479–504.

21. Franklin KA, Lindberg E. 2015. Obstructive sleep apnea is a common disorder in the population-a review on the epidemiology of sleep apnea. J Thorac Dis 2015; 7(8):1311–22.

22. Sateia MJ. International Classification of Sleep Disorders-Third Edition: highlights and modifications. Chest 2014;146:1387–94.

23. Mannarino MR, Di Filippo F, Pirro M. Obstructive sleep apnea syndrome. Eur J Intern Med 2012;23:586–93.

24. Alsufyani N, Flores-Mir C, Major P. Three-dimensional segmentation of the upper airway using cone beam CT: a systematic review. Dentomaxillofac Radiol 2012; 41:276–84.

25. Neelapu BC, Kharbanda OP, Sardana HK, et al. Craniofacial and upper airway morphology in adult obstructive sleep apnea patients: a systematic review and meta-analysis of cephalometric studies. Sleep Med Rev 2017;31:79–90.
26. Lenza MG, Lenza MM, Dalstra M, et al. An analysis of different approaches to the assessment of upper airway morphology: A CBCT study. Orthod Craniofac Res 2010;13:96–105.
27. Behrents RG, Shelgikar AV, Conley RS, et al. Obstructive sleep apnea and orthodontics: an American Association of Orthodontists white paper. Am J Orthod Dentofacial Orthop 2019;156:13–28.e1.
28. Mupparapu M, Shi KJ, Lo AD, et al. Novel 3D segmentation for reliable volumetric assessment of the nasal airway: a CBCT study. Quintessence Int 2020. https://doi.org/10.3290/j.qi.a45429.

Radiographic Diagnosis in the Pediatric Dental Patient

Jayakumar Jayaraman, BDS, MDS, MPed Dent RCS, FDSRCS, PhD[a],*, Angela Hoikka, DDS[b],
Maria Jose Cervantes Mendez, DDS, MS, FAAPD[a],
Evlambia Hajishengallis, DDS, DMD, MSc, PhD[c]

KEYWORDS

- Children • Radiation dose • Dental caries • Primary dentition • Permanent dentition
- Trauma • Dental anomalies • Cysts

KEY POINTS

- Children are susceptible to the deterministic and stochastic effects of radiation; hence, the risks, and benefits of ionizing radiation should be considered carefully prior to prescribing radiographs.
- Recommendations have been put forth for prescribing dental radiographs for children in primary dentition, transitional dentition, and permanent dentition.
- In routine dental practice, bitewing radiographs are useful to diagnose dental caries in proximal surfaces and monitor caries risk status.
- Panoramic radiographs are helpful to assess dental development and detect developmental anomalies.
- Computed tomography is employed as an adjunct to diagnose and treatment plan, certain dental anomalies, dentoalveolar infections, trauma, cysts, and tumors.

INTRODUCTION

Children have increased cellular metabolism and life expectancy and often a decreased willingness to cooperate. When prescribing radiographs to children, exposure settings are adjusted to accommodate a smaller physique and less calcified structure. The risk and benefit ratio must be justified, optimizing protection where dose remains as low as reasonably achievable and applying dose limits appropriate for the individual.[1] Mitotic cell activity in children is much higher than in post-pubescent persons of the same size, as is their life expectancy; this enables greater time and circumstance for tumor development or risk of exposure-induced cancer death.[2]

[a] Department of Developmental Dentistry, University of Texas Health San Antonio School of Dentistry, 8210 Floyd Curl Drive, San Antonio, TX 78229, USA; [b] Department of Comprehensive Dentistry, University of Texas Health San Antonio School of Dentistry, 8210 Floyd Curl Drive, San Antonio, TX 78229, USA; [c] Division of Pediatric Dentistry, University of Pennsylvania School of Dental Medicine, 240 South 40th Street, Philadelphia, PA 19104, USA
* Corresponding author.
E-mail address: jayaraman@livemail.uthscsa.edu

Dent Clin N Am 65 (2021) 643–667
https://doi.org/10.1016/j.cden.2021.02.009
0011-8532/21/© 2021 Elsevier Inc. All rights reserved.

Considering the potential greater effect of radiation in children, radiographs should be obtained based on the individual needs of a patient and calculated risk rather than determined by a general protocol. Radiographs commonly are prescribed in children for diagnosis and treatment planning of dental diseases and developmental abnormalities, monitoring growth and development, and assessment of dentoalveolar trauma. In an everyday dental practice, radiographs are obtained in children primarily for routine diagnosis for dental caries and assessment of growth and maturity. Some dental anomalies are identified as incidental findings during imaging. General dental practitioners should have adequate knowledge of diagnosing common developmental and pathologic conditions from radiographs to enable appropriate referral and timely management of those conditions. This article aims to describe radiographic diagnosis of common dental conditions in children.

DIAGNOSIS OF DENTAL CARIES AND PERIODONTAL CONDITIONS

A survey conducted by National Center for Health Statistics in the United States found that 23% of children ages 2 years to 5 years had dental caries in primary teeth. Similarly, 21% of children ages 6 years to 11 years had caries in permanent teeth. The prevalence was relatively higher in adolescents ages 12 years to 19 years, in whom 3 of 5 children had dental caries.[3] It is imperative for dental practitioners to identify the caries at an early stage to take necessary steps to restore the teeth and avoid further progression of caries.

Bitewing Radiographs

Although occlusal caries can be identified clinically, proximal caries requires further investigation. Proximal caries present on the distal surface of primary second molars increases the risk of developing caries on the mesial surface of the first permanent molars.[4] The importance of bitewing radiographs in diagnosing proximal carious lesions has been emphasized and a recent study has reported that 30% of caries in proximal surfaces of posterior teeth could go undetected without radiographic examination.[5,6]

The American Academy of Pediatric Dentistry recommends taking posterior bitewing radiographs on every new patient and at 6 months to 12 months intervals if the proximal surfaces cannot be examined visually or through probing the surfaces.[7] Several classification systems are available to record and score interproximal caries, and the most commonly accepted system was proposed by the International Caries Classification and Management System/International Caries Detection and Assessment System. Based on the extension of the caries and the location, they are ben classified as initial lesions (RA) when radiolucency is seen in the enamel or outer surface of dentine, moderate lesions (RB) when lesion extends into dentine, and severe lesions (RC) when the caries involves inner surface of dentine or pulp (**Fig. 1**).[8]

Anterior Occlusal Radiographs

Maxillary anterior teeth are affected most commonly by dental caries, in addition to the molars in primary dentition. This is due mostly to nursing habits and prolonged duration of exposure to milk and sugars from the nursing bottle in the maxillary anterior region. Anterior occlusal radiographs are useful to detect extension of caries into enamel, dentine, or pulp, so appropriate treatment could then be planned. Usually, mandibular anterior teeth are least affected by dental caries; however, in severe caries, occlusal radiographs may be indicated for mandibular anterior teeth. An adult-sized periapical radiographic detector, in horizontal position, usually is used to obtain anterior occlusal radiographs in primary dentition (**Fig. 2**).

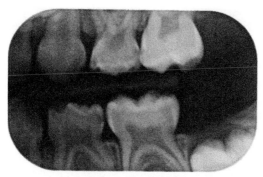

Fig. 1. Interproximal caries in a 4-year-old child in teeth #I, #J, #K, and #L with a score of RA2 and RA3, according to International Caries Detection and Assessment System classification.[8]

Periapical Radiographs

In primary dentition, periapical radiographs commonly are indicated to evaluate the patency in periapical region of the root canal following involvement of caries. Ideally, radiolucency can be detected first in the furcation region due the presence of accessary root canals in primary molars, and this can be observed in bitewing radiographs. Sometimes, this could be the first indication of caries progression in the periradicular region, prompting further examination using the periapical radiograph to analyze the extension of infection. In pulp-treated primary molars, it is common to see internal or external root resorption. Although this is a manifestation of inflammation, it should not warrant any immediate treatment, because most such presentations heal over a period of time based on immune response of an individual. It is strongly recommended to follow-up at update radiographs at regular intervals.

Clinical and radiological diagnosis may not always correlate; hence, both findings must be taken into consideration when planning treatment. Periapical radiographs also are used as a diagnostic tool to evaluate resorption pattern of pulp-treated primary teeth and development status of the developing permanent teeth (**Fig. 3**). In permanent teeth, a periapical radiograph is used to diagnose the presence of granuloma or a cyst that presents initially as widening of periodontal ligament (PDL) space

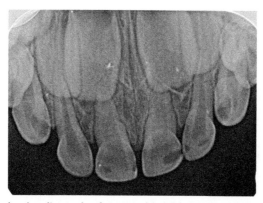

Fig. 2. Anterior occlusal radiograph of 4-year-old child showing caries in primary incisors and canines. Note the proximity of permanent incisors to the roots of the primary incisors.

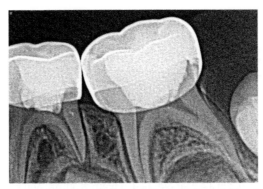

Fig. 3. Pulpotomy treated primary teeth #K and #L. Note the calcification in the distal root of tooth #K and the position of developing succedaneous premolars.

followed by development of circumscribed or diffuse radiolucency in the apex of the root. This occurs as a sequela of long-standing pulpal infection due to caries or trauma.

Extraoral Radiographs

Extraoral images, including panoramic radiographs or computed tomography (CT) scans, are indicated when the dental caries progress into a space infection. In the maxillary arch, it commonly is seen in the infraorbital region (**Fig. 4**), whereas in the mandibular arch, it manifests as submandibular space infection. Extraoral space infections should be attended immediately and aggressively. The imaging techniques provide an overall insight on the spread of infection originating from the infected tooth.

GINGIVAL AND PERIODONTAL CONDITIONS

It was found that 9% of children and adolescents showed some evidence of abnormal bone resorption in the molar region due to periodontitis, proximal caries, stainless steel crowns, and pulp pathology.[9] Most common gingival conditions in children do not warrant taking radiographs because the lesions are confined mostly to soft tissues. Periodontal conditions, however, like chronic aggressive and necrotizing

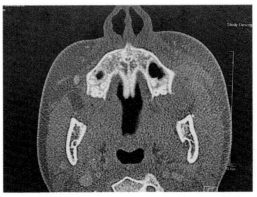

Fig. 4. Axial slice CT scan of 9-year-old girl of showing radiolucency and expansion of the cortical plate. The buccal space infection originated from dental caries in tooth #A.

periodontitis in children and adolescents present with bony changes that could be diagnosed from intraoral or panoramic radiographs. Generalized chronic periodontitis can be either localized or generalized and presents with loss of crestal bone surrounding all the teeth, particularly in a severe condition, when the clinical attachment loss in greater than or equal to 5 mm (**Fig. 5**). Refer to the latest classification of periodontal and peri-implant diseases.[10] Clinically, children and adolescents with aggressive periodontitis show severe interproximal attachment loss, categorized as localized aggressive periodontitis when 2 permanent first molars and incisors are involved and generalized chronic periodontitis when at least 3 teeth are involved other than molars and incisors. Periodontitis also can present as a manifestation of systemic disease in children, including diabetes, cyclic neutropenia, Down syndrome, hypophosphatasia, leukocyte adhesion deficiency, and Papillon-Lefèvre syndrome.[11]

DIAGNOSIS OF TRAUMA TO PRIMARY AND YOUNG PERMANENT TEETH

The prevalence of dental trauma is approximately 30% in the primary dentition and 20% in the permanent dentition. Particularly, in preschool children, oral injuries make up to 17% of overall bodily injuries.[12] For optimal treatment outcome, correct diagnosis of the severity of the injury is essential and should be achieved through a comprehensive history taking and clinical examination along with radiographic assessment.[13] In the event of trauma, radiographs serve as a diagnostic tool in the detection of injuries that often are not identified from clinical examination. Traumatic dental injuries based on both clinical and radiographic evidence enables making a better diagnosis than when based on clinical examination only.[14] A study found that 2.5% of trauma to primary incisors were observed from radiographic evidence alone without

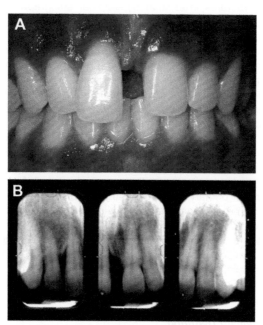

Fig. 5. A 17-year-old boy with localized periodontitis in maxillary anterior region (*A*). The condition has been diagnosed as periodontitis with stage 3 molar, incisor pattern, and grade C progression (*B*).[10] (Case courtesy of Dr. Swati Rawal, Marquette University School of Dentistry.)

any clinical evidence of trauma. Most recently, the International Association for Dental Traumatology has provided the most updated guidelines for clinical management in 3 separate sections for fracture and luxation injuries, avulsion injuries, and trauma to primary dentition respectively.[15–17] Trauma to the dentoalveolar region can be observed in both primary and permanent dentition, and management strategies vary between these dentitions.

Trauma to the Primary Dentition

Traumatic dental injuries can be distressing to both child and caretaker, and this might lead to difficulty in performing history taking, clinical examination, or radiographs. In addition to assessment of medical history, including immunization record, a systematic approach should be followed in deriving a diagnosis. Thorough extraoral and intraoral examination should be performed to identify any soft tissue injuries. Examination of all the teeth to identify fractures or mobility should be conducted, followed by radiographs as necessary. Trauma to primary teeth can directly affect the developing permanent teeth due to close proximity. Any disturbance to the developing permanent teeth could result to enamel defects, impaction, or ectopic eruption of permanent teeth. Of all the injuries, intrusion and lateral luxation injuries commonly are associated with developmental anomalies in permanent dentition.

Fractures of tooth fragments and impregnation into soft tissue could be identified by palpation of lips, cheeks, or tongue, and radiographs can be taken at low exposures to identify the embedded tooth fragments. For complicated fractures, a periapical radiograph using size 0 film or an occlusal radiograph with a size 2 film should be taken using paralleling technique.[17] Some root fractures may be obscured by the developing permanent tooth, so it is desirable to take several images at different vertical angles (**Fig. 6**). For alveolar fractures, in addition to periapical radiographs, it is recommended to take a lateral cephalogram to establish the relationship between maxillary and mandibular dentitions.

Concussion injuries usually present with pain on touch but without mobility or displacement. In such cases, no radiographs are required. However, in subluxation, extrusive and lateral luxation injuries where the tooth exhibits mobility and sulcular bleeding, a periapical radiograph or occlusal radiograph might be indicated for baseline record, this could show widening of PDL space around the tooth. Lateral luxation with lingual displacement of the root could affect the development or eruption of the permanent tooth. For intrusive luxation, it is recommended to take periapical or occlusal radiographs to identify the side of displacement. When the apex of the tooth is displaced labially, the tooth appears shorter than the contralateral tooth. In contrast, if the tooth is displaced palatally, the tooth appears elongated. A similar radiograph is required for avulsion of primary tooth to identify any displacement of the permanent tooth. Reimplantation is not recommended considering potential damage to the developing permanent tooth. Among all injuries, intrusive luxation and avulsion are likely to affect the permanent tooth to a greater extent. Sometimes, trauma to primary incisors could result in dark gray coloring due to pulp necrosis. In the event of absence of clinical or radiographic symptoms, it is advised to follow-up, and root canal therapy not always is indicated.[18] Follow-up radiographs are required for all traumatic injuries to primary teeth at designated time intervals.

Trauma to the Permanent Dentition

Several conventional and 2-dimensional images and angulations are recommended for traumatic injuries to the permanent dentition. Similar to the primary dentition, when soft tissue injury to lip, cheek, or tongue is evident due to trauma and the tooth

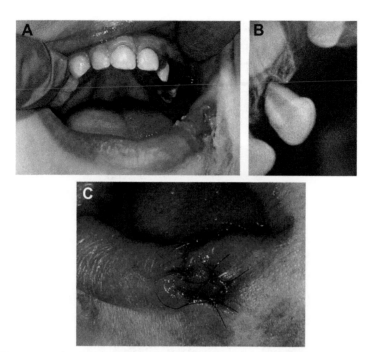

Fig. 6. Trauma to primary dentition and lower lip (*A*), periapical radiograph shows avulsion of tooth #H and root fracture in tooth #G (*B*); lip was sutured after ruling out tooth fragments in the lacerated tissues (*C*).

fragment is missing, radiographs should be taken to rule out any embedded tooth structures. For enamel and dentine fracture, and with pulp exposure, it is recommended to take 1 parallel periapical radiograph and additional radiographs based on the injuries. For crown-root fracture, root fracture, and alveolar fracture, obtain 1 parallel periapical radiograph, 2 additional radiographs at different horizontal and vertical angulations, and occlusal radiograph.[15] Cone beam CT (CBCT) additionally can be taken to visualize the direction of fracture in relation to the marginal bone and determine the crown and root ratio. Similarly, the same radiographic images are recommended for subluxation, intrusive, lateral and extrusive luxation injuries.

Avulsion is considered one of the most serious injuries to permanent teeth and it represents 0.5% to 16% of all oral injuries.[19] Reimplantation is the ideal treatment of choice and the success of the treatment primarily depends on the extraoral time and the stage of tooth development. The survival of reimplanted tooth is good if the PDL cells are viable with the extraoral dry time less than 60 minutes (**Fig. 7**). A periapical radiograph is indicated before reimplantation to evaluate the patency of the socket and to rule out marginal alveolar bone fractures and after reimplantation to verify the correct position of the tooth prior to splinting. Sometimes, root canal treatment might be indicated, and this should be initiated within 2 weeks. Radiographs should be taken based on the indicated treatment. Delayed reimplantation has poor prognosis, leading to replacement resorption, which present as ankylosis and infraocclusion.[16] The rate of ankylosis and resorption varies based on several factors; hence, clinical and radiographic examinations are required at regular intervals to initiate appropriate treatment (**Fig. 8**). Ideally, follow-up radiographs should be obtained for all traumatic injuries involving permanent teeth. Based on the extension of the injury, radiographs are

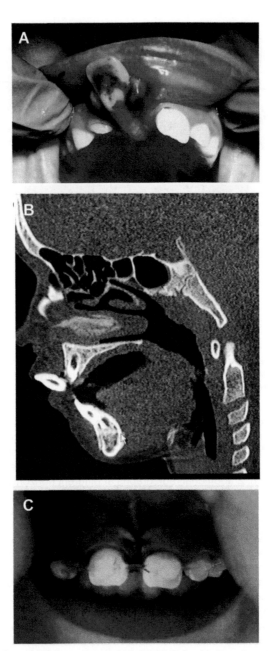

Fig. 7. Avulsion of tooth #8 in an 8-year-old child (*A*). Sagittal section of CT shows avulsed tooth attached to the gingival mucosa without root fracture. The alveolar socket was patent, and no signs of complicated alveolar bone fracture were observed (*B*). Tooth #8 was re-implanted and stabilized using 40-lb monofilament composite fishing line splint and resorbable sutures (*C*).

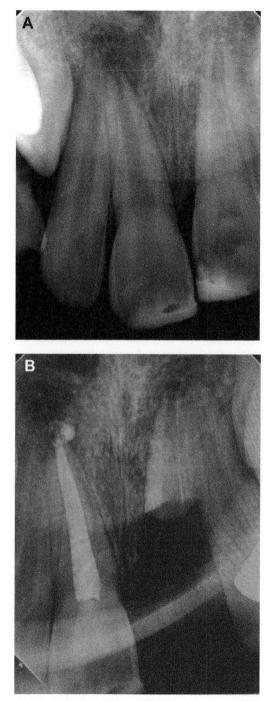

Fig. 8. Periapical radiograph showing periapical infection in tooth #8 and replacement resorption in tooth #9 following delayed reimplantation. Also, note infraocclusion in tooth #9 due to ankylosis (*A*). Root canal treatment was performed on tooth #8, followed by coronectomy and root burial of tooth #9 (*B*).

recommended at 2 weeks, 4 weeks, 6 weeks to 8 weeks, 3 months, 6 months, 1 year, and yearly for at least 5 years.[20]

Radiographic Imaging Following Dental Trauma

Extraoral images
Panoramic radiographs can help detect condylar fractures. If unavailable, reverse Towne posterior-anterior projection can be recommended. These images provide nondetailed images of teeth, hence cannot detect additional trauma to the dentition. In such cases, it is advised to take CT or CBCT, particularly in cases involving midfacial fractures.

Intraoral images
Based on the age of the patient and the stage of dental development, periapical radiographs (size 0–2) or occlusal radiograph (size 4) is recommended. Ideally, parallel images with positioning device are indicated for consistent repeated measurements. To detect root or alveolar bone fractures, it is recommended to take 2 horizontal or 2 vertical angulations. It is advised to project the central beam from +10° to −20° in relation to the normal angulation, which is perpendicular to the long axis of the tooth.[13]

DIAGNOSIS OF COMMON ORAL PATHOLOGIES IN CHILDREN
Odontogenic Cysts

Radicular cyst
As in cases of adults, radicular cysts are localized in the apex of nonvital permanent teeth of children. They usually are less than 1 cm in diameter and appear as well-defined round or pear-shaped unilocular lucent lesions with a well-defined cortical border (**Fig. 9**). If the cyst is secondary infected, the cortical bone may be lost.[21]

Dentigerous cyst
The dentigerous cyst is a slow-growing, benign, noninflammatory cyst rarely seen in early childhood because it is associated most often with the permanent dentition. It forms around the crown of an unerupted tooth and it appears as a unilocular radiolucency with a well-defined cortex. Its variable size ranges from only somewhat greater than a normal follicle to very large, involving the majority of the jaw. The small size dentigerous cyst is difficult to be differentiated from a large normal follicle. In general, a distance between the crown of the associated tooth and the cortex greater than 2.5 mm to 3.0 mm suggests a dentigerous cyst (**Fig. 10**). It resorbs the adjacent teeth and displaces the associated tooth in the apical direction.[22]

Buccal bifurcation cyst (also known as juvenile paradental cyst or mandibular infected buccal cyst)
The buccal bifurcation cyst is an inflammatory odontogenic cyst found at the buccal region of the first and second molars in children between 4 years and 14 years of age. Usually, it affects the second primary molars and results in delayed eruption of teeth and swelling at the affected area. It is characterized by a well-defined radiolucent area, often corticated around the roots of the involved teeth. The lamina dura of the affected tooth rarely is involved. CT in axial and coronal views may show buccal expansion and bone loss of the involved tooth.[23]

Odontogenic keratocyst (formerly known as keratocystic odontogenic tumor)
The odontogenic keratocyst is a noninflammatory odontogenic cyst usually found in the mandible of patients ages 20 to 30 years. Radiographically, it appears as a unilocular radiolucency with corticated borders, which can be scalloped around the roots of the teeth. It usually grows along the length of the mandible with minimal buccolingual

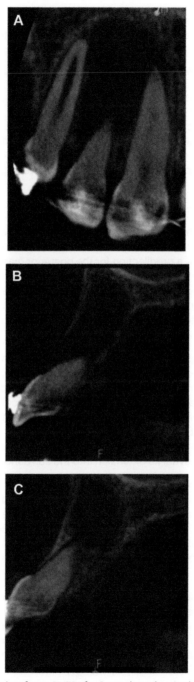

Fig. 9. Coronal reconstruction from CBCT of a 2-mm low-density lesion in the right anterior maxilla, highly suggestive of a radicular cyst developing around the apex of #7 with involvement of the apex of tooth #8 (A). Sagittal view of the lesion showing thinning of both buccal and palatal cortices with no interruption (B). The lesion is extending from the alveolar crest superiorly to reach the floor of the nasal cavity (C). (Case courtesy of Dr. Marcel Noujeim, Private Practice, San Antonio, Texas.)

expansion. It has an average size of 3 cm, may be associated with an unerupted tooth, and, if large enough, it may resorb the roots of adjacent teeth. Multiple odontogenic keratocysts are found in the basal cell nevus syndrome or Gorlin-Goltz syndrome (**Fig. 11**).[24]

Nonodontogenic Cysts

Nasopalatine canal cyst

The nasopalatine canal cyst is a well-defined, corticated, circular or oval in shape radiolucency of an average size of 1.5 cm in the anterior maxilla. If the shadow of the anterior nasal spine is superimposed, it can have a heart shape. It causes the roots of the central incisors to diverge and occasionally root resorption.[25]

Benign Tumors

Odontomas

Odontomas are odontogenic tumors, usually appearing in the second decade of life. Compound odontomas are found most often in the anterior maxillary region, whereas complex odontomas have a predilection for the posterior mandible. Radiographically, they are well-defined, dense, radiopaque masses that are surrounded by a radiolucent line and bordered by a radiopaque sclerotic border. In complex odontomas, the calcified mass does not resemble tooth structure, whereas in the compound odontomas they appear as multiple tooth-like structures in various sizes and shapes.[26]

Odontogenic myxoma

The odontogenic myxoma is a nonencapsulated tumor, which, although benign in nature, is locally invasive. It occurs in patients ages 8 years to 28 years of age and is localized, usually, in the posterior region in the mandible and in the premolar to molar area in the maxilla. Although it can appear as a unilocular or multilocular lesion, most often the form is that of a radiolucent tumor with fine, delicate or sometimes coarse trabeculae. It is an expansile tumor that causes displacement of teeth rather than root resorption. CT and magnetic resonance imaging (MRI) play a vital role in the diagnosis and surgical treatment because they reveal its extension into the surrounding tissues.[27]

Benign cementoblastoma

Benign cementoblastoma usually occurs during the second or third decade of life around the apex of the mandibular premolars or molars. It rarely is associated with primary teeth.[28] It appears as a well-defined radiopaque sunburst mass with a cortical border surrounding a well-defined radiolucent band. In contrast to condensing osteitis, the PDL is covered by the lesion.

Hemangioma

Hemangioma affects, more often, the posterior body of the mandible, the ramus, or the inferior alveolar canal. The radiographic appearance varies from presenting as a unilocular or multilocular lesion with various degrees of radiolucency. The periphery of the lesion also can vary from ill-defined (like a malignant tumor) to well-defined. Arrangement of linear bony spicules inside the tumor can look like spokes of a wheel radiating from the center of the lesion toward the periphery. The lesion may cause resorption of teeth as well as enlargement or early eruption of developing teeth. When the lesion involves the inferior alveolar canal, it results in an enlargement of the canal.[29]

Ameloblastoma

A majority of ameloblastomas occur in the posterior part of the maxilla and mandible, mostly occurring in the mandible in more than 80% of the cases. Although commonly

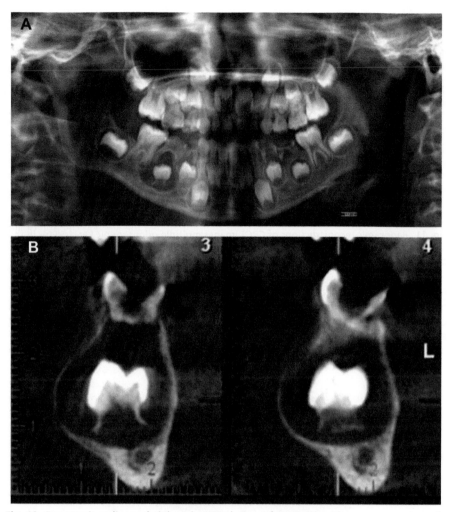

Fig. 10. Panoramic radiograph (*A*) and sagittal view of CBCT (*B*) with measurement markings on a 7-year-old patient. Patient had intraoral swelling and multiple decayed teeth, with area of concern in the right mandible. (Case courtesy of Dr. Marcel Noujeim, Private Practice, San Antonio, Texas.)

reported in adults, they also are seen in teenage children and young adults. They are slowly expanding lesions and are locally invasive.[30] Radiographically, they present as multilocular radiolucencies, and unilocular lesions commonly reported in children coinciding with unicystic ameloblastoma; however, the radiographic findings not always are related to histologic type (**Fig. 12**).

Malignant Tumors

Ewing sarcoma

Ewing tumor is a tumor of the long bones that is relatively rare in the jaw of patients in the second decades of life. When in the jaw, it is located most often in the posterior area of the mandible. Radiographically, it appears as a radiolucent, ill-defined, and

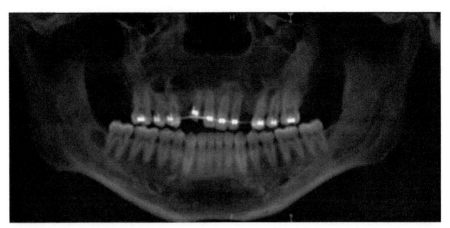

Fig. 11. Panoramic reconstructions of CBCT images multiple odontogenic keratocytes in the areas of teeth #4, #5, #8, #11, #18, and #32 were noted in a patient with Gorlin-Goltz syndrome. (Case courtesy of Dr. Marcel Noujeim, Private Practice, San Antonio, Texas.)

never corticated lesion. Destruction of the bone occurs in an uneven fashion. Periosteal reactions are variable, from onion peel appearance to a sunburst or spiculae pattern or a triangular lifting of the periosteum. Radiological findings of the adjacent structures include displacement or destruction of unerupted tooth follicle, advance eruption of teeth, loss of lamina dura, root resorption, eruption, widened canal, and so forth.[31]

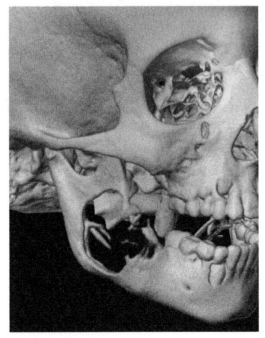

Fig. 12. Three-dimensional reconstruction of a CT scan showing ameloblastoma in right side of the mandible in a 17-year-old patient. Although benign, the lesion is locally invasive.

Acute lymphocytic leukemia

Panoramic radiographs of 63% of children with acute lymphocytic leukemia show changes that include loss of: cancellous bone, trabeculation, and lamina dura; thickened periodontal space; thinning of the crypts of developing teeth; teeth displacement; enlargement of the mental foramen; periosteal new bone formation; and disappearance of the radiopaque boarder of the mandibular canal. The molar and premolar regions of the maxilla and mandible are most commonly affected. These radiographic changes are related to both the activity of the disease and the anticancer chemotherapy.[32]

Bone Disorders

Simple bone cyst (also known as traumatic bone cyst, hemorrhagic bone cyst, and solitary bone cyst)

Simple bone cyst not a true cyst and usually found in the posterior area of the mandible of young patients during the second decade of their lives (**Fig. 13**). It appears commonly as unilocular radiolucency with ill-defined margins that scallop between the roots of the teeth, with no effect in the lamina dura or tooth displacement. Thinning of the mandibular cortex with osseous expansion also may occur.[33]

Fibrous dysplasia

The polyostotic form of fibrous dysplasia is associated with children less than 10 years of age. The zygomatic-maxillary complex is affected more often than the mandible.

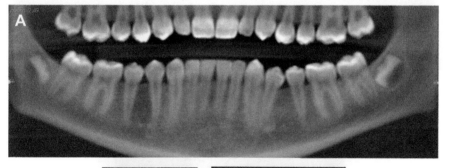

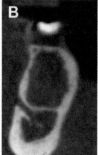
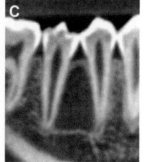

Fig. 13. Traumatic bone cyst in a child showing a triangular, low-density area interproximal to teeth #28 and #29 in a reconstructed panoramic image taken from CBCT (*A*). A sagittal view (*B*) and axial view of the area of interest shows it well-demarcated occupying the width of the alveolar crest with some irregular erosion of the lingual cortex and in contact with the lamina dura of teeth #28 and #29 (*C*). (Case courtesy of Dr. Marcel Noujeim, Private Practice, San Antonio, Texas.)

Depending on the stage of growth, it can appear as either radiolucent or radiopaque or a mixture of the both. The borders are ill-defined, and the internal bone pattern can be fingerprint-like, granular, cotton wool, or orange peel. CT and MRI scans help with the presence and severity of the disease (**Fig. 14**). It can cause displacement or interference of eruption of teeth.[34]

Cemento-ossifying fibroma (also known as juvenile ossifying fibroma)

Cemento-ossifying fibroma affects the maxilla more than the mandible. Radiographically, it appears radiolucent, radiopaque, or mixed radiolucent-radiopaque, with a well-defined sclerotic border.[35] The trabeculae form can present as a unilocular or multilocular radiolucency, with a variable degree of calcification manifesting as fine specks and occasionally producing a ground-glass appearance. Increase in radiodensity may be observed over a period of time. Root displacement is common and resorption, although rare, can occur. Also, the tumor may result in cortical thinning and perforation.

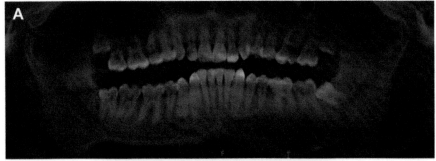

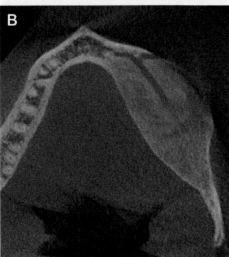

Fig. 14. Panoramic reconstruction from CBCT of a long-standing inactive lesion of fibrous dysplasia in the left body of the mandible of a young adult man (*A*). In the axial CBCT view on the same patient, a uniform expansion is noted on the buccal and lingual aspects in the body of the mandible, and the mandibular canal is situated slightly buccal, with no narrowing or interruption (*B*). (Case courtesy of Dr. Marcel Noujeim, Private Practice, San Antonio, Texas.)

Paranasal Sinus Abnormalities

The development of the sinuses is a dynamic process, which is completed around puberty. Understanding the radiographic changes occurring during growth is important to differentiate from pathologic conditions. For example, the maxillary sinus is undeveloped at birth and expands with pneumatization into the alveolar process with a growth rate matching that of the maxilla and developing dentition. Asymmetry in size and shape and opacification of the growing paranasal sinuses are normal until the age of 6 years. Paranasal sinuses are affected by a wide spectrum of conditions, including congenital abnormalities and inflammatory, traumatic, and neoplastic diseases.[36]

Temporomandibular Joint and Related Abnormalities

The anatomy of the pediatric temporomandibular joint (TMJ) is comparable to that of the adult at the time that children may need imaging. Imaging of the TMJ is important in the evaluation of TMJ because children may not exhibit TMJ symptoms. MRI is considered the gold standard of TMJ imaging because of its excellent soft tissue definition and lack of ionizing radiation. MRI imaging is important especially in cases of juvenile idiopathic arthritis because it can identify subclinical inflammation and thus contribute to early treatment and, therefore, prevention of TMJ destruction. Osseous changes are better seen with CT/CBCT imaging whereas plain radiographs can be used in the screening of the mandibular condylar morphology. Ultrasound scans also are convenient for identifying abnormalities and guiding therapeutic injections. The end stage of TMJ pathology looks similar in juvenile idiopathic arthritis, trauma, and infections.[37]

Salivary Glands and Related Abnormalities

Many lesions may occur in the salivary glands of growing children, and imaging techniques, such as Doppler sonography, CT, and MRI, may help in their diagnosis. Knowledge of normal salivary gland development, anatomy, and imaging appearance at various ages is important to differentiate normal variants from pathologic conditions.[38]

DIAGNOSIS OF COMMON DEVELOPMENTAL ANOMALIES IN CHILDREN
Anomalies in Number

Hyperdontia, hypodontia, oligodontia, and anodontia are anomalies in the number that arise during tooth development initiation and proliferation.

Hyperdontia has a prevalence of 0.3% to 0.8% in the primary dentition and up to 3% in the permanent dentition. Boys are more affected than girls.[39] Supernumerary teeth are found most commonly alongside the midline on the maxillary arch and are referred to as mesiodens. Radiographic diagnosis of asymptomatic patients is common. Possible complications include delay in eruption or impaction of the permanent maxillary incisors, formation of a dentigerous cyst, and root resorption. Surgical extraction usually is the treatment of choice; a patient's age, the position of the supernumerary, development of adjacent teeth, and patient characteristics all are factors to consider for a timely intervention, and the optimal age of surgical removal of mesiodens is determined between 6 years and 7 years (**Fig. 15**). Sometimes, supernumerary teeth are seen in premolar and molar regions (**Fig. 16**). Traditionally, the radiographic evaluation consisted of a series of periapical radiographs utilizing the parallax technique to localize the supernumerary position. With the development of the CBCT, however, this technique now is preferred. It provides the clinician a 3-dimensional image with accurate information on the tooth and the structures surrounding it. Cleidocranial

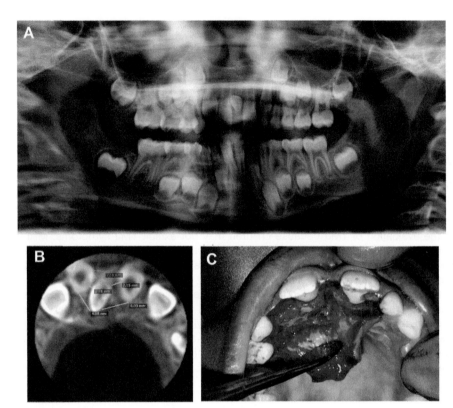

Fig. 15. Panoramic radiograph showing mesiodens between teeth #8 and #9 in a 6-year-old child (*A*). Unless symptomatic, mostly mesiodens are diagnosed as incidental findings during routine examination. CBCT was taken to locate the mesiodens (*B*). Because the mesiodens was inverted and causing diastema, it was surgically removed in office with oral conscious sedation (*C*).

dysplasia, Crouzon syndrome, and Gardner syndrome are among the conditions that have reported hyperdontia as one of their main oral characteristics.

Hypodontia, oligodontia, and anodontia all are terms that refer to different degrees of missing teeth. The prevalence in the permanent dentition varies greatly, 1.5% to 10%, whereas in the primary dentition, it is less than 1%, with a high correlation

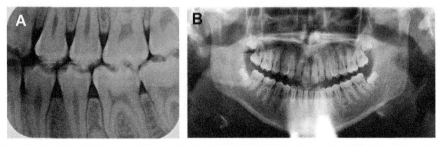

Fig. 16. Routine bitewing radiograph of a 15-year-old child showed calcified structure between teeth #29 and #30 (*A*). Panoramic radiograph revealed para-premolar (*B*). It has been decided to monitor the tooth periodically for any pathologic changes.

between missing a primary tooth and the succedaneous tooth.[40] Third molars are the teeth most frequently missing (10%–25%), followed by mandibular second premolars (3.4%), maxillary lateral incisor (2.2%), and maxillary second premolars (0.85%). More than 200 genes have been identified to express during tooth development, and mutations in several of these genes are known to arrest tooth development. MSX1 and PAX9 transcriptor factors are considered key in nonsyndromic oligodontia.[41] Ectodermal dysplasia is a heterogeneous group of inherited disorders with primary defects in 2 or more tissues derived from the ectoderm that has been associated with different degrees of hypodontia and teeth malformation (**Fig. 17**). The clinical diagnosis is supplemented with a radiographic evaluation utilizing periapical radiographs or panoramic films to evaluate the development and presence of the full dentition. Prognosis and treatment planning depend on number and location of the missing teeth and a patient's age.

Anomalies in Size and Shape

Dens invaginatus is the malformation of teeth resulting from the invagination of the dental papilla during tooth development that creates an infolding of enamel and dentin; it varies in morphology and severity, with a prevalence of up to 10%.[42]

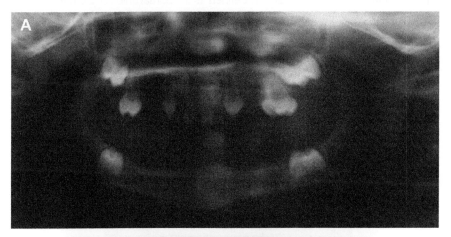

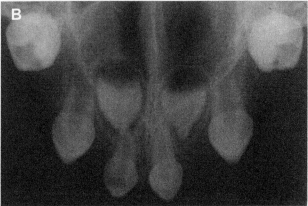

Fig. 17. Radiographs of a 5-year-old girl with ectodermal dysplasia showing multiple missing primary and permanent teeth (*A*), in addition to conical shaped anterior teeth (*B*).

Clinically it presents as an indentation or deep fissure in the cingulum of the tooth (**Fig. 18**). The tooth affected most commonly is the maxillary lateral incisor, but it can be present in other teeth, in particular central incisors. Periapical radiographs are used for the initial diagnosis of these lesions. The images can reveal radiolucent pockets surrounded by radiopaque enamel that may be confined to the crown and may involve the pulp or PDL. A periapical radiolucent image can be seen when there is communication between the oral cavity and the PDL. CBCT imaging is recommended for a more detailed assessment of the tooth morphology and treatment prognosis.[43]

Dens evaginatus is defined as a supernumerary tubercular structure that extends from the occlusal or lingual surface of the affected tooth. It consists of a layer of enamel and dentin and might contain an extension of the pulp tissue. The prevalence has been reported to be up to 15%, depending on race and diagnostic criteria.[44] The tooth affected most commonly is the mandibular second premolar, but it can appear on other posterior teeth and incisors. Radiographically, it can be identified in periapical radiographs and CBCT images that can assist the clinician in the early diagnosis and treatment.

Fusion and gemination are conditions that, although clinically can look similar, their etiology is different. Fusion of 2 teeth is defined as the partial union of 2 different dental germs, whereas gemination of 1 tooth is the incomplete division of a single dental germ. Dental fusion results in 1 tooth less than expected if the affected tooth is counted as 1, whereas gemination results in the standard number of teeth. Clinically, the affected tooth may have 2 crowns or a single larger crown with a notch or fissure. Radiographically double teeth can have 2 roots or a single root; the differences in morphology affect a tooth's prognosis and treatment plan.[45] Double teeth are more

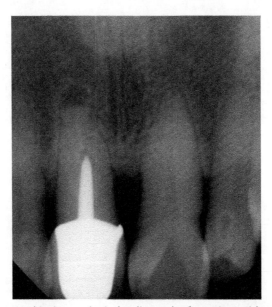

Fig. 18. Maxillary central incisor periapical radiograph of a patient with a history of trauma to the maxillary anterior teeth. Note the dens invaginatus (Oehlers type II) in both teeth #7 and #10. Tooth #8 shows prior endodontic treatment, a cast post and core, and a healed periapical lesion. (Case courtesy of Dr. Mel Mupparapu, University of Pennsylvania School of Dental Medicine.)

prevalent in the primary dentition than in the permanent dentition, with no sex predilection. The prevalence rate for double teeth in the primary dentition varies from 0.5% to 4.1%, whereas it has been reported to be 0.42% in the permanent dentition.[46]

Anomalies in the Eruption

Abnormal eruption patterns of the permanent dentition can cause malocclusion and loss of teeth and are most commonly associated with the first permanent molars and maxillary canines. A diagnosis of ectopic eruption can occur during routine radiographic examination or when suspected due to asymmetric eruption (**Fig. 19**).

Ectopic eruption of first permanent molars occurs in up to 3% of the population.[47] Bitewing and periapical radiographs of the impacted first permanent molar show a mesial angulation of the tooth and radiolucency of the second primary molar's distal surface due to external resorption. Approximately 66% of ectopically erupting molars self-correct; factors the degree and severity of resorption affect the prognosis and treatment options of this condition (**Fig. 20**).[48]

Impacted maxillary canines are present in 1.5% to 2% of the population.[49,50] A missing or peg lateral or the inability to palpate the canine's bulge should alert the clinician to recommend a panoramic or periapical image to assist with the initial diagnosis. The presence of an abnormal inclination of the canine and/or overlapping of the lateral or central incisor root, external resorption of maxillary incisors, enlarged follicle, or lack of resorption of the primary canine suggests an aberrant eruption pattern of the canine. Depending on patient age and radiographic findings, interceptive treatment most likely is indicated, and a CBCT image should be considered.

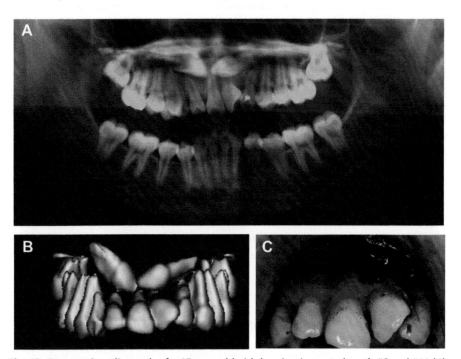

Fig. 19. Panoramic radiograph of a 15-year-old girl showing impacted teeth #6 and #11 (*A*). Three-dimensional reconstruction of CBCT shows orientation of the canines in relation to adjacent teeth (*B*). Both canines were removed surgically by sectioning under general anesthesia (*C*).

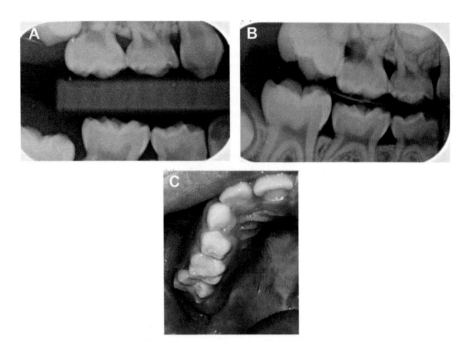

Fig. 20. Ectopic eruption of tooth #3 in a 4-year-old child (*A*). Note that the eruption of tooth #3 self-corrected in 1 year (*B*). Tooth #A clinically was asymptomatic, so was kept under review (*C*).

SUMMARY

Children present with unique challenges in the dental office, and routine, time-appropriate radiographic examination always is recommended to complement clinical examination. Radiographs commonly are prescribed for diagnosis of dental caries, followed by evaluation of growth and development. Dental practitioners should be aware of the long-term effects of radiation and be mindful when prescribing radiographs for children. It is recommended to follow established guidelines on the type of radiograph and based on the patient's age and dental developmental stage. Most of the dental anomalies are identified as incidental findings during routine radiographic examination, so thorough and systematic evaluation of radiograph is necessary. In traumatic dental injuries, additional images might be required to confirm the diagnosis. In complex cases, including cysts, tumors, and craniofacial anomalies, referral to an appropriate specialist is recommended for timely management of the condition.

CLINICS CARE POINTS

- The risks and benefits of ionizing radiation should be taken in consideration prior to prescribing radiographs in children.
- Bitewing radiographs serve as an excellent tool to diagnose interproximal carious lesions and the frequency should be based on overall caries risk assessment of the patient.
- Panoramic radiograph is useful in evaluating dental development pattern in children and in diagnosis of dental anomalies.

> • Clinicians must be aware of making appropriate and timely referral to Specialist for timely management of complex dental conditions.

DISCLOSURE

The authors have nothing to disclose.

REFERENCES

1. Ludlow JB, Davies-Ludlow LE, White SC. Patient risk related to common dental radiographic examinations: the impact of 2007 International Commission on Radiological Protection recommendations regarding dose calculation. J Am Dent Assoc 2008;139:1237–43.
2. ICRP. Statement on tissue reactions/early and late effects of radiation in normal tissues and organs, threshold doses for tissue reactions in a radiation protection context. Ann ICRP 2012;118:40.
3. Dye BA, Thornton-Evans G, Li X, et al. Dental caries and sealant prevalence in children and adolescents in the United States, 2011-2012. NCHS Data Brief 2015;191:1–8.
4. Vanderas AP, Kavvadia K, Papagiannoulis L. Development of caries in permanent first molars adjacent to primary second molars with interproximal caries: four-year prospective radiographic study. Pediatr Dent 2004;26:362–8.
5. Newman B, Seow WK, Kazoullis S, et al. Clinical detection of caries in the primary dentition with and without bitewing radiography. Aust Dent J 2009;54:23–30.
6. Daniels A, Owais A, Kanellis M, et al. Clinical versus radiographic caries diagnosis in primary tooth approximal surfaces. Pediatr Dent 2020;42:193–6.
7. Guidelines for taking radiographs in children. American academy of pediatric dentistry. Available at: https://www.aapd.org/globalassets/media/policies_guidelines/bp_radiographs.pdf. Accessed September 1, 2020.
8. Pitts NB, Ismail AI, Martignon S, et al. ICCMS™ guide for practitioners and educators. London (United Kingdom): King's College London; 2014.
9. Bimstein E, Delaney JE, Sweeney EA. Radiographic assessment of the alveolar bone in children and adolescents. Pediatr Dent 1988;10:199–204.
10. Caton JG, Armitage G, Berglundh T, et al. A new classification scheme for periodontal and peri-implant diseases and conditions–Introduction and key changes from the 1999 classification. J Periodontol 2018;89:S1–8.
11. Preshaw PM. Detection and diagnosis of periodontal conditions amenable to prevention. BMC Oral Health 2015;15:S5.
12. Andersson L. Epidemiology of traumatic dental injuries. J Endod 2013;39:S2–5.
13. Kullman L, Al Sane M. Guidelines for dental radiography immediately after a dento-alveolar trauma, a systematic literature review. Dent Traumatol 2012;28:193–9.
14. Holan G, Yodko E. Radiographic evidence of traumatic injuries to primary incisors without accompanying clinical signs. Dent Traumatol 2017;33:133–6.
15. Bourguignon C, Cohenca N, Lauridsen E, et al. International association of dental traumatology guidelines for the management of traumatic dental injuries: 1. Fractures and luxations. Dent Traumatol 2020. https://doi.org/10.1111/edt.12578.
16. Fouad AF, Abbott PV, Tsilingaridis G, et al. International association of dental traumatology guidelines for the management of traumatic dental injuries: 2. Avulsion of permanent teeth. Dent Traumatol 2020. https://doi.org/10.1111/edt.12573.

17. Day PF, Flores MT, O'Connell A, et al. International association of dental traumatology guidelines for the management of traumatic dental injuries: 3. injuries in the primary dentition. Dent Traumatol 2020. https://doi.org/10.1111/edt.12576.

18. Holan G. Long-term effect of different treatment modalities for traumatized primary incisors presenting dark coronal discoloration with no other signs of injury. Dent Traumatol 2006;22:14–7.

19. Andreasen JO, Andreasen FM. Textbook and color atlas of traumatic injuries to the teeth. Oxford (United Kingdom): Wiley Blackwell; 2019. p. 486–520.

20. Levin L, Day PF, Hicks L, et al. International association of dental traumatology guidelines for the management of traumatic dental injuries: General introduction. Dent Traumatol 2020. https://doi.org/10.1111/edt.12574.

21. Penumatsa NV, Nallanchakrava S, Muppa R, et al. Conservative approach in the management of radicular cyst in a child: Case report. Case Rep Dent 2013;2013:1231428.

22. Bhardwaj B, Sharma S, Chitlangia P, et al. Mandibular dentigerous cyst in a 10-Year-Old Child. Int J Clin Pediatr Dent 2016;9:281–4.

23. Ramos LM, Vargas PA, Coletta RD, et al. Bilateral buccal bifurcation cyst: case report and literature review. Head Neck Pathol 2012;6:455–9.

24. Ahlfors E, Larsson Å, Sjögren S. The odontogenic keratocyst: a benign cystic tumor? J Oral Maxillofac Surg 1984;42:10–9.

25. Nelson BL, Linfesty RL. Nasopalatine duct cyst. Head Neck Pathol 2010;4:121–2.

26. de Oliveira BH, Campos V, Marçal S. Compound odontoma–diagnosis and treatment: three case reports. Pediatr Dent 2001;23:151–7.

27. Harokopakis-Hajishengallis E, Tiwana P. Odontogenic myxoma in the pediatric patient: a literature review and case report. Pediatr Dent 2007;29:409–14.

28. Nuvvula S, Manepalli S, Mohapatra A, et al. Cementoblastoma relating to right mandibular second primary molar. Case Rep Dent 2016;2016:2319890.

29. Preethi B, Subhas B, Shishir R, et al. Radiologic features of intraosseous hemangioma: a diagnostic challenge. Arch Med Health Sci 2014;2:67–70.

30. Zhang J, Gu Z, Jiang L, et al. Ameloblastoma in children and adolescents. Br J Oral Maxillofac Surg 2010;48:549–54.

31. Krishna KB, Thomas V, Kattoor J, et al. A radiological review of ewing's sarcoma of mandible: a case report with one year follow-up. Int J Clin Pediatr Dent 2013;6:109–14.

32. Sugihara Y, Wakasa T, Kameyma T, et al. Pediatric astute lymphocytic leukemia with osseous changes in jaws: literature review and a report of a case. Oral Radiol 1989;5:25–31.

33. Scholl RJ, Kellett HM, Neumann DP, et al. Cysts and cystic lesions of the mandible: clinical and radiologic-histopathologic review. Radiographics 1999;19:1107–24.

34. Kochanowski NE, Badry MS, Abdelkarim AZ, et al. Radiographic diagnosis of fibrous dysplasia in maxilla. Cureus 2018;10:e3127.

35. Rao S, Nandeesh BN, Arivazhagan A, et al. Psammomatoid juvenile ossifying fibroma: report of three cases with a review of literature. J Pediatr Neurosci 2017;12:363–6.

36. Orman G, Kralik SF, Desai N, et al. Imaging of Paranasal Sinus Infections in Children: A Review. J Neuroimaging 2020;30:572–86.

37. Hammer MR, Kanaan Y. Imaging of the pediatric temporomandibular joint. Oral Maxillofacial Surg Clin N Am 2018;30:25–34.

38. Boyd ZT, Goud AR, Lowe LH, et al. Pediatric salivary gland imaging. Pediatr Radiol 2009;39:710–22.

39. Anthonappa RP, King NM, Rabie AB. Diagnostic tools used to predict the prevalence of supernumerary teeth: a meta-analysis. Dentomaxillofac Radiol 2012;41: 444–9.
40. Whittington BR. Survey of anomalies in primary teeth and their correlation with the permanent dentition. N Z Dent J 1996;92:4–8.
41. De Coster PJ, Marks LA, Martens LC, et al. Dental agenesis: genetic and clinical perspectives. J Oral Pathol Med 2009;38:1–17.
42. Hullsman M. Dens invaginatus: aetiology, classification, prevalence, diagnosis, and treatment considerations. Int Endod J 1977;30:79–90.
43. Gallacher A, Ali R, Bhakta S. Dens invaginatus: diagnosis and management strategies. Br Dent J 2016;22:383–7.
44. Lin CS, Llacer-Martinez M, Sheth CC, et al. Prevalence of premolars with dens evaginatus in a taiwanese and spanish population and related complications of the fracture of its tubercule. Eur Endod J 2018;3:118–22.
45. Bernardi S, Bianchi S, Bernardi G, et al. Clinical management of fusion in primary mandibular incisors: a systematic literature review. Acta Odontol Scand 2020;78: 417–24.
46. Gomes RR, Fonseca JA, Paula LM, et al. Dental Anomalies in primary dentition and their corresponding permanent teeth. Clin Oral Investig 2014;18:1361–7.
47. Yanseen SM, Naik S, Uloopr KS. Ectopic eruption- a review and case report. Contemp Clin Dent 2011;2:3–7.
48. Barberia-Leache E, Suarez-Claus MC, Seavedra-Ontiveros D. Ectopic eruption of the maxillary fisrts permanent molar: Characteristics and occurrence in growing children. Angle Orthod 2005;75:610–5.
49. Richardson G, Russell KA. A review of impacted maxillary cuspids- Diagnosis and prevention. J Can Dent Assoc 2000;66:497–501.
50. American Academy of Pediatric Dentistry. Management of the developing dentition and occlusion in pediatric dentistry. Pediatr Dent 2019;362–78.

Moving?

Make sure your subscription moves with you!

To notify us of your new address, find your **Clinics Account Number** (located on your mailing label above your name), and contact customer service at:

Email: journalscustomerservice-usa@elsevier.com

800-654-2452 (subscribers in the U.S. & Canada)
314-447-8871 (subscribers outside of the U.S. & Canada)

Fax number: 314-447-8029

Elsevier Health Sciences Division
Subscription Customer Service
3251 Riverport Lane
Maryland Heights, MO 63043

*To ensure uninterrupted delivery of your subscription, please notify us at least 4 weeks in advance of move.